WHEN DOCTORS GET SICK

WHEN DOCTORS GET SICK

Edited by

HARVEY MANDELL, M.D.

The William W. Backus Hospital
Norwich, Connecticut

and

HOWARD SPIRO, M.D.

Yale University School of Medicine
New Haven, Connecticut

Springer Science+Business Media, LLC

Library of Congress Cataloging in Publication Data

When doctors get sick.

Includes bibliographies and index.
1. Physicians—Diseases. 2. Physicians—Psychology. 3. Sick—Psychology. I. Mandell, Harvey N. II. Spiro, Howard M. (Howard Marget), 1924- . [DNLM: 1. Patients—psychology. 2. Physician Impairment. 3. Physicians—psychology. W 21 W567]
R707.W49 1987 616'.008861 87-14104
ISBN 978-1-4899-2003-4

ISBN 978-1-4899-2003-4 ISBN 978-1-4899-2001-0 (eBook)
DOI 10.1007/978-1-4899-2001-0

First Printing—September 1987
Second Printing—July 1988

Originally published by Plenum Press, New York in 1988
Softcover reprint of the hardcover 1st edition 1988

To
Marjorie Mandell
Marian Spiro

FOREWORD

When a doctor gets sick, his status changes. No longer is his role defined as deriving from *doctus,* i.e., learned, but as from *patiens,* the present participle of the deponent verb, *patior,* i.e., to suffer, with all the passive acceptance of pain the verb implies. From *passus,* the past participle, we get the word *passion,* with its wide gamut of emotional allusions, ranging from animal lust to the sufferings of martyrs. It is the connotation, not the denotation, of the word that defines the change of status. When a doctor is sick enough to be admitted to a hospital, he can no longer write orders; orders are written about him, removing him from control of his own situation. One recalls a sonnet from W.H. Auden's sequence, *The Quest,* which closes with the lines:

> Unluckily they were their situation:
> One should not give a poisoner medicine,
> A conjuror fine apparatus,
> Nor a rifle to a melancholic bore.

That is a reasonable expression of twentieth-century skepticism and rationalism.

Almost all medical literature is written from the doctor's point of view. Only a few medically trained writers—one thinks of Chekhov's *Ward Six*—manage to incorporate the patient's response to his situation. Patients' voices were not much in evidence until well into the twentieth century, but an early example is John Donne's *Devotions upon Emergent Occasions* (1624). Written over 350 years ago, it describes the feelings, perhaps recollected in tranquility, of an articulate Jacobean clergyman and writer with respect to an acute, febrile, life-threatening illness that struck abruptly in December 1623, when he was 51 years old.

Donne, ordained a priest in the Church of England in 1615, was appointed Dean of St. Paul Cathedral in 1621. Two years later he was suddenly taken ill. We know the onset was acute, because in the first of the twenty-three *Devotions* he writes, "This minute I was well, and am ill, this minute. I am surpriz'd with a sodaine change, and alteration to the worse." But an exact diagnosis remains unknown. Various writers have given such labels as "spotted fever," which merely indicates a skin eruption, "relapsing fever," which merely indicates that the fever was intermittent, and "typhoid fever," which in those days was not clearly distinguished from typhus fever. The last of these is not improbable; James I's eldest son is supposed to have died of it in 1612, and London's drinking water was hardly free from fecal contamination. However, Donne's "spots" seem to have developed late in the course of the disease and may well have been the petechiae of a rickettsial infection rather than the rose spots of typhoid, which characteristically appear late in the course of the disease. Establishing a precise diagnosis is not essential. What is important is Donne's reaction to his disease—how the patient felt. Apparently he made a few notes during the acute phase and wrote the set of *Devotions* while convalescing in the winter months of 1624. He comments:

> he feels that a *Fever* doth not melt him like snow, but powr him out like *lead,* like *iron,* like *brasse* melted in a furnace: It doth not only *melt* him, but *calcine* him, reduce him to *Atomes,* and to *ashes;* not to *water,* but to *lime.*

Donne seems to have been ambivalent about his physician; he had little faith in the medications:

> it may be that obvious and present *Simples,* easie to bee had, would cure him; but the *Apothecary* is not so neere him, nor the *Phisician* so neere him, as they are to other creatures.

He also complained of abandonment, suspecting that his physician was afraid of contagion:

> As *Sicknes* is the greatest misery, so the greatest misery of sickness, is *solitude;* when the infectiousness of the disease deterrs them who should assist, from coming; even the *Phisician* dares scarce come. *Solitude* is a torment which is not threatned in *hell* it selfe. . . . When I am dead, and my body might infect, they have a remedy, they may bury me; but when I am but sick and might infect, they have no remedy but their absence, and my solitude . . . it is an *Outlawry,* and *Excommunication* upon the *Patient,* and separats him from all offices not only of *Civilitie,* but of *working Charitie.*

Donne's *Devotions* contain many other passages a physician might well read to his advantage, especially to prepare himself for the time when he too will suffer from the ills to which the flesh is heir, but the climax is in the familiar passage in the seventeenth *Devotion:*

> Perchance he for whom this *Bell* tolls, may be so ill, as that he known not it tolls for him. . . . No man is an Iland, intire of it selfe . . . any mans *death* diminishes *me,* because I am involved in *Mankind;* And therefore never send to see for whom the *bell* tolls; It tolls for *thee.*

Donne's emphasis on the interdependence of making is not only one of the roots of medical care, why we minister to the sick, but also the root of any civilized society, and the day may yet come when, as a later poet wrote: ''*Alle Menschen werden Brüder.*''

For the present we have a book by some fifty doctors, each describing a sickness of his own. It would be easy to dismiss such a compilation as anecdotal but, in fact, what we know about medicine is the sum total of cases we have studied, and each one adds its increment to our knowledge. That is partly because each case is unique—''an Iland intire of it selfe''—yet all share in a common humanity. As individuals, each doctor's experience is unique and so is his insight. Assembled, they provide a rich variety of medical experience as seen through the eyes of patients trained in medicine, and in this way we learn from the experiences of others.

WILLIAM B. OBER, M.D.
Director Emeritus
Department of Pathology
Hackensack Medical Center
Hackensack, New Jersey

PREFACE

Doctors get sick even as other people do. We doctors have no magical immunity to ward off devils or germs, whichever you think causes disease. People may not know that we ever get sick because we tend to work just the same unless the illness is significantly debilitating. We physicians are in general a hardy lot and few of us stay home with the flu. This may not be good epidemiology but it helps to foster our superman and superwoman egos.

Most of us doctors are not neurotic about our health. Medical school and the years of internship, residency, and fellowship may lead us to the conclusion that if we can survive these programs we may just be immortal.

You will seldom find us admitted to a hospital or even having outpatient work unless we are very sick. Most of our medical "care" consists of a telephone call to a colleague, or a hospital corridor or doctors' parking lot consultation. Doctors' reactions to health measures otherwise seem to be, in general, rational and sensible rather than hysterical or obsessive. Few doctors smoke cigarettes and most, at least the young ones, seem always to be playing tennis or skiing. Running and jogging occupy the leisure time of many. Obesity at morbid levels appears to be less frequent among physicians than in the general public.

Most doctors know about illness only from their patients and journals and texts. Physicians who say the patient "has a low pain threshold" have probably not had the same disorder that is causing "the low pain threshold" patient to howl with agony at the passage of his ureteral stone. We have never heard a physician who has had a kidney stone or a "disc" belittle a patient's description of severity of pain. We have never known a migrainous doctor to make light of the discomfort of headache. How many physicians know firsthand the anxiety that accompanies the wait for a doctor's call with a report of a biopsy?

This leads inevitably to the question: Should doctors be sick with a painful or debilitating illness themselves before being permitted to take care of patients? Not very practical, and not likely to attract many volunteers even if the answer is yes.

We have shared both an abiding interest in physician behavior and an extraordinary delight in being published. Although one of us has had cancer surgery and the other no more challenging procedures than root canal and colonoscopy without anesthesia, we have often thought that physicians and others might be interested in reading about physicians who have become patients with serious diseases. This is, after all, a unique group of patients who have found in their experiences much to learn and much to teach.

We asked a few physicians who had been seriously sick if they would be interested in writing about their illness for a collection we hoped to publish. We asked the prospective authors how they discovered they were sick, how they chose their physicians and their hospitals, what it was like to be a patient and what the experience did to them as physicians and human beings.

The initial response was so promising that we began to search for physician-patients with increasing vigor, using acquaintances all over the United States and Canada and keeping a careful eye on the occasional anonymous pieces in the *Lancet* and the *British Medical Journal,* in which physicians in the United Kingdom described their illnesses.

The editors brought different viewpoints to the project. One of us, the cancerous one, is an obscure New England country doctor. He has spent his career in a community hospital, where the emphasis must always be on the practical management of patients who are acutely ill. The other is an amiable if peripatetic academic teacher and clinician among whose duties are thinking and ruminating. The collaboration has been amicable, and each editor is prepared to blame the other for any matters of concept or style that may irritate readers.

Since every physician cannot have every disease and since male obstetricians can never know firsthand the pain of labor and no female urologist can ever experience the pain and terror of torsion of the testis, we thought physicians might benefit, if not prosper, from the illnesses of their colleagues as related by those colleagues.

HARVEY MANDELL, M.D.
HOWARD SPIRO, M.D.

ACKNOWLEDGMENTS

All honor to our doctor-patient-writers who bared their souls in these essays as once they bared their bottoms in their hospital johnnies. A megathanks to Karen Hall, who pushed their manuscripts into the word processor and pulled them from the printer, performing bits of surreptitious editing on the way. Her rare brief snatches of testiness were more than compensated for by the excellence of her performance in all things. We thank Helen Markell Lewis, Chris Wajszczuk, Julie Sage, and Carrie Toth for their good efforts. Thanks to Janice Stern, who saw promise in the idea for the book and lured us to Plenum. Her enthusiasm and guidance gave us sustenance. We thank our wives, Marjorie Mandell and Marian Spiro, with their combined 72 years of monogamous marriage, for their love and their understanding of our preoccupation with this volume for the past several years.

H.M.
H.S.

CONTENTS

PART VI: CHRONIC DISEASES

PART VII: ACUTE AND/OR SELF-LIMITED DISEASES

PART VIII: AIDS

PART I

CARDIOVASCULAR DISEASES

CHAPTER 1

CORONARY ARTERY DISEASE AND CORONARY ARTERY BYPASS GRAFT

MAURICE FOX

In retrospect, I have lived most of my life with the certainty that a "big illness" was waiting for me. Not an ordinary illness, but something obscure. A medical education proved very helpful in giving substance to some of these ill-defined anxieties and I must have suffered enormously during second year pathology as the full panorama of disease passed under my microscope. I do not remember that suffering, however, and a preoccupation with illness may be more on my mind now than it was then. I did develop thrombophlebitis during my freshman year in college and Buerger's disease was diagnosed. My father took me to the Mayo Clinic, where I first developed significant antibodies to, and antipathy for, the role of patient. I stopped smoking, recovered, completed college, and found myself in medical school. Prior to that experience I think I was planning to become a writer. Afterwards, I found myself in premed courses. I suspect that somewhere along the line the idea developed and gradually matured that if "big illness" was waiting for me, then I was in a better position to deal with it if I were a physician. So, I became an internist, and luckily the choice was compatible with my interests and abilities, as well as my presumptive phobias. I enjoyed medicine enormously, and it kept me so busy that for 25 years I led a normally healthy life, except for several episodes of mycoplasmal pneumonia.

At times I wondered where my "big illness" was lurking, but most of the time I thought very little about my health. I worked long hours under great stress, sometimes drank too much, sometimes did not sleep well. My obligatory annual physical examinations were always normal. My cholesterol ran about 160 mg/dl, triglycerides about 70 mg/dl, and my HDL cholesterol was in the high 30s. I exercised very little, lived a very Type A life, and was constantly racing the clock.

DR. MAURICE FOX is a 53-year-old practicing internist and endocrinologist at the Palo Alto Medical Clinic. He is a clinical professor of medicine at Stanford Medical School and has served as regent and vice-president of the American College of Physicians.

My father, like me, had very low cholesterol and triglyceride levels and worried a lot about his health. He had chronic discoid lupus erythematosus that caused him great distress, mainly cosmetic and emotional. He was a very tense, emotional man who lived a hard life under great stress. In his mid-50s he suffered his first myocardial infarction. I remember sitting at his bedside during that episode. I was a medical student at the time and was very upset at how bad he looked and how primitive his care seemed in the small community hospital in Tennessee where my family lived, compared with the care available at the teaching hospital where I was studying. His illness may have raised anxieties in me about my own health, but I do not remember. When he died five years later of his second myocardial infarction, I had moved to the West Coast and my memories of that time are mainly of the sense of loss and transition engendered by the death of a father. I do not remember feeling personally threatened.

By the time my 49th year was under way, my schedule was close to saturation and my medical practice was very busy. In addition, I was director of the clinical laboratory at the large multispecialty clinic where I was a partner. I was on the executive board of the clinic and a trustee of the parent foundation, so most mornings were taken up with meetings. The anxieties that come with administrative responsibility were constantly with me. Periodically I would have to carve out some time to serve as attending physician on the teaching wards of Stanford Medical School. In addition, I was on the Board of Regents of the American College of Physicians and the Board of Governors of the American Board of Internal Medicine, so I was flying coast to coast once or twice a month. I thought I was enjoying myself. I knew I was enjoying the responsible jobs, associating with the most influential people in American medicine, and being involved in fundamental decisions affecting the profession and institutions I loved. My wife was understanding and busy with her own life. Our children were either in college or almost. The frantic pace came to be considered usual and customary.

Then on my return to Palo Alto from an ABIM meeting in Philadelphia, two weeks before my 50th birthday, the spiral unwound. I had not felt well on that trip, but in a nonspecific way. Maybe that is what patients mean when they complain of excessive fatigue. I was just more tired than usual. On returning home, I recall sawing some firewood with a chain saw. Then, while walking two blocks to the mailbox, I began to notice the unmistakable and, in spite of my best efforts, undeniable symptoms of angina pectoris. First there was a twinge over my left costosternal junction at the level of the second rib. Well, I thought, I sprained the joint with the chain saw. Then, as I walked faster, there developed a deep substernal rawness associated with some shortness of breath. I stopped walking. Gradually both discomforts subsided. I resumed walking and both discomforts resumed. The faster I walked, the more persistent and intense were the discomforts in my chest. I walked back home slowly and went to bed. I knew I had angina but was not yet ready to believe it. I had no trouble convincing myself that something else must be causing the distress and it would probably go away in a day or two. At rest I had no symptoms. Before I went to sleep, my wife asked if anything was the matter. I said, "No."

Over the next few days, the symptoms persisted. I was unable to climb even a few stairs without distress in my chest. The pain was not physically intense, but the emotional pain at the realization of what was happening was enormous. Denial was no longer an alternative when even mild exertion recalled the symptom complex. One diversion was the intellectualization afforded by my self-observation. I decided that much of what I had been taught about angina over the years was wrong. My initial discomfort was not in the center chest, but at a costosternal junction that was *tender.* On many occasions I had ruled out angina in patients in favor of musculoskeletal pain on finding a tender joint in the chest, but this joint hurt more on exertion. After two intense days of self-testing, my defenses were exhausted. Denial was no longer possible; it was not effective. I could not continue to work because of the recurring pain, weakness, and ever-increasing anxiety. Ultimately, I had to surrender to my greatest fear—not of death, which I considered without apprehension, not of disability, which I did not consider seriously enough, but fear of giving myself up to the doctors. It had to get very bad before I was willing to become a patient. I had to be quite desperate and afraid before I was willing to give up control of my body, my future, myself. That decision was very difficult. When I finally felt bad enough, I had to say to my doctors, "Okay, I give up. Do with me what you will." When I was able to overcome that hurdle, the anxiety level began to diminish and I assumed the role of patient, watching my case with some detachment. The worst of the fear and anxiety seemed to be over. It was no longer in my hands.

Needless to say, my doctors gave me excellent care. My anxieties at giving myself over to them had nothing to do with them; it had only to do with me. They treated me with the greatest respect and consideration, as well as the highest level of professional expertise, but neither they (nor I at that point) realized that my biggest battle was already over. I had made the decision to put myself in their hands, to relinquish the need to control my case and myself. I had become a patient and was enormously relieved.

The rest of the story gets less interesting as it gets more technical. My exercise EKG was positive. An attempted angioplasty failed. I then had bypass surgery, left the hospital on the seventh postoperative day, and recovered. I remember the ICU, being extubated, and the first steps to the bathroom. I do not remember any of the pain and discomfort. I recovered uneventfully, I take no medications, and I exercise at a YMCA rehabilitation class three times a week. I feel fine, and everyone says I look great.

As for the rest of my life, some things have changed and some things remain the same. Prior to surgery I considered myself a young man with everything ahead of me. Now I consider myself an older man with most of life behind me. I think of my prognosis in guarded terms—not with a palpable fear of death, but for planning purposes. Maybe that will change as the symptom-free years roll on. What has not changed is my basic self. I soon returned to a life-style of overwork, deadlines, tension, and anxieties. Jogging helps. Among other benefits from jogging is the reassurance that comes from the exertion itself. If I can run for this distance then I can't be in too bad shape. The basic patterns do not change much. I still avoid doctors and probably deny as much as ever. I will do almost anything to avoid being a patient.

CHAPTER 2

CORONARY DISEASE

MAURICE H. PAPPWORTH

Except for a ureteral stone, I had no important illness for the first 63 years of life. I am a nonsmoker, drink very little alcohol, and have never been overweight.

In 1973 I first experienced dyspnoea whilst walking about 200 yards up a fairly steep path outside my house. This was not accompanied by any definite chest pain, but there might have been a very slight pressure feeling in the sternal area, which I probably ignored, not wishing to contemplate its possible implication. I consulted a senior cardiologist, who reported that my blood pressure and heart were clinically normal, as were an EKG and chest X-ray. Having recently had domestic problems, I accepted his firm opinion that my symptoms were entirely psychogenic. The dyspnoea became no worse over the next few years, but it was a good excuse to curtail my working hours and stop doing everything at the double.

Later, with exacerbations and spontaneous remissions, I began to experience sharp pain situated variously in the lumbar region, along the sciatic nerve distribution, and in the neck. The neck pain radiated to both shoulders and along the clavicles to the sternoclavicular joints and, rarely, to the angles of the lower jaw. It was aggravated by walking, especially uphill or when carrying something. X-rays showed osteoarthritis of the cervical and lumbar spine. I appreciated that pain due to cervical arthritis may have a wide distribution, but I am now uncertain whether the pain, especially its occasional radiation to the jaw, was entirely due to the arthritis or at least partially to angina.

For many years I have had occasional bouts of mild epigastric pain, which is relieved by alkalies and occurs only after a large meal. But in

DR. MAURICE PAPPWORTH is a member of the Royal College of Physicians who has been a consultant physician in the National Health Service as well as in the private sector. In addition, he has tutored postgraduates working toward membership in the Royal College of Physicians. He is the author of numerous medical articles and three books entitled *A Primer of Medicine, Human Guinea Pigs,* and *Passing Medical Examinations.*

1980 I had three episodes of more severe epigastric pain occurring after dining and wining well outside my home and each time coming on only during a walk to my car but gradually subsiding with rest. An EKG was normal, and I chose not to think the pain was anginal.

In June 1981 I visited an acquaintance who lived 30 miles outside London whom I had not seen for many years and was quite excited about visiting. I had difficulty finding the house and was misdirected several times. There was no suitable parking outside the house so that I had to leave my car about 200 yards away. All this made me late and annoyed. Walking to the house I experienced mild but disconcerting retrosternal pain, which gradually disappeared when I sat down. That evening, after I had dined well, the pain recurred but with greater severity and persistence. I had a brandy and aspirin and 10 mg nitrazepam after my host had persuaded me to stay overnight. I slept fairly well and felt much better the next morning and, although worried, I drove home uneventfully. The next day's EKG showed changes not previously present.

I chose a cardiologist because his teaching hospital is near my home, he had qualified with honours from the same provincial medical school as myself, and, although he had but recently been appointed to the hospital, he had already developed a reputation as a sound practical cardiologist who was not primarily a research physiologist dabbling in clinical medicine. He found my blood pressure and heart to be clinically normal and repeated the EKG and chest and cervical spine X-rays. He was certain that I had angina. He inquired about my attitude to exercise EKG and coronary angiography. I informed him that I did not wish to submit to either because the results would not materially affect the diagnosis, because they are far from pleasant procedures and not without risks, and because, mainly on account of my age, I did not wish to consider coronary surgery. He, in my opinion correctly, said that in view of my opinion he would not attempt to convince me to change my mind or persist with the suggestions. He advised glyceryl trinitrate (GTN) not only to relieve any chest pain but also as a prophylactic prior to any undue exertion.

A comment on sublingual GTN may be of interest. A problem that I consider to be an important one, although it is but rarely mentioned or discussed by cardiologists, concerns deterioration of the tablets, with loss of efficiency. Those I have used have all been manufactured by the same pharmaceutical firm and the dark glass bottles have an expiry date on the label which has been usually about 12 months after I received them. Is that date a reliable guide that the tablets are still potent? I have discovered two essential signs of their activity; namely, they should cause a sharp tingling sensation in the tongue and visible and palpable temporal artery dilatation. But there are wide differences of opinion as to how long the GTN can be kept after the bottle has been opened. Many patients keep them in their trousers pocket, where the heat destroys them. This problem of GTN deterioration is often unfortunately considered to be too trivial to mention to patients.

My cardiologist also advised a beta-blocker, which I was not keen on taking because my blood pressure had always been well within normal limits and any lowering could be disadvantageous; my resting heart rate was always about 60 per minute and further slowing might possibly precipitate thrombosis in an atheromatous artery; and, finally, I was skeptical about the supposed value of those drugs in preventing subsequent myocardial infarction and regard the phrase ''cardiac protective'' as a sales gimmick. But I had made up my mind to be an obedient and compliant patient.

So I took the tablets, but after two weeks I felt continuously drained of all energy, with lassitude and inability to concentrate. I appreciated that those symptoms could be due either to my cardiac lesion or to the beta-blocker. So, rather than bothering the busy cardiologist, who might resent any suggestions of mine, I talked the matter over with a friend who was an excellent recently retired GP. We agreed, because the symptoms had been present only since the beta-blocker had been started and that my resting heart rate was only just over 50 and my systolic pressure had dropped from 120 to 100, that the drug should be discontinued. Two days later, on the 29th of July, 1981, although I spent the whole day sitting in my garden and later watching a long television programme on Prince Charles's wedding, I developed pain in the region of both sternoclavicular joints radiating to the shoulders. GTN did not relieve the pain, which gradually increased in intensity. For the first time in my life I had great anxiety about my physical condition and asked my GP friend to come and advise me. He thought that my pain was not cardiac but that I should take no chances and go to hospital. He telephoned the cardiologist, whom I had but very recently seen, who arranged for my admission to his coronary care unit (CCU) after being first seen in the Accident and Emergency Unit. It was about midnight when I arrived at the hospital accompanied by the GP and two members of my family. Seated in a wheelchair, I waited two and a half hours before I was seen by a doctor, although my medical friend kept reminding the nurse in charge to phone again for a doctor. During this wait I gradually felt much better and the pain ceased, so I tried to persuade my friend that it was all a false alarm and I should return home without waiting any more for medical attention. My request was flatly turned down. When finally a medical registrar of about three years' qualification did examine me and did an EKG and took blood for various estimations, he then insisted that the hospital routine before admission to the CCU was a chest X-ray. For that I was instructed to get off the couch and walk about 30 yards to the X-ray department, where the pictures were taken while I was standing. But on returning to the couch I suddenly experienced severe retrosternal pain which made me call out for help, and for the first time in my long medical career I appreciated precisely what physicians of a former generation had meant by the term *angor animi*. It was only then that the registrar told me that the EKG had shown changes pathognomonic of a myocardial infarct, although he himself had seen the tracing some 20 minutes previously. If my wits had been fully alert and if I had been told about the EKG before the chest X-ray, I might have objected to any X-ray other than a "portable" one. The registrar put up an intravenous drip very efficiently and through it inserted heroin, which fairly rapidly relieved the pain. It was nearly 3:00 a.m. before I was in bed in the CCU. That X-ray illustrates the folly of mandatory routine procedures done without regard to clinical judgment. I am willing to accept that the sudden stopping of the beta-blocker may have been a factor in producing the coronary thrombosis, but I have no doubt that the walk to the radiology department was harmful.

In spite of the bizarre surroundings, the noise of machines, and an uncomfortable bed, I slept well, but about 8:30 a.m. I was awakened by the cardiologist's senior registrar and his retinue of junior doctors and nurses. I was very dopey and had difficulty in concentrating on his barrage of questions but suddenly became more alert when he announced, "I want to twist your arm and get you to agree to a thallium scan." I wanted to cry out as Job had done, "Cease and let me alone." I inquired if there was any doubt about the diagnosis and if the investigation would alter my management in any way, especially when I had decided against submission to surgery. He answered no to both questions but maintained, "It would be interesting to see what it shows." I informed him that I have always been strongly opposed to submitting any patient to an investigation solely on the grounds that the result might be "interesting." When many months later I reported this crude and uncivil way of addressing any patient, especially an acutely ill one, my cardiologist informed me that although his junior had brusque manners resulting in a poor doctor–patient relationship, he was an expert at inserting pacemakers. I expressed my opinion that I preferred a genuine clinician to a medically qualified plumber.

I have always been a follower of the therapeutic advice of the Greek Celsus that an important aim in acutely ill patients should always be *Quies securitas silentium* ("rest of body and peace of mind"). Being awakened from much-needed sleep to be confronted with an unreasonable request and unnecessary questions could have been of no help but possibly harmful. Seriously ill patients are likely to be frightened by the paraphernalia of hospital admission. CCUs are not designed to reduce anxiety and their depersonalized atmosphere may be frightening. The apparatus for cardiac resuscitation was kept in the corridor outside my CCU room and the noise of the sudden scurrying of the staff and the ringing of alarms and telephones disturbed the slumber I craved. After transfer from the actual CCU to a single-bed ward I was put on a tranquilizer to be taken each evening at the same time as other medication. The drugs were handed out by the night staff but it was usually near 10:00 p.m. or even later before they got round to me. About 9:00 p.m. I was usually drowsy but had to keep awake for the medication. I often wondered if I had fallen asleep would I have been awakened for the tablets, including the tranquilizer? Amazingly, once a nurse woke me up at 6:30 a.m. with the incredible demand that I get out of bed to be weighed. I suspect that such peculiar antics occur in many hospitals but are not deemed to be the concern of senior doctors. Another feature militating against sleep was the pillows, which appeared to be stuffed with cement. Their plastic coverings accentuated the discomfort caused by excessive perspiration. I found great comfort from having my own down pillows brought in.

Only a few weeks after returning home I was struck by a bout of marked perspiration without fever but accompanied on this occasion by slight retrosternal pain. This again started in the early hours of the morning and my GP arranged readmission to hospital. On that occasion my wait in the A&E department before being seen by a doctor was one and a half hours. I was examined by a different registrar, who went into my history in great detail, most of which was completely irrelevant. Either the hospital notes were not readily available or he could not be bothered to wade through them. When he heard that I had had a ureteric stone 20 years previously he asked if I had had regular serum calcium estimations and expressed astonishment that I had never bothered to do so. Again, biochemistry had taken over from common sense. I was again admitted to the CCU for two days and the side ward for a further six days. Because my EKG had not altered and the serum enzymes were not raised, the label myocardial ischaemia was given to that episode. I was then put on isosorbide dinitrate, and a combination of potassium hydrochloride and cyclopenthiazide.

My third admission, on the advice of my GP, who had come to see me, was because I had been awakened with dyspnoea, palpitations, and chest discomfort. This time my wait in the A&E department before being seen by a doctor was only half an hour. I was examined by yet another registrar, who, probably because of my reputation as a teacher of bedside medicine, examined every part of my anatomy, including my testes, in spite of my obvious discomfort and anxiety. He was trying to impress me with his presumed thoroughness. His percussion of my chest and eliciting of my tendon reflexes were performed as though he had only the slightest acquaintance with sound techniques of physical examination. There must be such a thing in clinical medicine as being too thorough. We should heed the advice of Aristotle, "It is the mark of the educated man and proof of his culture that on every subject he seeks only such precision as its nature permits or the solution requires."

I insisted that the apparently mandatory preadmission chest radiograph be a "portable," and this was agreed to reluctantly. The EKG was unchanged but I was informed that the chest film showed gross pulmonary oedema. In the CCU I was given intravenous frusemide. I was not told that this was to be given, which was perhaps just as well because I had fairly often witnessed in elderly males the production of urinary retention by intravenous frusemide. This happened to me. My retention lasted for over 24 hours, by which time I could feel the upper border of my bladder well above the navel. I could not persuade any of the staff to do anything about it. During each of my five hospital admissions I had the greatest difficulty in passing urine whilst in bed, especially in the CCU, and the staff were reluctant to allow me to either stand or kneel by my bed whilst supported by a nurse. It was usually the most attractive nurse who agreed to that procedure, but several times this had embarrassing consequences which made urination even more difficult. On this occasion, after much delay, I was to be catheterized. Surprisingly, that was performed by an inexperienced male nurse instructed and assisted by a female nurse. The catheterization was finally clumsily achieved. Nearly two days later I had severe burning pain on micturition with marked frequency. When I complained about this to a junior doctor his only reply was, "We shall send a specimen to the lab for culture." Any treatment apparently had to await that result. For three days I painfully passed red-hot razor blades several times each hour. The culture was negative so I did not receive any medicinal therapy for the dysuria, which gradually cleared. Complete reliance and dependence on laboratory findings are nowadays common practice, and I find this approach to diagnosis and therapy disturbing.

In Britain, probably following U.S. practice, it has become the rule to depend on nurses, even very inexperienced ones, to record blood pressures. But nurses are often too busy to bother with all the essential details which should be scrupulously observed. Often they have been inadequately instructed. Moreover, their recorded results are rarely immediately checked by a doctor. When I was a patient in hospital I have been appalled to see slovenly techniques, including untidy placing of the cuff, often putting it far too low apparently in order that a stethoscope diaphragm can be tucked under it and so kept in place. Often I have seen the cuff wrapped over pajama, shirt, or blouse sleeves, which have often been hitched up as high as possible, ignoring the fact that this causes false readings. The senior nurse in the CCU where I was insisted on always taking the pressure in the left arm, claiming that that was essential. Taking blood pressures by nurses has often become the farce that routine repeated recordings of respiratory rates in all patients formerly was.

Whilst in the single-bed side ward I was awakened about 8:00 p.m. by a nurse and the same registrar who had previously wanted "to twist my arm" to be informed that I had ventricular tachycardia. This surprised me because I felt comparatively well and had no symptoms and my pulse rate was only in the 80s, in spite of the acute anxiety precipitated by that sudden announcement. I was shown the EKG only after much insistence and with great reluctance on the part of the doctor. It showed three ventricular extrasystoles but a subsequent long strip showed no further extrasystoles. I pointed out that if it was ventricular tachycardia the abnormality had lasted for only a fraction of a minute and the rhythm had spontaneously returned to normal. I was informed that arrangements were being made for me to have intravenous lignocaine over a 24-hour period to be done by a junior doctor. In fact it was about two hours before the apparatus and the doctor arrived. I pointed out that it was now over two and a half hours since the monitor showed the abnormal rhythm. I again pointed out that even if three consecutive ventricular extrasystoles constitutes ventricular tachycardia, which some expert cardiologists would deny, and the condition had spontaneously corrected itself, the use of lignocaine could be justified only as prophylactic against further such episodes, and its value for that was doubtful. So I, much to the consternation of a nurse and the doctor, refused the treatment. There was no attempt to get in touch with one of the senior cardiologists. It has always struck me that one of the weaknesses of CCUs is that urgent problems of diagnosis and management often arise in the early hours of the morning when senior cardiologists are very reluctant to come to the hospital and so many important decisions are made by a junior doctor who may be very inexperienced. In spite of never receiving such therapy my rhythm has remained normal for over three years.

My fourth admission to the CCU, again arranged by my GP, was because I was awakened by palpitations and slight retrosternal discomfort and feeling rotten. An EKG done by my GP showed gross changes which had not been present previously, but by the time it had been repeated in the hospital it had reverted to that which it had been ever since my discharge following my first hospital admission.

My fifth, and I hope the last, admission to the CCU was for a further bout of profuse apyrexial sweating accompanied by mild retrosternal pain which again started late at night. Again, the EKG showed no change and the serum enzymes were normal. I made a rapid recovery and was put on a calcium antagonist in addition to the other drugs previously prescribed.

I continued with the combination of drugs for over three months but gradually developed progressive marked lethargy, lassitude, and general weakness, and also anorexia, abdominal distension, constipation, and flushings. Again it was difficult to decide if those symptoms were due to the cardiac lesion or the drugs, and if the latter, which one or which combination. It was extremely difficult, if not impossible, to come to a decision on this, and I am sure that many patients suffer from symptoms due to drugs without realising this, believing they are caused by the disease being treated. However, because it was found that I had postural hypotension, the cardiologist agreed to a gradual discontinuance of the calcium antagonist. This produced a definite diminution of my symptoms, and one month later it was decided to also gradually discontinue the diuretic. Incidentally, I discovered that the long-acting vasodilator had a diuretic effect. All the symptoms disappeared and later the vasodilator was discontinued. During the past two and half years with only prophylactic GTN, I have remained better than at any time since the myocardial infarction in July 1981.

One of the main lessons I have learned from my illness has been the great difficulty, perhaps the impossibility, of differentiating clearly between symptoms due to drug therapy and those due to the illness being treated, especially when polypharmacy has been prescribed. Symptoms, especially gastrointestinal ones, vertigo, headache, lethargy, and inability to concentrate, are lightly dismissed by many doctors. But in my experience such symptoms can be important because they militate against feeling well and make the patient miserable and despondent and might delay recovery. Drugs can easily convert the most rational and intelligent of patients into hypochondriacs.

I wish now to consider the knotty question concerning the treatment of doctors as patients. The judgment of doctor-patients may be warped more often than that of other patients, but any doctor looking after another doctor, whatever the status of either, should allow for this and be attentive to the patient's opinions, comments, wishes, and even criticisms. Several GPs have told me that when they have been patients in hospital they have been treated as medical ignoramuses by the hospital doctors. That attitude is more galling when practiced by junior doctors. Doctor-patients should always be asked for their opinion on the diagnosis and investigations, and their comments should be carefully listened to.

I believe that physicians, when they are patients, should receive preferential treatment in every reasonable way. All important decisions affecting their diagnosis and management should always be made by a senior and never a junior doctor. Any surgery, including most importantly any emergency, should always be done by a senior surgeon. I myself was well looked after by both senior cardiologists themselves, but their juniors sometimes were not good. I appreciated the special privilege of having a single-bed room after each stay in the CCU proper.

When a doctor is admitted to a teaching hospital, his relationship with medical students should be a special one. Few doctors would refuse to be examined by a student provided that his or her permission was first asked and given. I am not in a position to give a firm opinion whether or not a female doctor or student should be expected to agree or even asked to allow a male student to examine her gynaecologically.

In submitting to investigations, my experience was not an entirely happy one. The hospital employed two phlebotomists who extracted blood very efficiently. But one day a medical student came to perform that task with me as a victim. It took her 12 attempts to get the blood, largely because she was inexperienced and nervous, which, she told me, was aggravated because she knew I am a physician. I found that this was her first few weeks of clinical work. The next day when standing outside my room I saw one of the senior physicians, who was not a cardiologist, and I showed him my arms, which were both black-and-blue from elbow almost to wrist, and I explained that this had been done by a completely inexperienced student. He informed me that it was a hospital rule that all patients, whoever they may be, are treated alike regarding all medical particulars. He showed not the slightest sympathy.

I would not expect a layperson to ask to be shown his or her X-rays or EKGs, but when doctors are patients, the attitude of the physicians and surgeons should be entirely different and a blank refusal to see the investigations should never be given. Nurses and junior doctors always refused any such request of mine. On one occasion late one evening, when apparently none of the staff of EKG technicians was available, a nurse who had shortly before taken an EKG of me came into my room accompanied by a junior doctor, and they were engaged in a whispered conversation, obviously about me. I asked for an explanation and was told that there was a gross change in the EKG. I had literally to implore them to show me the tracing, and when I finally saw it, I had no hesitation to point out that inversion of all the complexes in lead. I indicated that the leads had been incorrectly placed, and this could be proved by doing it again but with more care. I do not know what action they would have taken if I had not come to their aid. When I was admitted with acute pulmonary oedema my symptoms were far from severe, but I was admitted to the CCU on the insistence of my GP. There I was told by a junior doctor that I had acute pulmonary oedema and that this was confirmed by the chest X-ray but it was not shown to me. In fact, I immediately recalled the many patients whom I had personally seen in whom that diagnosis had been made virtually entirely on very questionable X-ray findings. But when two days later the cardiologist allowed me to see the films which showed gross lung changes, that was very important to me because it made me realise that my relapse, and consequently the restriction of my activities during convalescence, must be taken far more seriously than I had intended.

An interesting point is that when I was asked to contribute to this volume, I wrote to my cardiologist asking for permission to read through my hospital notes to refresh my memory. Surprisingly, he refused on the grounds that patients are not allowed to see their notes, even if the patient is a doctor. He did, however, agree to give me answers to any questions which I might ask about my stays in hospital and maintained there was neither secrecy nor anything to hide, and no comments in the records which adversely reflected on my behaviour as a patient. I accept that he was telling me the whole truth, but was his refusal justifiable?

There can be no doubt that I had had cardiac involvement for several months, perhaps even for years, before the actual myocardial infarction. If I have to justify any reluctance to diagnose my cardiac lesion myself or to have sought advice earlier, I can only plead the atypical nature of the pain and the coincidental presence of cervical arthritis and a long history of occasional dyspepsia. Moreover, I am by nature an optimist and have always regarded, until recently, my own aches and pains as of no significance.

Eight years ago I gave up my Harley Street consulting room and have since purposely seen only a very few patients at my home referred to me by GPs. During the past four years I have almost completely given up my postgraduate clinical teaching sessions. My principal medical activity during the past four years has been the preparation of the fifth edition of my *Primer of Medicine* and the second edition of my *Passing Medical Examinations*, both of which have achieved success. My hope is that reading and writing will delay senility, even though I have become the incarnation of idleness, always tending to put off all but essential activity. I keep reminding my friends, acquaintances, and family that to demand or even expect much activity from me is unreasonable. On the other hand, especially after each return from the hospital, I have had firmly to prevent the attempts by my family to cosset me, trying to prevent my walking upstairs except when retiring to bed, admonishing me when I carry even the lightest of objects, and wishing to impose on me all the nonsense concerning which foods are to be eaten and which to be avoided.

In spite of now doing so little work I have enough to eat and so far have escaped being eaten, even by the worms. I am now in the prime of my impending senescence and in full vigour of my incapacities. So, even as fools do, I grow one day older each 24 hours. Personally, I would not object in the least surviving many more years provided that I was not totally or near totally incapacitated.

I am usually regarded by my coreligionists as orthodox, and Jewish philosophy has taught me to be more concerned with the immediate future than any hereafter, and my orthodoxy has also inspired me to attempt to make this world, even to the slightest degree, a better place than when I arrived in it. Moreover, this will be itself a great reward, far more important than any possibility of an abundant reward in heaven for any little good done on earth. I believe that the truly religious person does not lay claim to any knowledge which he does not possess, and to me this includes any speculation about life after death. If forced to express any preference it would be the Sadducean notion of the immortality of the soul rather than the Pharisian belief in physical resurrection.

Because the British National Health Service is in many ways, in spite of its deficiencies, far superior to what I have seen in the United States, my five hospital admissions did not cost me a cent and would not have even if I were not a physician. Neither did I have to pay any fees to cardiologists, pathologists, or radiologists. I have myself seen professionally a large number of doctors and their families but have never charged them or asked for payment in kind. But commercialism is slowly dominating our profession and I know of quite a few consultants who invariably seek financial reward when they are consulted by doctors themselves or their immediate relatives. Recently I had reason to consult an ophthalmologist who is on the staff of a London teaching hospital, and he said after examining my eyes, "We must put this on a commercial basis. Normally my fee is X but in your case____." I immediately interrupted him, putting his "normal" fee in front of him, and left hurriedly. Doctors, their wives, and their children should never be charged for any medical services.

CHAPTER 3

CORONARY ARTERY DISEASE AND CORONARY ARTERY BYPASS GRAFT

BENJAMIN FELSON

It had a dramatic onset—a sinking sensation in my epigastrium that seemed to have ominous portent. The setting, too, was disturbing, if exotic: a hotel room overlooking the Indian Ocean in Mombasa, a resort city in Tanzania. An hour earlier, I had won my first set ever from Bill, had cooled off in the ocean, and had gone to my room exhausted but reveling in the triumph of a 63-year-old over a lad of 40.

My first thought was *coronary*, but there was no pain—merely a sensation of dysphagia that had quickly passed, and some palpitations. I felt my pulse and was startled by its slowness. Only 40 per minute! Poor clinician that I am, I could not distinguish between bigeminy and heart block, and couldn't recall which was worse. In either case, it was worrisome. I decided to wait it out, and soon my pulse returned to its normal 80, and I was "cured."

I remained well until a few weeks later when, back home playing tennis, I again noted the same feeling of dysphagia. I had no pain or pulse deficit, but a run of extrasystoles. The discomfort was quickly relieved by a drink of water. The dysphagia recurred on several occasions thereafter, usually on the tennis court but sometimes when I was not engaged in physical activity. I mentioned the symptoms to my brother, a retired internist, who insisted that I see a cardiologist. Thus was started a chain of events that I was never able to control.

My physical examination, laboratory tests, ECG, and exercise test were completely normal. The cardiologist put an electrocardiogram pack on my back and for a week I wore it constantly. It registered occasional extrasystoles, which I have had for years, but nothing more.

The pack reminded me of one of my colleagues, who, as part of a research project, collected his own colon gas in a backpack connected

DR. BENJAMIN FELSON is a 73-year-old professor emeritus at the University of Cincinnati College of Medicine, author of *Chest Roentgenology* and the paperback *Principles of Chest Roentgenology*, and editor of *Seminars in Roentgenology*.

to a tube that he had inserted in his rectum. Neither the container nor the researcher proved to be gas-tight, so by general agreement he completed the experiment during his vacation.

Though a nuisance, my own backpack functioned perfectly and was a lot less discomforting than the dreadful exercise test.

My cardiologist recommended a coronary arteriogram, but I was reluctant, for what I consider good scientific reason. As a young radiologist, I had once radiographed all 60 of the "normal" hearts in the formalin vat in pathology, looking for calcification. On reviewing the films, dissecting the hearts, and studying the hospital records of the individual patients, I learned that coronary artery calcification and narrowing were very common among unselected individuals over 50 years of age and that, despite severe coronary atherosclerosis, the myocardium often appeared relatively normal, and clinical and ECG evidence of coronary disease was often lacking. I was also aware of coronary arteriography studies in which the controls showed changes similar in degree to the symptomatic patients, albeit about half as often. So I knew that my coronary arteries would likely show distinct narrowing, whether or not my symptoms were of cardiac origin.

Since my cardiologist's diagnosis was "esophageal equivalent angina," he continued to press for coronary angiography. We reached a compromise: I postponed my decision but promised to temporarily give up tennis. My symptoms improved but did not disappear; they were sometimes relieved by a drink of water or a nitroglycerin tablet and sometimes not. In view of the diagnostic uncertainty, I decided to perform my own stress test—on the tennis court. It couldn't be any more strenuous than the cardiologist's. When he pointed out that emergency treatment was available in his department, I reminded him of the patient who had died on his treadmill only a few months earlier. He responded, with a sigh, "Doctors are such bad *patients*."

I tried doubles first; result: no symptoms, no extrasystoles. Next day came singles; result: no symptoms, no extrasystoles. The third day I ventured to the ultimate—singles on a hot day after a meal; result: dysphagia plus extrasystoles! I was finally convinced that I had coronary disease and accepted coronary arteriography. I tried to make arrangements for it in our own radiology department, but my colleagues were adamant in their refusal.

"No way. You're too close to us."

"But you've performed hundreds of coronary arteriograms without a serious complication."

"We don't want you to spoil our record."

Arrangements were made to have the angiography in a well-known institution in another city. A friend and colleague there, Dr. M., insisted on personally performing the procedure. I felt flattered and pleased since he was a world-renowned figure in this field. I was told that I must lose at least ten pounds in the six weeks before admission.

On the appointed date, exactly ten pounds lighter, X-ray film jacket tucked under my arm, I faced his administrative assistant, a very pleasant lady. She informed me that I would have to have new chest films. When I complained that mine were only a week old, she replied, "We have to have our own."

I said, firmly, "These are much better films than you make here! Tell that to your boss." She remarked, "You doctors are *such* bad patients!" She went into the inner office and soon I heard uproarious laughter through the door. Dr. M. came out to greet me. He was laughing as he accepted my films. I had won the first skirmish.

Next morning I was wheeled from my hospital room to the angiography suite, a large and incredibly well-equipped section with numerous rooms and a multiplicity of 35-mm cineangiographic units, undoubtedly the largest such collection in the world. Countless busy people—nurses, residents, technologists, and staff—in assorted but coordinated uniforms, were flitting about, some silent as ants and others noisy as bees. All conversation sounded staccato. I was transferred to an angiographic stretcher and a nurse came to describe the procedure. To save her time, I interrupted to point out that I had seen many of them performed. Annoyed at my interruption, she declaimed, "*Doctors* are such bad patients!" and stalked off.

Within minutes I was moved to the angiographic room, "prepped," and draped. Dr. M. appeared, talked to me a few moments, and went to work. He was quick and efficient with the catheterization and injection. The procedure was totally painless; the "heat" of the contrast medium was brief and mild, not unpleasant at all. I had a clear view of the television monitor and watched the contrast medium course through my coronary arteries. I could see the narrowed vessels even before Dr. M. pointed them out. There were three in all; I presumed the narrowest one was the culprit.

Afterwards, as I lay on the cardiac stretcher in an alcove, a persistent gnawing, sticking pain developed over my lower midsternum. I asked a passing white-coat whether this was significant, but he showed no concern. He was a nurse. Green was doctor-color, he informed me. The pain persisted but was not severe, so I tried to shrug it off. I asked several passing men-in-green about it. They too seemed unconcerned, hardly slowing their pace as they went on to other duties. Finally, the orderly came to move me to the ward stretcher. On sitting up, I became very dizzy and fell back to the pillow. A cardiology Fellow was quickly called. He took my blood pressure and appeared alarmed. I heard him whisper to the nurse, "90/70; get Dr. M." Within seconds there were six people surrounding my stretcher. They became even more concerned when my pressure fell further. I was given an injection; the pain soon lessened, my blood pressure rose a bit, and I was feeling pretty well. But as I looked from one hovering face to the other, I saw anxiety, alarm, apprehension, and even annoyance.

Who needs upset doctors? I decided to cool things off and spoke out, "Hey, who did the first coronary arteriogram ever done on purpose on a live human being?"

There was shocked silence at the incongruous question, but I pressed for an answer, and they started guessing. Several famous angiographers were named, including Dr. M. When I told them that my colleagues and I in Cincinnati had done it, they expressed disbelief, so I referred them to our article. The distractive stratagem proved successful—they seemed more relaxed. Nevertheless, I was wheeled to the surgical intensive care unit instead of to my hospital room. On the way, I thought to myself, "You fool. You didn't need any of this, and now you've gotten a coronary occlusion." However, the pain soon disappeared altogether and, since my ECG remained normal, my presumptive diagnosis seemed incorrect.

But now the heat was on. Dr. M. insisted that I remain in the hospital for immediate bypass surgery. I refused, pointing out among other reasons that I was to receive an important national award in two weeks. I offered to return for the surgery soon afterward. However, I hadn't reckoned with Dr. M. He went to the phone in the ICU and arranged a conference call with my wife, my brother, and my department chief. The call came through shortly. Since there was no extension (a bedside phone is *verboten* in the ICU), I had to get out of bed and walk barefoot to the nurses' desk. No one thought of moving the bed to the phone!

Dr. M. updated the Felson Decision Committee concerning my condition and findings and prevailed upon them to talk me into having the surgery now. He then handed me the phone. Since I make all such decisions for myself, I ignored the family entreaties in my right ear and the dire predictions from Dr. M. in my left. I pondered the turn of events with a series of self-interrogatories.

Question: If you don't have the operation, will you change your mode of life? Answer: Now that I *know* that my coronaries are narrowed, yes. I might give up tennis and other activities.

Question: Do you *want* to change? Answer: No, I'm enjoying myself tremendously!

Question: If you have the bypass operation, will you change your present life-style? Answer: No, the status of my coronary arteries will again be uncertain, as with anyone my age. I could go on as I have. *All* life is uncertain.

Question: Should you postpone the operation or do it now? Answer: Since I must have it, the sooner the better.

So, I decided on immediate surgery, with the proviso that I would absolutely refuse to have a postoperative angiogram and, thereby, recreate the blissful state of uncertain health I've always had. The hazard of the surgery never consciously entered my decision process.

I announced my decision, and my family, my boss, and Dr. M. were pleased with my decision and particularly with their convincing arguments that had led me to it. Dr. M. even suggested an intercity closed-circuit television hookup so that I could receive my honorary award while in the hospital. I refused on the grounds that his hospital was getting plenty of publicity and didn't need help from me.

The next morning my wife and brother arrived. We met my surgeon, a South American whose name I never did master. I was impressed with his "track" record: several thousand bypasses, nearly all successful. I wondered who kept the statistics but did not bother to ask about his mortality rate. It never occurred to me that I might be among the unlucky 1%. Hundreds of times in my life I have beaten 100:1 odds.

Two days later I awoke in the recovery room, groggy but alive. Soon a beautiful young nurse came over and explained the importance of coughing to keep my respiratory tract clear. I then tried it, only to suffer severe pain over my split sternum. Each cough was agonizing. My respiratory passages were completely dry, and I felt reasonably certain that for the moment coughing wasn't essential. Why torture myself? So I tried to fake it. But the nurse was too clever. "That's no cough," said she, and proceeded with the three C's: Cajoling, Convincing, then Commanding me to cough. I couldn't stand the pain, so she decided to pass an intratracheal catheter and suck out my nonexistent secretions.

I've passed many catheters into the trachea during bronchography, so I knew I was in trouble the moment she inserted this garden hose through my nostril without instructing me about breathing and vocalizing. The tube tip entered the back of my throat and was moving forward into my mouth, causing severe gagging, accompanied by excruciating stabs of sternal pain. I made several frantic gestures with my index finger toward my mouth, accompanied by guttural verbalization, which she failed to comprehend until the tube appeared between my teeth.

Her set jaw and steely glare marred her beautiful features. She indicated clearly that she was going to try again. I said, with commendable restraint, "My dear, I'll give you one more chance." I tried to time my breathing and voweling to the position of the catheter tip, but to no avail, and the same thing happened.

Preparing for a third pass, she seemed downright ugly. I said hoarsely, with a ferocity previously reserved for my wife, "If you try it again and I survive, I'm going to tell everyone that you don't know how to intubate, and I'll begin with the nursing office." She desisted. Subsequently, I made a few feeble attempts to cough, just to please her, but she no longer appeared to care whether my bronchi were stopped up or not. She merely mumbled, "Doctors are such *bad* patients!"

My first use of a bedpan and duck in many years also met with problems. The bedpan was difficult enough to mount, but a split sternum is not conductive to wiping and I was too embarrassed to ask for help. The duck was a lot easier, except that no one had warned me to keep the opening high, and I'm too old anyway. When the urine started to overflow, I panicked and spilled the whole damned thing. Now, you'd think such an event would be commonplace in the hospital, wouldn't you? That ugly bitch of a nurse—and this time with great conviction—hissed, "Doctors *are* such bad patients." I cocked one eye at her and, face flushed with embarrassment, said, "May your next patient be an incontinent camel!" She replied, "No difference," and walked out of the room.

On the second postoperative day, I was told to take a short walk. I was helped out of bed and weighed. I had gained ten pounds! Must be edema, I thought. My legs weren't swollen, so the fluid had to be inside me. My brother accompanied me as I slowly shuffled down the hall. About 30 paces along the corridor, I became extremely short of breath. My brother helped me back to my room and into bed and asked the nurse to summon a doctor. We both agreed that I probably had pulmonary edema.

A young cardiologist quickly appeared, listened to my chest, and commented, "Your lungs are clear. You don't have pulmonary edema, that's for sure." It so happened that my brother and I had done a study on the incidence of positive physical signs in pulmonary edema many years earlier. We reviewed 100 consecutive cases entering the hospital via the emergency room who showed the classical radiographic changes of pulmonary edema. Almost half of them had clear lungs on careful auscultation.

Now this young physician tells us that I don't have pulmonary edema when I probably do and urgently need treatment for it. How to convince him? "Then why have I gained ten pounds in two days?"

"You have? Must be edema in your legs. I'll give you a diuretic."

That's all I wanted to hear. The diuresis resulted in at least ten pounds of urine (who weighs it?) in the next two hours. Whether it came from lungs or legs is moot. Later I tried to educate him with a brief dissertation on the physical findings in pulmonary edema. He listened politely but, unimpressed, responded with, "Do you know why doctors are such bad patients? They lose objectivity."

Later on the second postoperative day I developed severe and persistent pain in my right acromioclavicular joint. Since my left arm was already sore from assorted intravenous and subcutaneous injections, I was virtually helpless and in considerable discomfort. I asked my resident, "Is A-C pain a common postoperative complaint or did something happen to my right shoulder in the operating room?"

The answer was in the negative on both counts.

It eventually occurred to my brother and me that I was probably having an attack of gout! Now, how could I convey this information to my doctors and get appropriate treatment instead of a skeptical "Don't be silly"? I gave the problem some thought and hit upon a plan.

Soon the chief surgeon of the hospital and his retinue of staff and house officers, making their daily rounds, single-filed into my room. I was flatteringly introduced as an eminent radiologist, which I acknowledged with a casual self-assured smile. "By the way," I asked, "do any of you know the causes of acromioclavicular joint disease?" They were obviously baffled by the surprising question. One of them mentioned trauma, but no other answers were forthcoming. I said, "Well, there are only a few conditions that involve the A-C joint with any frequency: trauma, hyperparathyroidism, lymphoma, rheumatoid arthritis, occasionally one of the granulomas," and I added, as an afterthought, "Oh, and gout." The head honcho asked, "Why all this interest in the A-C joint?"

"I've got gout in my A-C joint," I pronounced.

He responded as anticipated, "Don't be silly! Gout doesn't even occur in the A-C joint."

"Not so. Radiologists see it occasionally. I certainly don't have hyperparathyroidism, lymphoma, or rheumatoid arthritis, do I? Besides, I was taken off my gout medicine when I arrived here, and I haven't had any for almost a week. The pain started yesterday."

He looked surprised. "You do have gout?"

"Yes, I do."

"Oh! Well then, I'll call the orthopedist."

"Please don't. If anyone knows less about gout than the surgeon, it's the orthopedist."

"Well, what do you want me to do?" he asked, obviously annoyed.

"Just say it's okay for me to take my gout pills. They're in my trousers in the closet over there."

"I'll do better than that. I'll get them for you." He did, along with a glass of water. There was dead silence in the room as I took out the pills, tossed them down, drank the water, and thanked him. As they left, I heard him declaim to his colleagues, "Doctors are such weird patients!"

A few hours later an orthopedist arrived. He had never heard of gout in the A-C joint either, so I gave him a short dissertation on the subject. Later I saw an item on my hospital bill: "Orthopedic consultation." I wrote out a bill for an identical amount, "For teaching orthopedic consultant about gout," and sent it to the administrator's office with an explanatory note. The item was deleted—but I'm certain not without someone's commenting, "Doctors are such bad patients!"

On the third hospital day I was feeling great. One of the hospital radiologists dropped in to pay his respects and we talked for a short time. He got up as if to leave, shuffled his feet indecisively, and seemed to have something on his mind. I asked, "Is anything wrong?"

He replied, "I hate to ask you this, but the residents know you're in the hospital and asked me if I could arrange a teaching session with you."

"Fine. I'm bored stiff. Tell them I said okay."

He walked to the door, stuck his head out, and called, "Come on in fellas. He said okay."

Seven residents appeared, two of whom were carrying a four-panel viewbox, which they set up on my dresser. The others had brought radiographs for me to discuss. We were fairly noisy, and a steady stream of nurses, house physicians, and others congregated at the doorway to observe the unique "happening" in Room 3246.

Several hours later my wife was finally permitted to make her first postoperative connubial visit (in the broader sense). We had an emotional reunion, despite her annoyance at being upstaged by the radiology conference. She noted a band around my wrist and read it aloud, "Sensitive to horse serum." I recall having written this on my admission history questionnaire and was pleased that this important bit of information was available to all those entrusted with my care, including my veterinarian.

My subsequent recovery was speedy. Dr. M. decided that I could, after all, attend the national meeting and receive my medal. I refused politely, without explanation, knowing that he would never understand my reason: The tears of pity in the eyes of my colleagues as I doddered up the aisle and was lifted to the podium wasn't exactly an image that I wanted to perpetuate.

The award was granted in absentia, the ceremony was recorded on a cassette tape, and I received a personal copy. My hypopharyngeal lump and lacrimal effusion were my own private property and not for public display.

Just before my departure from the hospital, a young man-in-white came in to remove my leg sutures. Although some were in odd and obscure places, he seemed to know exactly where to find them. As he worked, I started to discuss a fascinating case of vascular ring I had recently encountered. He looked up, smiled, and said, "Sir, I'm not a doctor; I'm a surgical technologist."

"Oh, that's amazing. You seem to know so well where each suture is."

"I ought to. I put them in."

Some local friends drove us to the airport and we headed for home. It was the seventh postoperative day. Climbing the stairs to the plane was slow and painful, but I managed, preferring this to being conspicuously carried aboard.

Recuperating at home was pleasant. I received many calls from friends and was feeling beloved and important. However, I became dyspneic on climbing the stairs to my bedroom. My brother noted that I appeared anemic; my hematocrit proved to be quite low. We called Dr. M., who asked, "Have you been taking your iron pills?" I replied that there were no such pills among the ten bottles of medicine given to me when I left the hospital. "Oh," he said casually, "we must have forgotten. As a rule, we don't replace *all* the blood after cardiac bypass." The hemoglobin was soon restored to normal by injections of iron.

About three weeks later I was able to go to London. I had been instructed by my physicians not to do any lifting for three months. Since porters were seldom to be found, my poor wife had to carry all the luggage. Fortunately, one of our bags was lost, so she managed, with relatively little chest pain of her own.

On rereading this chronicle, I am forced to admit that *doctors really are bad patients*. But better bad than dead. Being a doctor may lower your risks in that most hazardous of places—the American hospital.

CHAPTER 4

MYOCARDIAL INFARCTION

ROBERT L. SEAVER

In December 1982, my busy practice of internal medicine and gastroenterology was rudely interrupted by a small inferior wall myocardial infarction. Because of persistent angina despite medication, this was followed a harrowing week afterward by a triple vessel coronary bypass graft. As I was recuperating from this technical tour de force some two months later, depression turned to restiveness. I cast about for something to occupy my time in case I could not resume my practice. I inquired of the local health planning agency if I could become a member of that august body. By law, the panel was to consist of a minority of physicians and other health care "providers." The majority were always to be "consumers." As I had just painfully consumed some $45,000 worth of health care, I asked to join as one of the latter group. The representative was visibly shocked. "Oh, no!" she replied, after a pause. "You can *never* be a consumer, only a sick provider!"

Physicians, especially practicing clinicians, face significant problems in dealing with their own serious illness, problems that are not shared by other groups. While there are some obvious compensations, it has been my experience that the mental and emotional mechanisms that we develop to permit us as professionals to deal with life and death issues in our patients may well prove a significant impediment in dealing with personal tragedy and pain. Of course, there is great variation among us, but insofar as any generalizations can be made, I believe this to be true.

What follows is not a treatise in psychology or a scientific analysis. Rather, these are personal and deeply felt observations, buttressed by

DR. ROBERT SEAVER retired from his practice of internal medicine and gastroenterology at age 45, disabled by unstable angina following bypass graft closure. He struggles now with only fair success to adjust to his new circumstances. He writes on medical subjects; eats pills, tofu, and fish oil; and counts chief among his blessings the time to watch his teenage son grow to splendid manhood. Dr. Seaver hopes fervently that the boy will see his father achieve a degree of contentment and accomplishment for a considerable time to come.

a 20-year experience in caring for the acutely and chronically ill in a busy practice of internal medicine. These views necessarily reflect my own socioeconomic and familial background, and are colored by personal philosophic and somewhat inchoate religious views. Nonetheless, it is expected that these remarks will strike a responsive chord in those who have undergone a similar ordeal. Sooner or later, most of us will have had to face such a trial. If I can furnish no transcendental answers, perhaps I can alert others to anticipate the sometimes unique fears and frustrations of being ill while being a doctor.

I was 42, obese, and a chain smoker when I became short of breath after lifting furniture. Light-headed and weak, I lay down. I had had chest pains on and off for several years, but unrelated to exertion and, thus, not classic for angina. These I rationalized to myself as chest wall pain, "smoker's angina," and esophageal reflux and spasm. (I am, after all, a gastroenterologist.) I swallowed antacids and never mentioned the pain to other physicians. I reassured myself that I was neither diabetic nor hypertensive. My intense and compulsive personality was well suited to the pressures and responsibilities of my work. I had not missed a day of work in 20 years because of illness, managed quite well on self-medication (who, after all was better qualified than I to handle my minor medical problems?), and had only reluctantly consulted the cardiologist down the hall when bouts of frequent premature ventricular contractions had frightened me several years before. A normal EKG, a diagnosis of "benign premature ventricular contractions," and a stern lecture on the evils of obesity, smoking, and coffee did not dissuade me from my self-destructive behavior. I was, after all, young, becoming affluent, and going to stop smoking "any day now."

When bands of steel suddenly encircled my chest, I found myself enumerating all the reasons why it was *not* a heart attack. Something, however, was *very* wrong. I yelled for my wife to run for the car even as I snuffed out my last cigarette. I had never permitted myself to seek attention before, but my body screamed in panic what my mind dared not accept. We raced to the emergency room, as I begged my wife to ignore the red lights.

"It's probably only bronchospasm," I told the ER staff, even as I ran to lay myself on the cardiac bed by the crash cart. "Take an EKG stat," I told the ER physician with whom I had so often worked, "but please don't tell me it's an MI." When he studied the strip and stammered before replying, I knew before he spoke. At once, my terror, shame, and guilt were overwhelming. The unthinkable was happening to *me*. I wondered (as had how many before me?) if the last sight I was to see on earth was the stain on the emergency room ceiling.

It was not to be the last time I lay upon that stretcher, but I shall always remember that first terrifying certainty of mortality and the attendant despair. My first thoughts were of my wife and 11-year-old son. How would I tell them, and how would they react? What would become of them if I were to die? It was my night on call, and, incongruously, I worried that my partners would be inconvenienced, and even angry at this inexcusable dereliction of duty.

Suddenly, drastically, everything had changed. My life had reached a blank wall. There was to be no future, the past had no meaning. Here, now, all ended.

As the oxygen hissed in my nostrils, and a technician poked endlessly at my veins, I felt the utter futility of all the skills and knowledge which I had acquired, and of which I was so vain. I had trained for so long, and all the effort and ambition, hopes and expectations were now totally irrelevant.

I remembered now the hypochondriasis of my years in medical school, when learning each new disease evoked subliminal fear of contracting it. Subsequent years had strengthened my denial, and I marveled at my seeming immunity to all the disease to which I was daily exposed. I had, I now realized with awful clarity, come to regard myself as having entered into a pact with God. I would devote myself and my energies to care of my patients, relieving pain and suffering in others. By dint of sheer intelligence, a willingness to work long hours, and competitive striving with my peers, I had proved that I could daily save lives. If I abused my own body with endless cups of coffee, donuts, and cigarettes consumed at late-night sessions writing orders in intensive care, did I not sacrifice myself in the noblest of causes? Was it not written in the Torah that "He who saves a single life, it is as if he had saved the whole world"? Surely divine Providence would preserve me as its instrument in my good works. I enjoyed the respect of my colleagues, and a modicum of financial success. Was this not proof that I was destined to continue at my tasks to a ripe and honored old age? Now, the contract had been broken. My illusion of moral and intellectual superiority was shattered. Nitroglycerine and morphine had relieved the pain beneath my sternum. The rage and anguish were not to be so quickly allayed.

Foreknowledge is the scourge of the physician-patient. Within moments of the onset of my symptoms, I knew what was to become of me if I survived. I was young, and my prognosis was less favorable. If I did not recover without angina, the cardiologist was going to insist upon cardiac catheterization, which I feared. In this heyday of the coronary artery bypass, surgery would be inevitably recommended. It had not yet been proven that surgery increased survival, and the prospect of a painful, dangerous operation in which my brain was perfused by a pump while my heart lay in asystole in the hands of strangers was less than appealing. Years before I had delayed repairing my intermittently incarcerating hernia because of my fears of anesthesia and loss of control. (It had not escaped me that the only people I knew who still wore trusses were surgeons with hernias.) The prospect of this major operation of debatable efficacy for palliation of progressive fatal disease was horrible. Statistics, complications, my experience with my own patients with similar disease—all ran endlessly through my mind.

Meanwhile, my doctor urged calm. He offered practiced reassurances. "Don't worry about it; one step at a time," he urged. I was being asked to play the game—and I had the misfortune to know all the rules. If I lived, I would have to give up my three greatest addictions: food, tobacco, and stressful work. If I died, I would be proven a failure to my family, my art, and myself. I cursed the injustice. My too-small hospital gown could only try to conceal my nakedness. I was surrounded by my associates and assistants in the hospital that had been my subservient domain for a decade and a half. With family at my side, and my parents en route, I was, nonetheless, alone. Ultimately and crushingly alone.

In fairness, there are advantages to being a doctor even in life-threatening circumstances. As a group, we are obsessed with security. Thus, we have adequate incomes and (prodded by legions of voracious insurance salesmen) at least some disability protection and life insurance that blunts the impact of financial disaster.

Professional courtesy dictates that we are cared for at no cost, or that fees in excess of medical insurance coverage are rarely charged. If, as I was, you are hospitalized in your own institution, you are likely to exercise considerable clout. The best available room, prompt and efficient service, and more than sympathetic attention by the nursing staff are your due. Knowing just what to expect in the way of routine procedures and the familiarity of the surroundings ease many common anxieties. But if there is greater comfort in demystifying the hospital experience, there are also great penalties to be paid for your "privileged" status.

Privacy, no matter how zealously protected by "do not disturb" signs and "release no information" orders, simply does not exist. We are a professional community bonded by interdependence, shared confidences and crises, and no little curiosity. Among paraprofessionals, technicians, your partners, your doctors, and their partners, your chart is virtually an open book. After my catheterization and bypass (performed in an adjacent community), half the people in the hospital and a significant number of my patients and friends knew the anatomy of my coronary circulation better than I. What wasn't already common knowledge was the subject of conjecture.

This can prove painful later as you wrestle with recovery and, subsequently, return to work. Physicians whom I had encountered daily in the corridors or with whom I had shared cases for years were to stop me weeks later. With a bluntness that they would not dream of inflicting upon their own patients, they would ask, "Has your angina recurred yet?" or "Why do you want to continue to work with double vessel disease?" Others offered horror stories about other colleagues who had fared badly with similar disease.

Some took pains to remind me that I had, after all, only myself to blame for smoking and overeating. I prided myself as best I could upon the extraordinary effort it had taken to survive, to stop smoking, and return to full-time practice.

I struggled to rebuild a practice that was eroded by a three-month absence from work. It was excruciatingly painful to have a colleague remark casually after rounds, "Gee, we were just discussing the rumor that you had announced your retirement!" All protestations of my recovery were met with visible skepticism. I had committed the cardinal sin of the consultant—being unavailable. I was slow to regain the confidence of some referral sources. It was as if to many, I had already died.

I noted a related phenomenon in a few of my long-time patients whose devotion and gratitude I took for granted. Finding that they had left me for another physician even though they had not been acutely ill, I was astonished that they returned reluctantly or not at all. It was not that they preferred my replacement or even doubted my skill. (Indeed, their cards and notes were laudatory and sympathetic.) It was that I had proved to be fallible and mortal, even as they. The therapeutic magic, the constancy of care, and the implied assurance that I would always be available to ensure their welfare had been disrupted. I was no longer to be completely trusted.

With financial considerations no barrier, and with a more or less intimate knowledge of the abilities, style, and availability of hundreds of doctors, we physicians would seem to be in an enviable position to select the most qualified people to attend us. Instead, I submit that precisely because of this surfeit of options, we tend to choose our doctors in an even less rational manner than do our patients.

The central issue is one of control, the great reluctance most of us feel to abandon our own training and ego, knowledge and pride, to the power of another. Each of us has feet of clay, shortcomings of knowledge or personality. We must knowingly surrender our autonomy to men no better than ourselves. As patients we yearn for the magic of the shaman, the wisdom of Maimonides, the omnipotent kindness of our mothers. Such people do not exist, but the frightened and vulnerable patient finds this difficult to accept without resentment.

Furthermore, in the very act of naming your own physician, you cannot escape beginning the process of unconscious manipulation. We cannot help but know whether the doctor we choose is aggressive or nihilistic, empathetic or authoritarian, cool or emotional, scientific or intuitive in his approach to medicine. Thus, the spectacle of colleagues selecting as their doctors men of distinctly mediocre credentials, so that they may assert their autonomy. Their choice is seen, usually unconsciously, as posing no threat to their ego. Yet other doctors confronted with serious health problems immediately seek care in distant communities to protect their privacy and minimize the impact on their business, at the sacrifice of convenience for themselves and their families. Still other physicians, who would not dream of losing a patient of their own to a distant medical center, flee at once to the halls of academe and the tertiary care hospital at the first suspicion of serious illness. Only the full professor in a university hospital will be adequate for their personal needs.

Most of us self-treat (or ignore) our minor ailments. When forced to seek attention, we seek most often friends (usually specialists or subspecialists) in self-referral. To some, economic or social considerations are of great importance. The surgeon who brings his illness to the medical man who has been his major source of referral, despite the latter's less than enviable qualifications, is such an example.

For other, equally valid reasons, I firmly believe that it is wise to avoid using a partner, no matter how great your respect for his skills, if only to avoid the inevitable conflicts that arise. Your partner must be privy to your most personal affairs in order to be effective. He has, by definition, great personal stake in your recovery. His judgment necessarily suffers. He cannot be impartial in assessing your disability without also affecting his livelihood.

Mindful of this, I chose a local cardiologist of unquestioned ability, though of a temperament very different from my own. Naturally, he was on vacation. Thus, my initial care fell to his associates. These were highly qualified men who were not primarily cardiologists. Since they were anxious to afford me every bit of expertise, their discomfiture in having to treat my persistent postinfarct pain in the absence of their subspecialist partner was all but palpable. Their care was excellent, but their relief was evident when I accepted transfer to the cardiac surgical unit in the neighboring community. There, a team of cardiologists and cardiac surgeons assumed my care. Responsibility became diffuse, and the machinery of the large institution took over.

It is flattering to be asked to take care of one of our own, but it is no small burden emotionally, intellectually, and sometimes financially. We tend to treat each other with hallway consultations, keep poor records, adopt short-cuts, and display poorer judgment than we do with laymen. There is always the implicit fear that our doctor-patient may know more than we do, and there is the virtual certainty that he will ask difficult questions and make demands that the ordinary patient will not. In our desire to extend the professional courtesy that our oath and training demand, we often commit excesses of both omission and commission. In seeking to avoid manipulation and to maintain our objectivity, we may become more authoritarian than is our normal practice; similarly, a sense of identification and heightened concern not uncommonly leads to excessive compliance with the patient's wishes even when they are inimical to his best medical interests. It takes a very rare doctor to be able to treat a colleague with both empathy and dispassion.

There is a great tendency to assume that the physician-patient needs little coaching or advice when in fact he may need more instruction in the management of his illness than others. Or, the patient may find his doctor seemingly condescending when he restates the obvious. If it is difficult to communicate with any patient, the problems are compounded when the therapist and the patient share the same basic knowledge and often similar personality traits.

The conventional wisdom that doctors and nurses make the worst patients has basis in fact. It is axiomatic that if complications and diagnostic dilemmas arise, they will occur in such patients. Whatever you, the attending physician, do for your fellow professional, he will have at least two physician relatives (usually in another state) who will pointedly question your judgment and your actions.

Knowing this, I strove to be a model patient. I was quiet (withdrawn, my nurses said), uncritical, or wryly sardonic when plagued by the innumerable small errors and absurdities that occur in every hospital every day. I took pains to praise all and sundry for small favors, and bit my tongue when awakened for sleeping pills, disturbed to have my blood pressure taken 30 minutes before and 30 minutes after the change of shift, or other needless annoyances. Insofar as my anxiety permitted, I strove not to abuse my status, lest I antagonize those who held my life in their hands. I was not without peccadillos of my own, after all. The staff, I found, is quick to bristle if their routine or their authority is challenged, and becomes even more upset if criticism is justified. I, too, had reacted in this fashion.

An example springs to mind. In the course of a subsequent bout of angina, I was again in my own emergency room. A nurse, well known to me, was pressed into service in place of the regular EKG technician. She strapped the electrodes to my chest, visibly nervous. Suddenly I noticed that the precordial electrode was misplaced by almost four intercostal spaces. The result would be an erroneous diagnosis of new necrosis. I told her (quite gently) of the error and indicated the correct spot. "Don't you tell me my job, Doctor!" was the reply. Insulted, she turned on her heel and stalked out. Within moments the head nurse was at my bedside, chastising me for intimidating a good employee. I protested that I had not been abusive but could not let the error pass uncorrected. I pointed to the suction mark six inches from the proper location. She admitted the error but was still reproachful. "You must understand that taking care of doctors makes everyone nervous." This was to be a recurrent problem. Though they tried to conceal it, many of the people upon whom I was now dependent were made uncomfortable by caring for me because of what I was. Uncomfortable people make mistakes—and I was the potential victim.

Suffering had sensitized me to the human condition. I would salvage much of my experience and turn it to value in my career. If I had not been afforded any cosmic revelations while standing at the brink of the abyss, at least I would become more compassionate toward others.

Gradually through the years I had become increasingly somewhat inured to the spiritual as well as physical pain of my patients. Now I would use my own reprieve to advantage and soften this psychic shell.

As a patient, I was reminded once again of the truism, for example, that the nurses and not the doctors determine the quality of a hospital stay. I had known but forgotten how important to the patient is the provision of adequate, timely analgesia, a kind word, a bed bath. Soft stool, a decent mattress that gives no backaches, and an effective bedtime hypnotic are *important* to us when ill. The doctors' vital choice of an antiarrhythmic or antibiotic is virtually invisible to the patient unless it produces unpleasant side effects. As physician, I would never again forget the promised laxative, the requested diet or room change. A supportive word and attention to the little comforts were critical, not minor accouterments of my treatment.

Also, I could deal in very practical terms with my patients who had undergone similar surgery or suffered ischemic heart disease. There was a camaraderie. Our problems and concerns were mutual and our rapport enhanced.

But rather quickly other, more ignoble, reactions to my illness became apparent. I was, after all, a "cardiac" patient now. Stress was to be avoided where possible. My threshold of tolerance became very low for some hostile, litigious, and otherwise "undesirable" patients. I yearned to get rid of them, for the sake of my own health. Was I not entitled to spare myself avoidable tensions that could kill me?

One morning at 2:00 a.m. I was attending a filthy, abusive, and indigent drunk with no redeeming qualities whatever. I was seething with anger. Was this the reason I had been spared—to minister to this unappreciative, unregenerate lout so that he might live while my chest ached with fatigue and resentment? Guiltily, I only redoubled my efforts not to moralize, but to perform the duties to which I was sworn. Inwardly, I raged.

Still another painful consequence was the aversion I felt to learning anything new or even remotely pessimistic about my disease and its complications. How I envied those among us who sublimate their own fears by avidly reading about their disease and immersing themselves in it! I now avoided, or sat only with dread through, medical rounds and meetings that had as their title "Sudden Death in Ischemic Heart Disease" or "Surgical Cure of Angina—The Fad That Failed."

When *The New England Journal of Medicine* published an article clearly demonstrating accelerated atherosclerosis in bypassed coronary vessels, I could not bring myself to open the cover. It was as if I were required to read my own death warrant.

It is a doctor's job to search diligently for the worst. The *patient* hopes eternally for the best. When they are the same person, the conflict becomes extremely difficult (perhaps impossible) to reconcile.

A corollary of this is the compulsion to identify too closely with patients having similar disease. The objectivity and detachment we all cultivate is virtually destroyed. There is a constant urge to measure yourself against your patient. His success and survival becomes a harbinger of your own. His relapse or deterioration is the mark of your fate. His death portends your own. Not surprisingly, I noted that my patients with ischemic heart disease, and particularly those who had undergone the same operation (by the same surgical team), were watching *me* with equal intensity. I had become not only their doctor but their example. If I seemed in good spirits, they brightened noticeably. If I expressed confidence, they were reassured. When I was depressed, their complaints increased. It was only a week after my resumption of practice that I had occasion to give full-scale resuscitation to a man of about my age who had arrested after an inferior wall infarction. As I pounded his chest and barked orders, my knees were trembling. I had done this hundreds of times with skill and a certain morbid pride. Now, however, no longer was it an exercise of my craft, but a confrontation with my future. Not "There but for the grace of God go I," but instead "Here *I* go." The resuscitation was unsuccessful and I finally called it off. Had I persisted too long because of my own fears? Had I given up too easily because I could not bear the anguish? I am not sure.

A routine visit to a nursing home to pronounce death had become traumatic for me. Viewing the corpse in that bare, still room in the early hours of a winter morning, I stared at the sunken eyes and rigid, oval mouth. The face I saw was my own. The awful mystery of that moment had not struck home since seeing my first cadaver a quarter of a century ago. What bored and tired doctor with a black ballpoint pen would all too soon be signing *my* death certificate?

There is a good case to be made that one who has a chronic illness may not be wise in continuing in an environment where death and suffering are daily occurrences. Do not people in other walks of life typically deny their illness and seek refuge in idyllic or distracting settings where the more joyous and positive aspects of life are reaffirmed? Is it not a form of masochism that compels the physician to immerse himself again in a job in which he is graphically confronting his worst fears, now made immediate? Misery loves company, but continuing to make a career of it requires a great deal of emotional sacrifice or the development of psychic armor.

Medicine itself becomes a religion to many of us. The sanctity of life, the endless struggle to preserve it, the dedication that we bring to the task are hallmarks more of religion than of vocation. Sudden severe illness can make a mockery of that devotion, as we have seen. At such times, we often turn to the faith of our fathers.

As a Jew, I am not very observant of the ritual mandated by my religion. Nonetheless, I try hard to believe in the God of the Bible and to honor the tenets, if not the trappings, of my faith. As I lay upon the OR table, I prayed sincerely if not proficiently in a language thousands of years older than my fears.

It is cold in the cardiac surgical suite on Monday mornings. The heat is off on Sunday to conserve energy, then kept low because of the bypass pump and its associated equipment. Naked and with eyes covered, I shivered despite the preoperative medication. Arterial and venous lines made me miserable as they were threaded into the groin, arms, and neck. The "coldness of the grave" was no longer simply a cliché. I thought achingly once more of the loved ones I fully expected never to see again. Finally, someone said mercifully, "Ready, let's put him to sleep."

As consciousness dimmed, I recited the central prayer of the Jewish faith, the "shema." It is a simple prayer which asks for no mercy and promises neither heaven nor hell. It simply affirms the existence of "God" and His unity. As the anesthetic took effect, the words seemed appropriate and conforting.

"Hear, O Israel, the Lord is our God, the Lord is One."

It would suffice.

CHAPTER 5

CARDIAC ARREST

LEWIS DEXTER

In 1969, when I was 59 years old, I made a diagnosis of angina pectoris on myself in curious circumstances. My wife and I went swimming in Antigua, where the water is warm and balmy. Instead of plunging in, I waded in. When the water reached the level of my PMI, I developed classical distressing substernal pressure. I headed for shore, and on the way in the discomfort disappeared. I repeated this performance—same result. I ran rather gingerly down the beach. After about 50 steps, the discomfort reappeared. Incidentally, the following year I had no angina while swimming in similarly warm water in the Virgin Islands. Collaterals were presumably doing their bit.

Having angina disturbed me. My life-span had once seemed infinite and now I had to come to grips with the realization that I might die in just a few years or, come to think of it, suddenly at any time. To make things worse, I am a cardiologist.

On returning home, I checked in with my physician, who, except for the symptom of angina, found everything to be normal, including an EKG and an exercise tolerance test. For the next ten years I had stable, unchanging angina on effort. Sick sinus syndrome with a variety of atrial arrhythmias was well controlled with propranolol. I was able to live a satisfying life walking, swimming, sailing, rowing, chopping wood, digging in the garden, raking leaves, and the like.

My initial depression and worry over the presence of coronary disease became modified with time. At first, I wondered whether I would be alive next spring. And then what a joy it was to see the crocuses, not only for the crocuses themselves but for the fact that I had survived

DR. LEWIS DEXTER is an emeritus professor of medicine at the Harvard Medical School and an emeritus visiting professor of medicine at the University of Massachusetts Medical School. His career was spent in internal medicine and cardiology at the Peter Bent Brigham Hospital, now the Brigham and Women's Hospital, where he was chief of the Cardiac Catheterization Laboratory from 1944 until his retirement in 1976. His activities combined practice, teaching, and research.

to see them. As the years went by, I became less and less worried. In fact, I became quite resigned to the fact that I was going to die one of these days, that there wasn't much I could do about it, and while life lasted I might as well live it to its full enjoyment.

After ten years of stable angina, things began to change. Angina appeared on less and less activity, but I didn't do anything about it because there were two medical meetings in rapid succession I wished to attend—one in Bermuda, the other in Holland. As long as I did not walk up hills, I was comfortable. I enjoyed the medical meetings and the countryside.

On my return home I planned to see my physician, but before I knew it, I was in all sorts of trouble. Walking up the incline at the entrance to the Peter Bent Brigham Hospital, I became very short of breath. I wrote out a requisition for a chest film, which revealed classical acute pulmonary edema. Before I could protest (because I had rounds and a lecture to give), I was whisked away to the EW and then to the Levine Coronary Care Unit. EKGs showed changes suggesting an apical infarct. Pulmonary edema disappeared rapidly with therapy. Coronary angiography was postponed until my condition should become stable, which it did not do. I continued to have angina. It came without provocation. It occurred at night, waking me from sleep. During the attacks, the EKGs showed changes all across the precordium, and my doctors thought I probably had a critically narrowed left main coronary artery. After about a week of instability, it seemed as though something definitive had to be done.

My illness should have ended fatally. My survival at first glance seemed miraculous. But it wasn't. Webster defines a miracle as "an event or effect in the physical world beyond or out of the ordinary course of things, deviating from the known laws of nature or transcending our knowledge of these laws." In my case, there was no mysterious intervention of the Almighty, but, instead, a whole series of fortuitous events.

The first fortuitous event for me was that as I lay in the Coronary Care Unit talking with the chief of the unit, my eyes rolled up and I became unconscious. (From my point of view, everything from now on is hearsay.) If any of you who are reading this decide to have a coronary occlusion, please arrange to have it in a coronary care unit. The doctors and nurses promptly discovered that I had electromechanical dissociation, often considered to be a good reason for discontinuing CPR. The second fortuitous event was that since I had trained, directly and indirectly, most of the physicians in attendance, they were reluctant to discontinue CPR until (third fortuitous event) the cardiac surgeon came to see me. No one expected him to be willing to operate because there were no coronary angiograms. To everyone's amazement, he said, "Let's operate." CPR was given continuously for about 40 minutes during the time of transfer from the Coronary Care Unit in elevators and along corridors to the OR.

The fourth fortuitous event was that in the OR, a surgical team and an extracorporeal pump team were awaiting the arrival of another patient for coronary bypass surgery. The teams were scrubbed and the pump was all prepared. The other patient's operation was postponed, and I was slipped into his place. Thus, there was no delay and I was put on bypass in five minutes. This, together with expert CPR, has resulted in my still having a brain.

Since there wasn't time, I was put on bypass without anesthesia. After five minutes of no perfusion, brain function deteriorates rapidly. I like to think that I was one of those iron men of yore who could have his sternum sawed down the middle and maintain a stiff upper lip, but I have to admit that I was unconscious.

At this point, you might wonder why the surgeon was willing to operate blindly, as it were, without benefit of a coronary angiogram. There was no precedent. His decision, however, was logical: (1) Coronary occlusions occur in the proximal parts of the coronary arteries which lie on the surface of the heart where the surgeon can see them and palpate them. There is about a 60% chance that the smaller distal vessels will be normal. (2) The surgeon always examines these proximal vessels to determine the best site for making the bypass anastomosis. (3) He needs an angiogram not so much to determine the distribution of lesions, although this is very useful, but to determine their severity. In my case the severity was obvious—complete wipeout of the left ventricle as indicated by electromechanical dissociation.

The surgeon put in two bypass grafts—one to the left anterior descending branch and one to the circumflex. An aortic balloon assist was used for a short time postoperatively until heart function and rhythm stabilized. From then on convalescence was routine. Despite the fact that I awoke from anesthesia, was to all appearances making sense, and seemed well oriented to time and place, I actually had complete amnesia for ten days. Then, over the course of 48 hours, memory returned, and I was perplexed to have a lot of pain from broken ribs and to find scars running with interruptions from the sternal notch to the left knee. As I later reported jokingly to the Human Subjects Committee, of which I was a member, "All of this happened as a result of a simple vasovagal syncopal attack." They never obtained consent to operate. They did not bother to do a coronary angiogram and, therefore, did not prove I had anything wrong with my coronary arteries. They operated without anesthesia. They gave me an experimental drug, nifedipine, not yet approved by the FDA, to keep me from having a "stone heart." However, I recommended to the committee that not only should my physicians be forgiven, they should be heartily commended.

I thought I was a very good patient, but few agree with me. For example, I did not seek medical advice when my angina was worsening. In retrospect, I should not have gone to Bermuda and Holland but, instead, should have been hospitalized for elective angiography and surgery. I denied too much and tended to look after myself—a historically bad, bad thing to do.

From all that I have described, I think it is clear that I received very special treatment. I received a lot of TLC and my convalescence from surgery was routine but not uncomplicated. My broken ribs from CPR really hurt at first and healed over a period of six weeks. Since then I have treated pain of all sorts more aggressively than before.

I had the usual postoperative fatigue syndrome, which lasted in fairly severe form for six weeks and then progressively disappeared over the next three months. I do not know why we patients are practically never forewarned of this complication. It can be mild, moderate, or devastating for weeks and months. It consists of transient negative nitrogen balance and of continuing weight loss, anorexia, insomnia, restlessness, and a form of fatigue unlike that due to excessive exertion, which a night's sleep corrects. This postoperative fatigue is just as severe on awaking as on going to bed the night before. Every activity is an effort, be it physical or reading a book or carrying on a conversation. There is a real element of discouragement and of depression. Since then, I have warned all my patients undergoing surgery, and their spouses too, of what to expect. I remind them that eventually they are going to recover their energy. One can put up with a lot if one knows what to expect. I eventually got back my energy and have not had any angina. I am now as physically active as most healthy 75-year-olds.

I am sure that my illness has made me a better physician and much more effective in dealing with patients with heart disease. I don't mind at all telling them of my illness when and if there is reason to do so. At times, I think it can be reassuring to them.

The main effect of my illness within the family has been to create closer family relationships—more realization on their part that Dad needs to be protected from heavy burdens and realization that he will not be around forever. This is not outwardly displayed very much but is apparent on the basis of many little things that they do. This applies not only to me but to my wife as well.

I was reared in a religious atmosphere. My father was an Episcopal minister. I am a vestryman of the Episcopal Church of Our Savior in

Brookline, Massachusetts. But this does not mean that I am a particularly good Christian. There are a number of teachings of the Church that I do not believe in and there are many that I do. I wish I could say that my illness has deepened my religious beliefs and faith, but it really has not. I wish I could say that during the 40 minutes of cardiac arrest, I had profound religious experiences as others have described, but if I did, amnesia erased the memory.

My illness has given me plenty of time to consider my inevitable demise sometime in the next few years. I'm probably not as prepared as I like to think I am, but only time will tell.

CHAPTER 6

VIRAL MYOCARDITIS

HASTINGS K. WRIGHT

I have always ignored my own symptoms, and not without good reason, for they have always gone away without benefit of diagnosis or treatment. Abnormal signs, such as a generalized urticaria finally traced to penicillin allergy acquired as a surgeon, or a dislocated finger, are another story, and I have always seen to them promptly.

Thus, I finally came to realize with trepidation that some disquieting symptoms were not going to disappear in July 1984. I had had a one-week bout with bronchitis earlier in the month. A chest film suggested a resolving viral pneumonitis, but I took a week's course of erythromycin suggested by an anesthesiologist and a cardiac surgeon who had similar symptoms. I did not quit work for even a day, and carried on an extremely busy schedule caused by summer vacations in my department.

About a week after the bronchitis ceased, I began to notice mild dyspnea when walking on flat ground from my car 500 feet or so to my office. I thought little of this and learned to stop halfway at a men's room to comb my hair and rest for a minute. I then found myself unable to climb a very small hill to the faculty club at Vanderbilt in Nashville while attending a son's graduation from business school. This seemed strange, since I have hiked and climbed in the mountains of New England every summer, and had done so in May and June of that year without any symptoms whatsoever. This worried me, not because the symptoms might signify some major underlying problem but because they suggested possible severe curtailment of vacation plans to climb extensively in the White Mountains in August.

I then found that my shirts were a tight fit, and I began to leave the collar undone to avoid crushing my trachea. I could not understand this sign but my wife certainly did. She accused me of surreptitiously

DR. HASTINGS WRIGHT is a general surgeon on the faculty at Yale. He is also an avid outdoorsman and mountain climber in his spare time.

gobbling fast foods and proved her point by demonstrating with our bathroom scale that I had gained 15 pounds in less than three weeks. I couldn't believe this measurement and bought a new scale, which corroborated the original observation.

I really never put two and two together in those three weeks, and I did nothing until I had two-pillow orthopnea and dyspnea at rest the final weekend before seeking help. Finding help was a problem, for I had no internist or family doctor. Medical problems had always been specifically self-diagnosed and self-referred to a superspecialist who ignored all other organ systems to concentrate on the specific problem at hand. I actually had to ask a wise and experienced nurse whom to see, and when, and she had me in a doctor's office in the next 30 minutes.

I walked into the internist's office at 11:00 a.m., fully expecting to be seeing a busy surgical clinic myself at 1:00 p.m. the same day. My wife was away on a business trip, and I was in charge of a voracious team of family pets who couldn't be ignored for more than 12 hours. Thus, I was not prepared for more than a brief consultation.

It took the internist 30 minutes, and the X-ray department plus electrocardiogram and chemistry services another 20 minutes to make a specific diagnosis: I was in gross congestive failure with an enlarged heart, atrial flutter, bilateral pleural effusions, and peripheral edema. The presumptive cause was viral myocarditis, since I had no signs suggesting arteriosclerosis or valvular heart disease. This initial impression was corroborated later by evidence that a Coxsackie virus titer had risen astronomically from the time of the presumed viral pneumonia to the time of diagnosis of the myocarditis, but I soon discovered that this simple and unitarian diagnosis made within an hour by a competent internist was to be questioned and then only painstakingly reaccepted after an exhaustive 36 hours on a university hospital medical service.

The problem seemed simple enough: Get me out of atrial flutter, diurese off the 25 pounds of fluid accumulated in the last month, do something prophylactically to prevent further arrhythmias, and then proceed to rest and recuperation as the presumed myocarditis subsided. Accordingly, I was sent to the hospital for conversion of the atrial flutter, a process that I was assured would require only two or three hours of use of an inpatient facility prior to return to the infirmarylike intermediate setting used for most inpatient care by my HMO—an inpatient facility run by the HMO internist without benefit of house staff.

I walked into the emergency room expecting to meet the consulting cardiologist and anesthesiologist who were to supervise conversion of the arrhythmia, and was never on my feet again for the next 36 hours.

Before the consulting cardiologist could even get down to see me, the medical house staff had placed me on oxygen, put me on a 10-lead cardiac monitor, inserted a central venous line, plus peripheral lines, and started rapid digitalization. A history and physical examination were performed sequentially in the emergency room by a medical student, a medical intern, an assistant resident, and a cardiac fellow (to be repeated by two more house officers and the cardiologist after transfer to the intensive care unit). I had eaten breakfast six hours previously, which raised the possibility that my stomach was not empty enough yet to make anesthesia safe. In addition, the intern had elicited on admission that I took seven or eight Gelusil tablets a week for heartburn, and he promptly made a presumptive diagnosis of reflux esophagitis, which would, of course, compound the risk of the stomach being partly filled.

It seemed obvious to everyone but me that I had to come into the hospital for several hours, and that the most convenient site would be the medical intensive care unit. Now, there is one rule that has governed my self-care, and my care of patients, and that is *to stay away from university medical services at all cost unless a definitive diagnosis has already been made and accepted* by all. The only reason for admission must be treatment. I have observed such medical services for 30 years and understand their voracious need to do differential diagnostic work-ups, never accepting the referring physician's impression until the diagnostic armamentarium of the university hospital has been exhausted. But I had lost control of the situation already.

After arrival in the intensive care unit, I was seen within three hours by cardiologists, gastroenterologists (that heartburn again!), pulmonary disease experts, infectious disease experts, immunologists, and anesthesiologists, all of whom were attended by numerous fellows and junior house staff. At least ten attempts were made by assorted types to convert my atrial flutter by carotid sinus pressure. Only the arrival of my internist and cardiologist put events back on course, even though everyone deemed it necessary to honor my status as a chief of service by going to a major operating room for conversion rather than staying in the Intensive Care Unit (that heartburn again with the possibility of aspiration pneumonitis, although by this time, I had not eaten for almost 11 hours).

It was now 10:00 p.m. and the senior staff disappeared. I was now in the vulnerable position of being in the hands of the house staff. Despite conversion, I was still mildly dyspneic. Ah ha! Could the diagnosis of myocarditis be wrong? No problem. The entire diagnostic armamentarium of a world-class university hospital was within 100 feet of me, and most of it was simply lying fallow at this time of night.

Could I have had multiple pulmonary emboli? No matter that there was not a shred of evidence that this could be so. A phone call from a medical intern and I was to have a pulmonary scan at midnight, the soonest that the technical staff in radiology could be mobilized—probably at double pay. No matter that such a diagnosis could not be acted on even if made. In addition, Lasix had been started, and I was to void 8 liters in the next six hours, most of it in the X-ray department while attempting to hold my thorax still for two hours for the scan (negative).

I went through the night without possibility of sleep since the medical intern assigned to me finally got around to doing a two-hour definitive work-up starting at 2:00 a.m. Other consultations proceeded through the night, supported by two portable chest films and the application of skin tests ordered by immunology.

In the next 24 hours, with no sleep and no food, I underwent a transfemoral myocardial biopsy, cardiac catheterization, and isotopic scanning of the heart. Everyone who had seen me the previous day, of course, came by again. My hospital chart was already the size of the New Haven telephone book, and all the evidence pointed directly to the diagnosis made in the quiet of his office by my internist after a simple phone call to my cardiologist. There seemed to be nothing else to do to me, although the epidemiologists were summoned in the hope of getting at least some public health good out of my case.

My internist and cardiologist finally rescued me and personally pushed my bed out of the intensive care unit to a quiet room in the coronary care unit. I never again saw any of the house staff or consultants who had so frantically worked on me in intensive care. I doubt that any of them ever obtained any follow-up on my case except those who saw me later in the faculty lunch room. Two days later, in the hall, I saw the intern who had applied the skin tests, and suggested that he give me a quick curbside consultation on my immune status. Nothing was to be seen, and he had forgotten where he had applied the tests at 4:00 a.m. In any event, he was involved in a new medical diagnostic crisis in the intensive care unit and had forgotten my problems. Two days later, I left the hospital.

In retrospect, I could have avoided the whole scene if I had been smart enough to self-diagnose my case, or at least to have seen a physician before going into frank congestive failure and triggering atrial flutter. Once this occurred, I had to pass through hospital doors, and the diagnostic events that then occurred had a momentum of their own that even my internist and cardiologist had little control over. I was swept like a log in a swollen stream through rapids which bumped and bruised me but which did little else to add to my diagnosis. My own doctors remained in charge of treatment, befitting Wright's rule that the only reason to be in a hospital is for treatment, but how could they control all else when diagnosis is an art as well as a science?

When the shouting stopped, I proceeded home to my wife and pets for six months of enforced rest. I counted every oak leaf that fell outside my window in the fall of 1984. A year later, I still do not know how I could have controlled events, but I am finally back at work with no immediate medical appointments to keep, and no diet, no drugs, and no evidence of that Coxsackie virus.

PART II

ORTHOPEDIC–NEUROMUSCULAR DISORDERS

CHAPTER 7

GUILLAIN-BARRÉ SYNDROME

DENISE BOWES

The illness was one that I had always found fascinating—Guillain-Barré syndrome. I was 33 years old, healthy and fit. It came on so suddenly—putting me in hospital for three months, taking a summer out of my life. All I had to do was wait. That's what they all told me. I had never been a patient person. I did everything in a hurry. I had graduated from medical school at 24 and at 26 had started a practice in the village where I now work. I had a busy, successful practice, lots of close friends, and a significant relationship with a man who was very supportive of my career. I was a very lucky woman.

While on call for my family practice group in emergency one night, I noticed before lying down at 11:00 p.m. that I had a mild ptosis of my right eyelid. By 1:30 a.m. I had developed diplopia and began to worry why. I continued my work and had a chance to sleep from 3:00 to 7:00 a.m. By then I was slightly ataxic and had problems going downstairs. I phoned my family doctor at 8:00 a.m. and was seen immediately. I was very calm at this point. My first concern was a brainstem tumour, since I had recently had an 8-year-old patient develop a brainstem glioma with the same presentation, although slower in onset. After seeing an ophthalmologist who candidly discussed the possibilities of a postviral illness or a tumour, I was upset and crying with fear. I was referred to a neurologist at the nearest tertiary care centre, 50 miles away, because I needed a CAT scan. I could not eat lunch because of my anxiety. I saw the neurologist at 2:00 p.m. the same day, and by then I was so ataxic I could not walk without assistance and had developed tingling in my hands and feet. I chose the neurologist I would see because he had been a clinician of mine when I was a medical student, many years before in another city. I usually referred my patients to him

DR. DENISE BOWES is a 36-year-old practicing family doctor in Athens, Ontario, a rural community. She has found considerable satisfaction in sharing her practice and working a more limited part-time schedule since returning to work after her illness. She has helped to establish a support group for other Guillain-Barré patients.

for consultations and found him to be both kind and clever, with a sense of humour, approachable as opposed to "godlike." Unfortunately, he was not admitting that month, and I saw him very little after that initial assessment. The other neurologists I had known little of but felt quite confident in their care.

I was admitted to hospital undiagnosed owing to the rapid progression of symptoms and signs, with weak abdominal muscles and absent deep tendon reflexes my only additional findings. I felt very tired and developed a tension headache. Someone told me that evening that I had Miller-Fisher syndrome—previously unknown to me—and that I would *not* develop the peripheral weakness or paralysis of classical Guillain-Barré syndrome. I decided that I was being given the name of a nonexistent illness to hide the fact that I had a brainstem tumour. The CAT scanner was out of order for four days, during which I became almost completely paralysed. By the time I knew the CAT scan was normal and believed it was Guillain-Barré, I was off to the intensive care unit. But in the meantime, the day I woke and was unable to move in bed or to feed myself, I changed my mind and decided I had multiple sclerosis. I cried again as I showed the resident how helpless I had become and said I was going to be an invalid. He brought in the staff neurologist, who reassured me that they were being honest and not hiding anything.

A lumbar puncture had to be attempted three times before it was successful. Every subsequent procedure through which I was awake—starting intravenous lines, arterial line, subclavian line, oral endotracheal tube, and nasal endotracheal tube—had to be done repeatedly. I don't know whether this is due to an increased anxiety level on the part of the staff doing them, or just my bad luck, but it seems to be a common experience for doctors as patients.

I began to feel like a "patient" only when I was brought into my first hospital room. I was so tired I realized I needed to lie down, so I changed into my nightgown, put my clothes away in a drawer, and lay down to rest. Taking off my clothes seemed to make me a "patient" suddenly. A nurse admitted me. Two more neurologists came in, took my history, and examined me. Later the intern arrived to do it all again for the fifth time that day. I told him to come back tomorrow.

Two anecdotes point out that the physician-patient *is* different—he is treated differently and his response to illness is different, probably less submissive and with more attempts to maintain control over his body than the lay patient.

A medical student who developed Guillain-Barré syndrome before the time of respirators was given artificial respiration by teams of medical students organized by the dean of medicine. He survived.

A physician attending the 50th anniversary celebrations at the Montreal Neurological Institute began to have early symptoms of

Guillain-Barré syndrome while at the M.N.I. He was assessed and advised to fly home to Minnesota. He drove home, his illness progressing along the way.

For me, an important and obvious difference from nonphysician patients was that I knew most aspects of the care I should get, what complications might develop, and what errors in treatment were made. Once I was given two conflicting medications together (Heparin and vitamin K) because the previous order for vitamin K had not been cancelled when the Heparin was started. Since I was unable to talk or write at that time, I had no way of communicating the mistake. It made me feel angry, helpless, and frightened. I waited anxiously for the error to be repeated, and it was, but by then I was able to write and told the nurse not to give the vitamin K and to have the order cancelled, which she did.

Often student nurses asked how to do some aspects of my care. I doubt this would have happened if I had not been a physician. It did not inspire my confidence in my nurse for that day. I wished that she would go away and find out from someone responsible for her how to do the procedures.

I was not a particularly "good" patient, although I worried about being too demanding. I wanted to be assertive enough to ask for what I needed, and that meant making some demands. For example, it was important to me to do my physiotherapy routine the prescribed number of times daily and I needed an assistant to do the passive or active assisted exercises. I insisted on this kind of help because I felt it would help me improve faster. I did not insist on unnecessary care, such as hair washing, which did not affect my outcome. I often complained directly to the person who did something harmful. If my call bell (when I was well enough to push it) was left outside my bed where I couldn't reach it when I was put to bed for the night so that I had to find some way of making a noise to attract attention (I couldn't talk), I vented my anger directly at the person who forgot to pin the bell to my sheet, hoping that she would not forget if she looked after me again.

I did have some input into my treatment because of being a physician. For example, when I was able to swallow fluids, I asked to take liquid iron and a liquid stool softener orally to correct my iatrogenic anemia and my constipation.

Neither a neurologist nor a critical care specialist, I had never followed a patient with Guillain-Barré syndrome. I think there was some tendency on the part of physicians to assume I knew the answers and, therefore, to explain less. When I developed a severe headache lasting two days and finally realized that it was a result of my anger and depression about such a sudden and severe illness, I wrote a note describing my feelings to my nurse. I asked her to pass it on to the doctors so they would know how I was feeling. At my next meeting with them, they said, ''We've been waiting for you to become upset and expecting it and wondering why it was taking you so long.'' It might have facilitated my awareness of those feelings earlier if they had talked about it with me sooner. Also, I felt they sometimes waited for me to ask for what I needed without initiating treatment first. For example, I went through weeks of a very limited diet of fluids since my slowly recovering cranial nerve palsies prevented me from being able to move semisolids or solids to the back of my mouth to swallow them. Later, when my tracheostomy tube was removed, I talked with a strong accent. I privately wondered about speech therapy but assumed my speech would recover in time without it as my muscles strengthened. At least two weeks later, a resident asked me if I usually talked like that and ordered speech therapy. The therapist was horrified that I hadn't been having speech therapy at least six weeks before when I started swallowing to encourage progress in the swallowing muscles and faster improvement in my speech patterns. I think this was an example of everyone's assuming that the others would arrange treatment if it were really necessary and not knowing enough about it to know it was necessary. I took speech therapy for over four months until my speech returned to normal.

I felt some fear of reprisals if I dared to complain too much—reprisals that could easily have been life-threatening for me in my position. It was all too easy for a nurse to casually lay a gauze square over my tracheostomy opening so that I couldn't breathe as she did my ''trach care,'' or to empty the water from the hose carrying humidified air to my tracheostomy by disconnecting the wrong end of it, thereby pouring the cold water into my tracheostomy. So I usually vented my anger to the psychiatry resident who came to see me every day as I recovered. I had all the expected anger about ''why me?'' and also a lot of anger about my care. I was successful in restraining some things, but one can't hold back everything.

Being discharged from hospital became a big goal. I was elated by progress on a daily basis, seeing it all as leading up to leaving the institution. My first steps were overwhelming emotionally. During my three weeks on a rehabilitation ward, I continued intensive physiotherapy as well as occupational therapy concerned with building my endurance and helping me improve at activities of daily living. Making a simple recipe in the kitchen took me many times longer than it normally would have, and I was exhausted by it. On one hand, that helped me realize that I was not ready for discharge, but I also began to fear that I would have to be able to jog again in order to be released. If I went out for a day on the weekend, I had a strong feeling that the staff believed I overdid it, even if all I did was ride in a car and sleep.

They seemed to be looking for problems where there weren't any, like overprotective parents with an adolescent who has separated from them emotionally but is not yet ready to leave in physical terms.

After being home for several months I was terrified to resume practice—afraid my patients would be too demanding of my time and my energy. I had been off work eight months. I was afraid "part-time" practice would mean half days every day and knew I wasn't physically able to do that. I was also a strong believer that one couldn't do "part-time" family practice. In primary care one can't say "no" when patients perceive the need to see their physician. My physiatrist suggested I keep my locum on and start back to work for a two-hour morning once weekly, increasing every two weeks by another two-hour morning. When I was working five two-hour mornings, I could start adding two-hour afternoons, and I was to keep up the swimming I had started three months previously in order to help increase my endurance. This schedule worked exceptionally well. In time I found an associate with whom to share my practice and I now do so, working about 20 to 25 hours weekly, including some hospital rounds. My associate does my night call, emergency shifts, and obstetrics. This positive arrangement has helped me see my practice differently; i.e., it *is* possible to work part time in family practice.

Surprisingly, I am content to work part time and feel I am earning enough to live comfortably, which is all I need. My patients were very understanding. They were glad to see me return and concerned that I take it easy and not work too hard too soon. Even more surprisingly, it was my colleagues who seemed less understanding. They were not doing any extra work for me and so were not anxious to have me working full time in order to relieve them at all, but often I was asked if I was back to full-time work in a way that implied I should be. "You look okay" was a frequent comment. My feeling was that they chose to see me return to my previous workaholic schedule as rapidly as possible in order to be reassured that should anything similar ever happen to them, they would know that they could return to work as fast as possible. Also, there is a possibility they may have thought I was depressed and that a full return to work as fast as possible would be "good for me." Fortunately, I had made contacts with other Guillain-Barré patients and, therefore, knew how long and slow the return to normal endurance is and that 18 months to two years to return to normal is about usual. By 18 months I do not consider myself disabled, but I still require more sleep than I previously did.

I was already an empathetic physician before my illness, but I did learn much about illness and hospitalization that one perhaps cannot learn without being a patient. I feel I am now a good resource person for many neurological patients and more aware of rehabilitation and recovery processes. This helps me plan care and graduated return to normal life-style for patients. I initially had difficulty listening to respirators, but now they are just a reminder, causing a little "ache."

I am quite willing to share any and all of my experiences during my illness with patients and colleagues and with other GBS victims. I have had feedback that this has been quite helpful, so I feel it is worth the loss of privacy.

Religion was not important to me before or during my illness. I feel that we must help ourselves, with love and support from others. I was very much a "fighter" during my illness, trying my hardest to get better as fast as possible. I was concerned that I might later be impatient with my patients who did not try to get better as hard as I had. However, I can see that not everyone responds to illness in the same way and that my way was to try to get out of hospital fast. Someone else who feels more nurtured by the hospital environment may want to take longer to get better.

I feel strongly that I do not have to be functioning as a physician available 24 hours a day for all my patients' needs in order to like myself or to feel that I am a worthwhile, useful person, contributing to the health and healing of others. Being seriously ill and off work for a long time has helped me to come to terms with that. I was surprised by how much I enjoyed being at home. My values have changed somewhat. Work was so important to me for many years, but now it has a lower place on the list of what is important to me—after my significant relationships and my life; my abilities to see, talk, hear, walk, and eat; and my own needs for self-fulfillment, leisure, rest, and privacy. The ability to make decisions about myself and to act on them, to be responsible for myself, and to have some autonomy over my own life is too important to be taken for granted.

Now I am healthy and fit again, after a lot of waiting and hard work and a lot of extraordinary support from my mate and my friends and family. My illness brought most of us closer and gave me a few months of time to renew old relationships. I take life a lot slower now. I try not to put things off, since I never know what tomorrow might bring.

SUGGESTED READINGS

Denise Bowes, "The Doctor as Patient: An Encounter with Guillain-Barre Syndrome," *Canadian Medical Association Journal* 131 (1984), pp. 1342–1348.

CHAPTER 8

MENIERE'S DISEASE

WILLIAM D. SHARPE

It began innocently enough like a spring cold—pressure in my left ear, the blahs, and an occasional sniffle. My left ear gradually began to feel fuller, and I was constantly aware that I *had* a left ear. This annoyed me but was not really painful. It felt as though air were trapped in it or some water remained after swimming. I thought, "Eustacheitis. No problem, a little Benadryl." But it didn't get better, and two or three days later a cacophony of unpleasant noises began—ringing, buzzing, water flowing. My hearing began to fluctuate wildly and reminded me of the radio when I was a boy, as remote stations came in and out of range always interrupted by static. Then I began to be nauseated, dizzy, and depressed. One day I stood up, lost my balance, and fell to the left and slightly forward, breaking nothing but frightening the kitten who had just adopted me. Something was obviously amiss, perhaps seriously so. I had recovered from a mild Bell's palsy a few months earlier, treated at home with aspirin and hot towels by my loyal Filipino internist, Dr. A., one of the few who makes house calls. Obviously this was not a good year for my cranial nerves. I was concerned enough to go through a differential diagnosis. I didn't think a vascular problem likely and—being a pathologist—was left with the choice between a cerebellar tumor and an acoustic neuroma. Dr. A. suggested Meniere's disease and advised that I see an otologist, "preferably a good one." I made up my mind then and there that if I had an acoustic neuroma, the chisel and rongeur boys would get one shot at me, but that a cerebellar tumor would have to run its course.

Dr. S., the otologist, saw me a few days later and ordered a spate of skull films, laboratory tests, tomograms, hearing tests, and the like—CAT scans were not then easily available. I had the tests done as an outpatient, and I paid for most of them. These were extremely worried days, but life went on. I was dizzy, tended to stumble, and was

DR. WILLIAM SHARPE is a pathologist in Manhattan who has concluded that most of what he can't hear probably wasn't worth hearing in the first place.

morbidly depressed, and my hearing kept going up and down. Finally, Dr. S. ran me to the ground and said, "Congratulations, you don't have a tumor. You have Meniere's disease."

"What the hell is that?"

"Nobody knows."

"Will it get better?"

"No, but you'll get used to it and think that it is."

"Will it get worse?"

"Possibly."

"Will I get totally deaf?"

"In one ear, possibly."

"Will the dizziness get better?"

"It will come and go."

"Can I do anything about it?"

"No."

"Should I worry about it?"

"No."

"What do I owe you?"

"Don't be silly."

I decided, like Dorothy Parker, I might as well live. Despite this decision, there followed 18 remarkably miserable months. I was tired, dizzy, wobbly, and short-tempered; my left ear hurt; I was wretchedly depressed; and I came to the point that I really wanted to assume the fetal position, stay in bed under the covers, and feel sorry for myself. I had thought that Meniere's was a trivial disease. I was wrong. I was not prepared, for example, for sudden flashes of nausea as I moved slides too rapidly around the microscope stage, for the fatigue, or for the constant annoyance of fluctuating hearing: "What's that?" "I'm sorry, can you repeat that?" "I didn't hear you." The telephone, an instrument I've detested since my internship, became hopeless—all connections were bad, all lines were affected by interference, every caller mumbled. The complex series of sounds that make up multiple-digit numbers proved particularly vexing, and until I understood that I did not fail to hear sounds so much as misinterpret them, I had real problems with being where I was supposed to be when I was supposed to be there. Unless I walked on a broad base—like the proverbial drunken sailor—I stumbled and, at first, often ran into people on my left. I forgot the extent to which we locate ourselves in space by hearing, and I had to learn to navigate by sight rather than by faith.

Hypersensitivity to noise persists and can be almost physically painful; large cocktail parties are peculiarly awful. The New York subway system is impossible: I cannot hear socially underprivileged youths who may be creeping up on me, their ghetto-blaster radios are torture, and the noise level of the cars is intolerable. Certain tones achieved by female announcers on defective public address systems are irksome. Problems with my sense of balance are worrisome, but if I stumble, the direction and trajectory can be anticipated. I avoid sharp turns, especially to the left. Peculiarly, bowing during church services is extremely difficult. I keep away from the edges of station platforms. I am very careful descending the steep staircases of my old house, and because I topple over so easily, I get dressed sitting down. I have given up live theater, opera, and ballet because my hearing is so unpredictable.

Treatment has been disappointing. A low-salt diet doesn't help, though I neither salt food nor use salt in cooking anything. Various drugs and vitamins proved worthless, although I have the impression that a small dose of phenobarbital and belladonna extract at bedtime (¼ grain) reduces my wobbliness. Postural imbalance is aggravated by tension and fatigue; upper respiratory infections make the discomfort and noise in my left ear worse. A little alcohol goes a long way, and red wine goes farthest. Hearing fluctuates: Some nights I can hear the whirring noise that my case clock makes before it strikes the hour; some nights I cannot even hear the hours strike. I can *feel* my cat purr, but I have never *heard* her purr—curiously, she consistently meows into my *right* ear, never my left, when she wants to awaken me to let her out in the morning.

Deafness and dizziness have not really affected my practice very much: I administer the department and do autopsies but am extremely slow at signing out surgical cases. My three colleagues have been incredibly loyal and supportive. During the first two years, routine chores took so much time that I fell behind in research and writing and gave up several consulting positions. Meniere's has affected my social life in that a quiet, middle-aged, bookish bachelor has become quieter, more middle-aged, more bookish, and much more withdrawn—almost reclusive. I go out socially only when I absolutely must. I eat at home because restaurants are so noisy. Air travel is very hazardous—if I fly, I have to allow a clear day on each side of the meeting to let things settle down, and a flight will occasionally precipitate an acute exacerbation.

I make no bones about having Meniere's disease. I detest the term *hearing-impaired*: I am *deaf*.

When a significant illness is diagnosed, patients are supposed to go through a complicated series of emotional responses. Once Dr. S. gave me the diagnosis, I was, of course, glad that I need not undergo that chain of indignities known as modern treatment. I was annoyed in the sense that any grit in the cogs of orderly existence annoys me (late trains, lost luggage, rude people), but I doubt that denial, anger, or plea-bargaining entered my mind. Nor did religion affect my reaction.

I now avoid going out, and this has made me only an occasional churchgoer. The clergy of my vexed and troubled denomination are now so relevant, so concerned with South Africa, with sexual reform, and with liturgical innovation that they aren't worth a damn as pastors, and even during the few days that I worried about having a lethal brain tumor, it never occurred to me to discuss my worries with them. My internist, Dr. A., himself legally blind in one eye from macular degeneration, merely pointed out that if Helen Keller could make it through life, I should have no problem.

Autonomy and paternalism are the sorts of vague concepts that social workers yatter about. So far as paternalism goes, I never treat myself. I found an excellent otologist, did what he told me to do, and am not fool enough to think that I know more about his business than he does. If I didn't trust him, I'd go elsewhere. Autonomy? Country boys who grew up where I did when I did were expected to be self-sufficient and to keep their worries to themselves. Though it is sometimes difficult to get to work and I may leave half an hour early, I have managed. And expect to.

In summary, Meniere's disease is a chronic and supremely unpleasant disease. I wish I didn't have it. Scarcely a day passes that I am not reminded of its existence. It could have been worse. And may yet be.

CHAPTER 9

MALIGNANT FIBROUS HISTIOCYTOMA AND LIMB AMPUTATION

HUGH L. DWYER

The events I am about to describe took place seven years ago when I was 61 years of age. I was, at that time, a practicing internist in a community that is the site of a major medical center. I was on the clinical faculty of the medical school and the staff of its major teaching hospital. My wife, a radiologist, was a member of the radiologic department in the same hospital where we both had received most of our training.

During the winter of 1978, I became aware of a slight discomfort in my left forearm. This discomfort was provoked only by using the forearm to move an object such as a door when I was carrying something in the left hand. Since this was not a common combination, the experience was infrequent. After some time, with repeated episodes, I began to examine the left forearm. I could not palpate anything, and I could not elicit an area of sensitivity. Over a period of several weeks, however, without other symptoms, I gradually became convinced that I could perceive, in profile, a slight elevation of the soft tissue on the extensor surface of the left forearm. In the ensuing few weeks I consulted several colleagues in the corridors of the hospital and was, with some difficulty, able to convince them that there was, indeed, a slight elevation of the soft tissue in this area. For the most part, none of them was alarmed, and one or two suggested that he would be happy to explore this surgically if I wished him to do so. No one seemed to feel that there was anything urgent about doing this. I finally convinced myself, however, that, indeed, a tumefaction of this sort required a histologic diagnosis and removal. In 35 years of practice I had not encountered anything of this type so that a differential diagnosis did not occur to me. This seemed to be true of most of the surgical colleagues whom I consulted.

DR. HUGH DWYER is a retired internist who practiced in New Haven and served as a member of the clinical faculty at Yale Medical School. He was a member of the staff of Yale-New Haven Hospital and a trustee of that hospital at the time of his retirement.

As I look back upon it, I realize that I was comfortable in acting as my own primary physician. I had exhibited the slight swelling and described the slight sensitivity to at least three colleagues and finally reached the point where I was prepared to have someone explore it. On this occasion I seemed to be concerned less with the significance of the character of the lesion than with the preservation of function in the left forearm. As a result I chose a plastic surgeon, also a close friend and colleague, because I felt he would handle muscles and tendons with the utmost delicacy. Up to this point I had not seriously considered the possibility of benign or malignant lesion, though, like any experienced physician, I was aware of the fact that a swelling that justified surgery was possibly malignant. By this time, perhaps three or four months had ensued since the initial sensitivity and some half of that time since the awareness of tumefaction.

In the period before choosing a surgeon, I had briefly, but not seriously, considered the possibility that amputation might be ultimately required. I had, I am reminded, stated to my wife that I would not consider this option. I do not believe that this particular possibility occurred to my physician-friends and I do not recall that those who examined me, both prior to surgery and upon admission to the hospital, were sufficiently concerned to have made a very careful examination of the axilla or epitrochlear area. So I entered the hospital some months after the initial symptoms and was prepared for general anesthesia and what I presumed to be removal of the soft tissue lesion. I thought it might well be a benign lipoma.

Shortly after I regained consciousness, I was visited by my surgeon and was a little surprised to learn that only a biopsy had been carried out. This was probably his intention prior to surgery, but I was not aware of it. He informed me that frozen sections had revealed a malignancy, as yet undefined. Further surgery was scheduled within the next two or three days, presumably for total removal of the tumor. Immediately following the surgery for attempted removal, I was told that cleavage lines of this tumor were not easily identified and that, after presumed removal, biopsies from the bed of the surgical field had revealed residual malignancy in all areas.

Within an interval of a few days, the permanent sections revealed that this tumor was a malignant fibrous histiocytoma with myxomatous change. This was a lesion with which I had no familiarity. I discussed it with the surgical pathologist on the telephone and was told simply that this lesion was treatable by total removal. I found a reference to this lesion in extremities and, while still in the hospital, requested that the chief of the surgical service allow me to borrow his copy of the journal describing it. He was a little reluctant to allow me to see it but soon recognized that this was unavoidable. The information here revealed that this was not as uncommon as I had assumed and that the information I had received from the pathologist was quite accurate. The pathologist had assured me that the lesion was treatable by total removal, and I had the impression, confirmed by my reading, that it was not characterized by early distant metastases. When the pathologist also recommended a second opinion, my wife took the slides to a New York medical center, where the diagnosis was confirmed. While in the pathology department she happened to encounter an old friend, the former chief of our radiology department and a well-established radiotherapist. He confirmed the diagnosis and suggested that amputation would be the treatment of choice. This information was brought to me promptly and was compatible with the information that I was receiving from my surgeon, our chief of radiotherapy, and others. While I had expressed a strong rejection of amputation prior to the biopsy, like most people who do not have to face the problem squarely, I promptly abandoned this point of view. Being in a medical center, I found it easy to consult many specialists, all of whom were eminent surgeons, radiotherapists, or oncologists. I soon established the fact that radiation was not likely to be the best treatment. My limited consideration of chemotherapy was abandoned after consulting an old friend in a distant medical center who had considerable experience with perfusion chemotherapy of extremities. He was familiar with the lesion and confirmed that amputation would be the best choice of therapy. So the impact of considering an amputation as the curative treatment came in stages to me and, perhaps, was easier to accept than if it had been immediately recommended on biopsy.

I then had to made a choice of a surgeon to carry out the amputation. I was acquainted and friendly with a number of orthopedists, but I elected one of my older friends who was chairman of the department, and he responded promptly. Surgery was to be carried out shortly thereafter, and I was allowed to spend a weekend at home before readmission. During the weekend at home I discussed the final decision with my children and my siblings in another city. I remember that during the phone discussion with my brother, a physician, I had difficulty finishing the conversation because of an emotional reaction. This happened again when I was phoned by a solicitous cousin. On each occasion I had to hand the phone to my wife to complete the conversation. I was quite aware of the fact, on this weekend, that this was my last with two arms. I elected to play my final round of two-handed golf, which concerned my wife enough to prompt her to get the approval of the orthopedic surgeon. I entered the hospital late that Sunday afternoon prepared for amputation the following morning.

My surgeon had, by this time, discussed with me the nature of the amputation and the nature of the phantom symptom and the phantom pain, which I emphasize as being quite separate problems. He did not minimize this but assured me that it was temporary. I had no previous experience with this subject nor any familiarity with the literature or proposed treatment. Through no fault of anyone I was ill-prepared for the next series of events.

I accepted amputation with reasonable equanimity. I was neither depressed nor apprehensive. Following surgery on Monday morning, I awakened in the early afternoon in good spirits. I was aware of pain but expected this. It was unlike anything that I had previously experienced, which was very little. I had much attention, many visitors, and many distractions. I felt well enough to have a surreptitious martini prior to the evening meal and promptly rejected it. The following day I was out of bed visiting two or three patients that I had referred for surgery who were residing on the same corridor. Some colleagues who came to see me were surprised to discover that I was out of my room and in such good spirits. On the fourth postoperative day I was to be discharged and a nephew came to visit me and drive me home. My car was in the hospital parking lot for this short interval, and I felt quite able to drive myself home. I returned to my office for resumption of practice within less than two weeks and shortly thereafter I returned to the golf course to learn a new form of golf with one hand.

From this point on, my activities were resumed in a more or less normal fashion. I resumed driving the car without difficulty. I took a relicensing examination and passed easily. I visited a mutual friend in a nearby community who was, himself, an amputee, having lost his arm in a wartime accident. He helped me by showing me how he managed certain simple activities such as tying shoes, knotting a necktie, and other commonplace daily experiences. He was a person of awesome resources. He not only drove a manual shift car but was also able to fly an airplane despite a comparable handicap. Curiously, he had no experience with phantom pain.

For the next year my chief preoccupation was the phantom pain. For those who are not familiar with it, I make a sharp distinction between phantom sensation, or the feeling of the existence of forearm and hand, and phantom pain, which is a steady burning, rather severe pain extending into the phantom hand, present at all times without significant variation. This bothered me more than the handicap of the loss of the extremity. In fact, in some desperation, I accepted the suggestion of a colleague to visit a distant medical center where there was an orthopedic surgeon with a special interest in amputees. He had developed a unique clinic for their care and rehabilitation. I did not investigate comparable help locally. My wife and I embarked to this medical center, where we spent about a week. The physician who had been recommended could not have been more concerned or considerate. I stayed in a motel across from the medical center and daily went to his clinic. The physician and his assistants seemed to be anxious to prepare me for a prosthesis. I was so concerned about the pain, even though having been assured that it would not be permanent, that I was more anxious to have some temporary relief from this than to secure the prosthesis. I had not even considered this subject prior to my visit to this clinic. A number of things had been attempted in my own hospital, including nerve block and even stellate ganglion block, neither of which eliminated the pain. A small battery-operated gadget for counterstimulation was tried through the kindness of my colleagues, but it proved to be of no avail. This was again tried in the clinic while preparing me for a prosthesis. About the end of the week the prosthesis was finally fitted and adjusted. Up to this point I had not taken a stand as to whether or not I wished to wear a prosthesis. I felt fairly adequate with one hand except for some minor personal experiences with daily activities, and these were usually things that I could adjust to or for which I could seek assistance. After a very short experience with the prosthesis, I convinced myself that I would never wear this. My professional and other activities did not require it. Only constant wearing would afford me the skill necessary to use it. It seemed unnecessary and in the way in driving a car and practicing medicine, so I did not even bring it home with me.

I was pleased with the way my problems were handled but disappointed that I had not been relieved of pain. At this point I could see living with ease with no left arm but could not tolerate the prospect of indefinite continuation of the pain and had hoped and anticipated that this distinguished center for amputees would have been able to provide some relief. By this time suggestions that I visit other medical centers or undergo acupuncture fell on deaf years, and I was satisfied that I would simply have to wait for the spontaneous recovery from pain.

The next year was one of constant pain, relieved only to a limited degree by distraction and activities, and occasionally testing my patience. I remember the observation that this pain was relieved by attaining sleep. Since it had not been affected by nerve blocks and so forth and no medication had an effect, I was fascinated by the clear relationship between pain and sleep. Another observation was even more fascinating. Upon awakening in the morning, frequently if not invariably, there was a short period of somatic wakefulness but an interval of a few seconds when the pain did not immediately reappear. I was reminded of the condition experienced by some victims of narcolepsy in which consciousness is attained in waking from sleep, but there is a total paralysis of the neuromuscular system until a stimulus, sometimes physical, can awaken it. This fascinating subject has always interested me and is known as sleep paralysis. Since sleep was so effective in relieving pain, I occasionally came home in the afternoon hoping to get some temporary relief. After a short nap I would awaken a little depressed at having had to give in to this and, fearing falling into this habit, did not allow myself to continue it. After about a year I became aware of the fact that this pain was not as severe, and I was able to assure my surgeon that I was aware of its diminution and disappearance within a very short period of perhaps two weeks. The phantom sensation has been with me unabated and easily tolerated. It is occasionally accompanied by brief surprising shocks of pain as though I were stimulated by a disagreeable electrical impulse in the phantom areas, but these occur in flurries and are largely absent when I am busy or distracted.

At this writing, some seven years after surgery, I am two years into retirement. The retirement was not related to the handicap. While there are some limitations, I seem to have accepted the handicap without continuing emotional impact. Occasionally I am a little sensitive about my appearance, usually preferring to wear a jacket with an empty sleeve rather than a sweater or polo shirt. I accept the latter in recreation and in sports activities. I continue to play golf with considerable pleasure and enthusiasm, finding it even more challenging than before. I have some difficulties with small things, such as writing a check or signing a small piece of paper without requesting that someone hold it for me and particularly in handling paperback books. I continue to have an interest in gardening, and I can plant, weed a garden, edge, spade, transplant, and other such chores. I find pruning very frustrating and usually avoid it. I cannot say enough for the sympathy I received from patients and my helpers, as well as my wife. My children have been supportive. I do not believe that my practice was significantly altered by my handicap. My patients were quite accepting of the compromises that I made with the assistance of my office nurses in carrying out physical examinations and treatments. I made no attempt to continue pelvic examinations, for obvious reasons, and I would not consider my capability in examining the breast to be equal to that of a person with two hands, but most of my patients were capable of consulting gynecologists and other physicians for this purpose.

Having accepted the amputation as the treatment of choice for this malignancy and having been assured of its characteristics as well as the fact that lymph nodes in the epitrochlear area were negative for malignant cells, I have not been concerned at any time about recurrence or the appearance of metastases.

In summary, I acted as my own primary physician, having the advantage of a very supportive and professional wife and being in a medical center where I had access to unlimited expertise from colleagues. I do not believe that there was unnecessary delay in seeking attention for treatment. I could not have asked for exploratory surgery in the forearm for the first month or two when there was no convincing evidence of tumefaction. While the initial acceptance of the handicap of surgery was not without its emotional impact, I believe that the reaction was minimal and that, with the help of others and with a certain amount of determination on my part, I accepted what had to be done with as much fortitude as one could expect. I continue to enjoy life and, almost without exception, the activities that interested me before the amputation, sometimes with more satisfaction, perhaps because of the increased challenge.

CHAPTER 10

LYME DISEASE

DAVID B. BINGHAM

"If ya got cows, they're gonna git out."

This is a fact of life, as stated by a local farmer to my dismayed wife the first time our heifers got into our neighbor's garden. Having been raised in the country, I've spent many hours rounding up straying farm animals, but Annie never has quite accepted my excuse that no matter how much time I spend mending fences, sooner or later the cows will find a way through, over, or under whatever fencing is there.

The cows are especially adept at escaping when they are "in heat." One Sunday in April 1979, it was my good fortune to be home, so Annie wasn't left alone to try to herd the stubborn, unpredictable, and lovesick young animals back into our pasture. They had eluded me successfully by reaching a swampy area, and it took several hours of slogging around through the muck before the two stubborn animals finally decided enough was enough and agreed to head back to the barn for some grain.

I worked in the yard and vegetable garden throughout the afternoon, so it was not until evening that I showered and changed my clothes. After removing my blue jeans, I noted an itching sensation on my right thigh and while scratching the area felt two tiny bumps. The bumps were two pinpoint black dots on the skin, which turned out to be ticks approximately one-half the size of a flea. They came off easily between my fingernails, which I used to crush them before flushing them down the drain.

Although I had lived in the area all my life, I had never seen ticks this small before. Wood ticks (the size and shape of an apple seed) and dog ticks (pea-sized and gray) have always been found in the area, but

DR. DAVID BINGHAM practices ob/gyn in Norwich, Connecticut, and is politically active in behalf of reproductive freedom rights and tort liability reform.

I had never seen any so tiny. It is in the first few molts of the tick that it is apparently most infectious for Lyme disease.

The following day I noticed a red, well-circumscribed, slightly raised, and very sensitive patch around each of the tick bites, almost 10 cm in diameter. This appeared so much like a streptococcal cellulitis that I picked up some Keflex samples from my office the next day. I forgot to take the medication, however, and when I awoke the next morning the rash was gone. How fortuitous, I thought to myself. If I had taken the antibiotic I would have thought that the rash cleared up because I had treated the infection, and I would have been obligated to continue the medication for several more days. Now I could get by without any further medication—how wrong I was!

About a week later I began having midthoracic back pain while chopping wood. Over the next few days the pain seemed to move to various levels, including the cervical and lumbar spine areas, with different degrees of intensity and duration. By now I had temperature elevations up to 102°, headaches, and general malaise. By this time the probable diagnosis was evident. My hometown of Salem is adjacent to Lyme, Connecticut, where the constellation of symptoms was first noted by residents of a single street who prompted the investigation leading to the discovery of Lyme disease by the team at Yale University School of Medicine.

Since there was information about the disease in the local newspaper indicating that it was carried by a newly discovered tiny black tick, caused polyarthritis, and frequently was accompanied by a rash and fever, I felt fairly confident of the diagnosis and did not seek any further medical care at that time. I did read the information that was then available in the literature, which indicated that antibiotics did not seem to prevent the symptoms from occurring, and that the only treatment recommended was to use aspirin or other antiinflammatory agents.

It was disconcerting to learn that several neighbors had ended up with prolonged hospital stays, some with neurological symptoms including facial and other peripheral nerve paralysis, heart block, and major joint complications. On the other hand, it appeared that most patients had eventually recovered from the disease, sometimes in months, but usually in two to three years.

Since most of the neurological and cardiac complications of Lyme disease occur as early sequelae, and since my course over the next few months consisted only of mild and intermittent joint pains, I had no particular concern about the disease at the time.

Six months after the onset, I experienced my first severe pain. I awoke with swelling and tenderness in the left temporomandibular joint and had difficulty opening my mouth to brush my teeth. For the next ten days I subsisted on liquids or semiliquid foods put through the blender. I relived the glorious days of infancy and rediscovered the joys of applesauce and hot cereal. Trying to chew ever so gingerly brought involuntary tears to my eyes, and Annie finally succeeded in getting me to seek medical consultation.

I was fortunate to be able to have nearby one of the principal investigators of the disease and an associate professor of rheumatology at Yale to confirm the diagnosis. His thorough evaluation, including the usual university hospital battery of blood tests, inspired confidence that we were in fact dealing with Lyme disease, although at that time there was no specific serology as there is now to confirm the diagnosis. He suggested larger doses of aspirin as long as I tolerated it and filled me in on the vagaries of the disease.

At the time of the initial tick bite, I developed a lymph node in the right inguinal area which had gradually subsided in size but which even six months later was still palpable. I told him of my initial impression that the rash looked suspiciously like a bacterial cellulitis, and that there might be bacteria in the lymph node that could possibly help lead to the discovery of an etiologic agent. I would have been happy to let him remove the lymph node if he thought it would be helpful. At that point there had been numerous attempts at culturing affected areas, without any success, so my offer was declined. I was disappointed not to be able to play a significant role in the study of my disease. In retrospect, it is unlikely that the spirochete that causes Lyme disease would have been discovered in this node without the special staining and culture techniques that were later used in identifying the organism, even if it had been present.

I went home with a large bottle of aspirin and learned my first big lesson from having this disease, which was an appreciation for what a good drug aspirin is. During acute flare-ups of the arthritis and fasciitis, it substantially diminished or completely alleviated my pains. I was later to find that when aspirin failed, the newer nonsteroidal antiinflammatory agents work even better, but for most of the inflammatory pains aspirin was sufficient and inexpensive.

I have subsequently learned that when I tell patients aspirin can be an effective pain-killer, they rarely seem to believe me. It has the stigma of being cheap and readily available without a prescription. When patients reach the point of seeing a doctor, they seem to want a medication that only the doctor can provide, perhaps to feel that the consultation was worth the cost. But I appreciate that my physician was cautious about using what were then relatively new antiprostaglandin drugs on the market and gave me the encouragement to stick with a tried and true drug as long as it was effective.

During the next two and a half years the polyarthritis was intermittent but occasionally severe. My knees at times were so painfully swollen that I had difficulty walking and crutches were needed. When the swelling was at the point where I had difficulty getting into my car to get to work, I was willing to have the knee tapped and drained and had cortisone injected into the joint. The immediate effect of this was truly remarkable, gave lasting relief of pain for weeks, and made me appreciate being in a modern era of medicine to have such a drug available. On the other hand, there was the nagging worry that if this had to be done often, there might be some permanent damage to the joint. I was determined to get through this disease without any permanent effects, so it was only when it reached the point where I feared I would not be able to go to work that I would submit to the injection. Fortunately, there were only three times when this was necessary, and no permanent changes have occurred.

One of those episodes, however, was particularly frightening. My knee was extremely swollen in the morning, so much so that I had difficulty putting my pants on. I had been using elastic stockings to keep the swelling down with only moderate success. While making rounds in the hospital in the morning, hobbling around on crutches, I felt a sharp increase in pain in the calf of my leg. By late morning the whole leg was swollen as large as my knee and tender throughout. I was reluctant to leave my partner with a ward full of patients in labor and an office appointment schedule that was filled to overflowing. But both of us looked at the leg and decided it was time to head back to Yale. I really thought that this might be a deep venous thrombosis and that for the first time in a year and a half of the illness I might have to take some time off from my practice. I dared not even think about the threat of pulmonary embolism.

It turned out the change in the leg was due to a rupture of a Baker's cyst behind the knee and that heat, elevation, and a cortisone injection would do the trick. By the next day I was able to return to work and was relieved that I would not have to burden my partners with a change in the "on call" schedule, which, for a busy obstetrical practice like ours, would be devastating to our precious family life. It turned out to be the only day that I missed work, despite many episodes of pain, fever, and poor mobility, during several years of illness.

The biggest change in my life was my inability to participate in sports. Running, hiking, tennis, and ice hockey have been a central part of my life. I continued to participate as much as I could, despite the admonitions of my physician, who felt that activity might make the joints worse. In general, my experience was just the opposite. If the pain was tolerable, I continued to play. There seemed no relationship whatsoever to new joint pains or any particular activity. Frequently, after using my joints, they seemed better the next day, and certainly the exercise made me feel better and "more normal." I was delighted to find that ice skating did not cause any "jarring" of the knee and that the smooth use of the knee joints felt as therapeutic as swimming or bicycling. The conventional wisdom still seems to be that if a joint hurts, rest it. But I was determined that as long as I could tolerate the pain I would lead as normal a life as I could, and in retrospect, this attitude certainly got me though the worst of the disease in relatively good spirits and the time seemed to pass quickly.

Nevertheless, I was definitely less mobile than before. There was one very positive effect of this inability to get around as far as I was concerned. While it probably tortured my family, I spent a good deal of time trying to learn how to play the piano and got a great deal of pleasure out of it. I still can play a couple of tunes and wish I could spend the time I did in those days to get in more practice.

Over the next three years, evidence began to accumulate that antibiotics were effective in treating Lyme disease. The initial reports considered only the acute early phase, however, and it was not clear whether antibiotics would work to help in long-term cases such as my own. It was felt that many of the symptoms could well be due to immune mechanisms rather than to bacterial infection. Yale was offering a double-blind study of injectible antibiotics, in conjunction with placebo, to patients like me with chronic recurrences.

At about this time, I had an elbow swollen the size of a grapefruit and had difficulty tying a necktie. Fortunately, I was able to deliver babies at arm's length and do surgical procedures, but I could not brush my teeth or button my shirt except with my left hand, because I simply could not bend the elbow beyond a right angle.

Although I believe strongly in double-blind studies, I was getting concerned that I might not be able to operate if things got any worse. I therefore decided to go ahead and take penicillin on my own, in relatively large amounts (500 mg q.i.d. for a month), even though there was no medical literature to support the efficacy of my self-medication.

After a week of medication there was no change whatsoever in my elbow, and it was clear that if antibiotics were effective, there certainly was no dramatic effect. Nevertheless, I continued the medication for the whole month. The elbow gradually subsided in pain and swelling over the following several weeks.

If there was an effect from the antibiotic, you would not have been convinced at the time. But since then, three years have gone by, and I have not had a single significant joint pain! I run five miles regularly several times a week, play ice hockey, and give thanks to penicillin whenever I get a chance! The literature now supports the use of a large amount of antibiotic for longer than usual courses, and it looks like that was what cured my case as well.

In looking back over the several years that I was ill, I do not recall any particular depression and few moments of anxiety. Compared to the emotional distress caused by malpractice litigation which has affected our practice, the physical distress and pain that I suffered from Lyme disease was negligible. Those years were happy years in terms of my relationships with wife, children, and colleagues, and my life was full despite my physical disability.

Perhaps the most striking change in my relationships with patients since the illness has been my decrease in tolerance for patients who wish to get out of work because of various pains and complaints. I am often asked to sign a letter to an employer stating that a patient cannot work because of a pain in a muscle or a joint, even when the work itself bears no relationship to the pain and will not cause any injury. In the past, it was hard for me to know whether or not a pain was "bad enough" to warrant staying home at rest. From my own experience, however, the time passes more quickly, and life is more meaningful, when one has a job and a specific purpose.

Perhaps one might say that a job as a physician may seem a lot more meaningful than a job in a factory or typing in an office. Nevertheless, most physicians would concur that much of the work in their day becomes routine after a while. It is not until one has done many operative procedures that one becomes an excellent surgeon, but by this time the newness and excitement have gone. The emotional rewards come more from the challenge of doing a good job rather than from the idealistic and naive notion that a gynecologist is something more than a highly specialized plumber.

Many physicians have written in the past that being sick has made them more sensitive to the complaints of patients. But when these complaints take the form of "I can't do this" or "I can't do that" because of pain, I find myself bristling. It is harder for me than it was in the past to be kind and compassionate when such patients fail to respond to encouragement and reassurance. I want to be able to say that I know what pain is, and it didn't keep me from working long hours, and that by doing my job, I felt good about myself and my lot in life. But I'm afraid most of them would look at me with complete lack of comprehension or perhaps consider me a masochist. So I swallow my angry thoughts and try to be patient.

In closing, I am reminded of the philosophy of Norman Cousins in his *Anatomy of an Illness*,[1] which emphasizes the importance of good humor and a positive approach to pain and disability. In my own case, without the benefits of aspirin, cortisone, and penicillin, I would have suffered far more and might well still be disabled. But the good humor and encouragement of those around me at home and at work were the best medicine of all. The physical pain, acute as it was, could never match the rewards of a caring environment or compete with the joys of exploring our wonderful and fascinating natural world with an inquisitive mind. I have at times wondered whether I could psychologically survive a serious handicap such as spinal injury or loss of vision. My illness convinced me that physical handicaps are only physical, and the emotional pursuit of happiness need not be impaired by pain or physical disability.

While my experiences may have at times triggered impatience toward those who use their disease as an excuse to withdraw from active participation in the chores of day-to-day life, they have also given me confidence that caring and encouragement can go a long way in helping to maintain emotional health and a positive attitude, despite significant illness.

REFERENCE

1. Norman Cousins, *Anatomy of an Illness* (New York: Norton, 1979).

CHAPTER 11

PROSTHETIC HIPS

JOYCE L. DUNLOP

As well as enjoying my full-time job, large house and garden, and three teenage children, I played competitive tennis for a local team until my mid-40s.

In the summer of 1981, my forehand drive seemed to deteriorate and I, who had been renowned for "getting everything up," missed easy shots and felt generally clumsy. I put it down to "age" but felt a bit aggrieved when I remembered that my father had had an unreturnable serve well into his 60s. Throughout the following winter, walking became increasingly tiring. I had no pain then, but my legs felt "odd." It was particularly noticeable over the weekends when I stood a lot, shopped, or gardened.

I visited my family doctor with my nebulous symptoms and, not surprisingly, he found "nothing wrong." All that winter and throughout the following year, I became increasingly restricted and began to feel a complete fool since nothing resembling a "textbook picture" emerged. What was particularly odd was the daily pattern. I was "completely normal" on getting up, a bit stiff at breakfast time, struggling by lunchtime, and hardly able to stagger by teatime. This led to a certain amount of denial during the night. Each morning I was hopeful the improvement would continue. It did not. My family affectionately described my gait as that of a "ruptured duck." I began to worry about my job and to sleep badly, which was most unusual for me! I lost about two stone in weight; one was probably a good idea, but not the second one. My doctor sent me for X-rays, which were "normal" apart from "minimal arthritis in both hip joints."

I came to the conclusion that if I was not suffering from multiple sclerosis, my symptoms must have a hysterical basis. I somehow felt

DR. JOYCE DUNLOP is a general adult psychiatrist practicing in a mixed urban and rural area on the east coast of Britain. She tries to preserve what is best among the older physical treatments (e.g., medication, ECT) and combine them with the newer "therapies" to give a "two feet on the ground" approach.

ashamed of being ill, which I knew was illogical, isolated, which I was not, and uncertain of everything. When symptoms become chronic, it is particularly difficult to reach the point when you "cannot take any more."

Matters came to a head in the spring of 1983 when I was unable to straighten up after interviewing a patient in the cells at the local police station. What the police thought of the duty psychiatrist I can only imagine!

My doctor asked me who I wished to be referred to: an orthopaedic surgeon, a neurologist, a rheumatologist, etc. I did not know. All I wanted was to be told what was wrong and what should be done about it. I saw a general surgeon and a physician, who found "nothing wrong" apart from an ESR of 86. The choice of orthopaedic surgeon was my family doctor's. It was the man to whom he referred all his patients with suspected orthopaedic problems. I was happy to leave this choice to him, and, as things turned out, I have no regrets. (I used to seek a "father figure" for my medical attendant, but the older you get, the harder this is to find!) This surgeon was considerably younger than I. On reflection, this is a good idea because he will be around for a long time should anything further ever be required! I can understand how patients hero worship and become overdependent on their surgeons. I found myself noticing if his car was in the car park and when he was away on holiday—really quite ridiculous. At that time he examined me and took further X-rays, commenting that there was bilateral absence of joint space with bony changes on the left side. Joint replacement was suggested for the left hip.

There was a great feeling of relief once something definite was found. This was something tangible, something I could get my hands round, something we could fight, and, most important, an illness that something could be done about. As expected, initial relief was short-lived. Soon I was asking the questions "Why me?" "Why a doctor?" "Why so young?" (the pathology was probably caused by congenitally poor positioning). There is a natural recoil from major surgery, and female vanity dislikes the thought of two long scars. All television programmes at that time portrayed leggy women with high-cut bikinis. There is unreasonable distaste at the thought of incorporating lengths of metal and polyethylene sockets into your body. All the above worries need to be faced and worked through. The anxiety state so common after emergency surgery probably results from lack of time to do this. As for me, when you cannot walk and modern surgery offers an escape, there is no alternative.

I had my left hip replacement during the first week of July 1983. I was admitted to a single room off the main ward in a National Health Service hospital, my surgeon commenting that he could "keep an eye" on me best there. I felt very fortunate being able to choose the date, appreciating the long waiting lists in many areas. The date selected was after a conference I wished to attend and when a locum could be found, although the latter was something of a disaster since the unfortunate man was admitted to the coronary care ward the weekend following my operation.

Being at the receiving end is a useful, if somewhat undesirable, experience. It impressed upon me the importance of communication and also the unrealistic ideas and emotional lability that bedevil all patients. Probably owing to pelvic tilt prior to operation, the "new" leg appeared considerably longer than the other one. I had an uncanny feeling of having to "tuck in two or three inches" and had visions of walking with elevated boots like children in the 1930s who had suffered from polio. My long-suffering surgeon produced a tape measure, but I remained unconvinced. An unguarded remark from my nearest and dearest, who normally gets back as good as he gives, resulted in a flood of tears. I was desperate to try out the new "me" and found myself becoming upset if I was not taken for my "walk" on time. I was terrified I might be "forgotten." It seems silly now, but each day appeared vital.

For the first day or two after a replacement, movement at the hip is discouraged, and thereafter it is impossible for a bit. This should be emphasized to all patients lest they wonder in horror what they have sanctioned. Each day after this brings its own rewards as individual groups of muscles realise they can now move metal as easily as bone. A Zimmer frame is a great comfort for a day or two while you feel your way. Sticks tend to wobble at first. You are allowed two walking sticks only for the next day or two and then only one, to be used in the opposite hand to the operated side. It was reassuring to be told that the new hip had been taken to 90° in the theatre, so you know that anything less than this is unlikely to cause problems. It also helps to be shown the postoperative X-ray and, particularly, an identical joint with its range of movements, how it might dislocate, etc. When I qualified in 1957, artificial joints had not been invented. Patients should be warned about the increased heat under the scar; otherwise, they may worry about infection.

I have been asked why I did not choose a senior anaesthetist. This never worried me. I was more than happy to have the one that always did the "list" with the surgeon, feeling their working together as a team was most important. I appreciated his pre- and postoperative visits and feel that he, like the surgeon (who visited me every day, weekends included), did much more than what was strictly necessary. Waking with an accessory nipple (from the cardiac monitor) impresses upon you the care and trouble colleagues have gone to that you are not aware of. I was less happy receiving blood and had to remind myself that the acquired immune deficiency syndrome was at that time mainly confined to the far side of the Atlantic!

Within a month my new hip became the better one. Because of my age and a family history of longevity, I was advised to try and get further "mileage" from my second hip. Men always seem to describe things in terms of motorcars; even my milkman commented that I seemed to have failed my Ministry of Transport test!

My right hip seemed to deteriorate rapidly after the left was done. I do not know whether this would have happened anyway or whether supporting the first hip accelerated it. Before three months were up I was struggling again, and this second hip, with its lack of bony changes, caused considerable pain. It seemed to lock when I walked and this happened after about ten yards but eased with rest, rather like intermittent claudication. A new worry was that I would damage the hip that was already done as I toppled sideways coming down stairs. At this time I was driving my car and parking outside my wards. I tried to do home visits early in the day and dreaded finding patients in bed upstairs. Slopes were impossible; there appeared to be a great number that I had never noticed before at entrances and exits to hospitals. I found myself going wide detours to try to find steps with a handrail. The entrance to one of my wards had steps but no handrail. I crawled up them on all fours and on occasions my patients looked out for me and manhandled me up them, not the most dignified way for a consultant to arrive on her ward. I tried antiinflammatory drugs, but they only produced a facial rash; dihydrocodeine tartrate helped when I had a social commitment or was on call.

I found it difficult to get clear guidance and to accept advice. Both my surgeon and my husband, whom I knew I should listen to most, thought I should wait before having the second hip done. I think they worried mostly about the long-term prospects, and maybe there is a natural reticence toward advising a colleague or a spouse. There was never any doubt in my mind. I felt strongly that I wanted my life "now" and might be dead from something else in 20 years' time. I wanted to shop with my children, attend Sports Days, entertain occasionally, and do my job competently. I felt somehow a bit "cheated" that I had been through major surgery but was only "half well." I eventually got support from two greatly respected sources. One was a retired anaesthetist who had trained both me and my husband. She took the attitude that the way I was was unfair to my family, and particularly, it was no pleasure for my husband, still comparatively young; to go anywhere with me. The other was a retiring orthopaedic surgeon, who remarked to my family doctor, supposedly out of my hearing, that he did not know why we were not going ahead with the second one. Another general surgeon did confide in me that no surgeon likes to operate until "pushed"! Once a patient is in possession of all the facts, the final decision is up to him or her. Looking back, I think that my advisers were right to fight to save the second joint. I might have felt that they were "knife-happy" if they had gone ahead at once as I initially requested. I think, also, patients need a few months for the first hip to take over as the "good leg."

The second hip was replaced five months after the first. This time I was much happier. I had a good working "partner" who would look after our "patch," I knew that problems tended to be temporary, that each muscle would eventually work, if not to Olympic standards then certainly to competent doctor-housewife-mother ones. I knew that I would get off my stick within a fortnight from the six-week checkup, that stairs would cease to be a problem a few weeks later, and that I would be back at work eight weeks after the operation. Driving a car you need to have a slightly quicker reaction in the right leg than the left. "Embolic stockings" were very helpful in preventing ankle oedema after the second operation, but I feel perhaps they should be called by a more attractive name! A sheepskin blanket also made a great difference preventing sacral pressure, though perhaps the winter generally is a better time to have an operation (I had hit a heat wave the previous July!). An overhead handle on a fracture bed helped early movement after the first operation and was useful for improving the micturition angle, but an ordinary bed, as I had on the second admission (if a hospital bed can ever be called ordinary), was certainly easier to get in and out of. Each time, the importance of early movement impressed me. I now think hard before I allow any patient of mine to remain immobile, even for a few days. Early swimming was a great boon, and I was lucky in having a sports centre very near my home. I attended the "disablement night" once a week. This had the added advantage of making you ashamed of ever complaining as you continued to improve whilst most of the other swimmers remained the same or deteriorated.

Physiotherapy is a vital part of rehabilitation. It is very important that people do not assume that doctors know what to do. I was reminded of a horrified midwife whom I had asked many years ago to show me how to bathe a baby. I was just as ignorant then, in this sphere, as I was doing physiotherapy 20 years later. The best advice I received was from a physiotherapist friend who told me to exercise my feet postoperatively for "ten minutes out of every conscious hour." I was determined the second time round to keep both knees bendable because of being so stiff the first time, but in spite of this resolve, the operated quadriceps, probably because of two short-term drains, was initially too painful. Remembering how light-headed I had been the first time when put from lying flat for a week to standing, and still being forbidden to sit, I dangled my legs over the bed, unobserved, to try and get at least some circulation going. I had taken Nitrazepam on my first admission, but it had not improved my sleep and caused some rebound anxiety, so I did not repeat this experience. My ESR quickly returned to normal following the second operation.

My only contact with an occupational therapist was a shy little man who brought me my toilet seat and "stocking gutter" at the time of discharge. He was covered in confusion when I asked him if the latter would work as well "with pants." No "lady" had ever asked him this before, but it worked very well!

I think what I found most difficult to cope with was my dependence on other people. It is most frustrating not being able to do things when you want—pick up things, bathe, tidy your kitchen, garden, etc.—without having to ask someone to help. I hope as I get older I will learn patience, but I find this difficult. The only really unpleasant bit was the removal of one drain that appeared to have got stuck. It felt like having a ball of string unwound from around the joint.

Progress often seems slow. As a doctor, one expects to be able to grit one's teeth and walk away, but this does not happen.

You learn all sorts of dodges with a stick. I became adept at filling my washing machine with it, but was unable on one occasion to stop three pints of milk slipping off the doorstep and emptying themselves down the garden path. I found a short stick with a hook at one end and a rubber stationer's thimble at the other invaluable for light switches, television knobs, etc., and feel this should be routine equipment for all patients.

I found the nurses on the whole very pleasant and helpful. The hospital tended to be short-staffed, particularly at night, and employed some part-timers. Elderly people might be a bit upset at seeing new faces. Nurses are initially a little in awe of doctor-patients, but this soon disappears. The only indication I got as to whether I was a "good patient" was one that commented how they always came at once when I rang because I "never called unnecessarily"! Perhaps junior doctors also treat you somewhat warily. They particularly like to get into a vein the first time round! I was fortunate in that one of the junior doctors wished to study psychiatry after his surgical job, so he was particularly attentive to his future "boss"!

The reaction of other patients to doctors in a similar predicament is interesting. I once heard two of them outside my door discussing whether a doctor would "look like the rest of us when ill." I invited them to come in and see for themselves! One of my colleagues sent a "get well" card enquiring how my new "ball" (and socket) was progressing. This inevitably led to comments such as "So you're the psychiatrist who has come in for a sex change!"

Perhaps one needs an experience of this sort to really appreciate the support of one's family. I feel one's spouse has great difficulty with such emotional involvement in offering constructive advice. It probably is quite unfair to expect them to give you firm guidance. After surgery, intercourse is something that is just not discussed. Everyone seems to hope that you will ask someone else and assume that ''abduction'' is all that is required. You worry about damaging the new joint, and I found it took almost six months before abduction, flexion, and external rotation could be enjoyed simultaneously without worry! I never had any difficulty lying on either side, possibly owing to the preservation of trochanteric integrity.

As regards neighbours, I felt I carried a responsibility to do well, to be a ''good advertisement'' for the medical profession.

I think sick doctors do differ from other patients. I still have the ridiculous notion that somehow we should not get ill, that we must appear ''fit'' when treating patients. I was horrified when someone suggested that I do home visits with a walking stick. I was particularly stupid in not wanting my colleagues to know when the diagnosis was uncertain. I felt ashamed and inferior and the usual lunchtime jokes were not funny anymore. I think they, too, found it difficult. If I was obviously in pain they did not know what to say or suggest. Their kindness and concern once I was admitted affected me. My room was so full of cards and flowers that a cleaner asked if ''the Queen Mother is in there''! I think doctors worry more about diagnosis and dread particularly the uncertainty and ''loss of control.'' I did not worry about developing a pulmonary embolus, though this is a continuing worry with this type of surgery. I suppose nondoctor patients would not be invited to scrutinize their X-rays. This can be a mixed blessing. Viewing mine at my final appointment, taken for future reference, caused some depression for a few hours. I seemed to be nothing but solid metal from the waist down! But, after all, metal is what X-rays detect better than anything else, and it is well buried in other material, as confirmed when you glide innocently through the metal detector at inefficient airports. I wonder gunrunners have not learnt to wrap their weapons in raw meat!

It is easy to develop a limp following hip surgery. Concentration is required, particularly when you get up from sitting. I was particularly conscious of having to ''do well'' when lunching with colleagues. I attended a meeting with three-quarters of the local doctors ten days after my second operation together with my stick, so it was only too obvious that I had had problems, and again, their support and encouragement was much more evident than their curiosity. Perhaps it would be nice to be nonmedical and have unlimited confidence in acrylic cement. Unfortunately, we know that it is purely a ''grouting agent'' that has caused many problems in the long term in the past. Like other patients, we have a dislike of injections and suffer "anxiety" going for X-rays and other examinations. I think this is partly due to a feeling that, in some way, we have to put on a superior performance. We are terrified of being made a fool of, of letting the side down; knowing that this is irrational and that we are as much entitled to physical or, indeed, mental illness as anyone else does not really help.

I was brought up in a Quaker/Church of Ireland family. By current British standards, I am told that I am "very religious," although I certainly do not see myself as this. I attend the local Methodist church once or twice a month. The minister from this church visited me several times whilst I was in hospital, and, although we discussed general topics, I would have been quite at home if he had wished to say a prayer. Similarly, it was easy for me, prior to my operations, to leave myself "in God's hands" in the same way as I would if I was facing any unpleasant or difficult situation. I do not think my experiences have altered my faith in any way or made me any more or less "religious." I am very aware of my deficiencies but feel they are a personal thing. I have never felt it was any part of a doctor's brief to preach to or try to influence his patients. On the other hand, I believe you portray a sort of quiet confidence if your own faith is fairly solid.

On the whole, I am happy to share my experiences with others, but one is afraid of boring people, probably because of the hours spent listening to long-winded patients who recount their experiences in great detail. I only originally went into print to suggest alternative ways of bathing and showering to a local professor who found he could do neither. I was amazed at the response I received to an article in the *British Medical Journal*. I received letters from people in all walks of life who suggested that it would be helpful to other patients if I wrote in magazines, etc., a suggestion which I declined.

I feel several things could add to the comfort of patients having hip replacements. Some form of hammock would be wonderful if it could turn so you could lie on your face occasionally. One gets very tired not being allowed to turn over for six weeks. Younger patients would greatly benefit if some form of cement could be found that would allow a more active life where sport is concerned. As the "age limit" progressively gets younger, the idea of numerous revision operations is daunting. Many centres continue to develop cementless joints, but so far there is little indication that they do better than the more old-fashioned ones.

I feel an explanatory booklet might be useful for younger patients, explaining the dangers of early dislocation, increase in weight, etc., and suggestions on intercourse, exercises, etc. Medical and nursing staff should check for postoperative nausea, monitor laxatives for each patient, and perhaps think about the final appearance of their handiwork. Half the scar can be hidden under a bikini, and a curved incision avoids a pucker at the top.

I think I am now more sympathetic toward other patients as a result of what has happened, perhaps particularly toward those who complain of "pain" for which no organic cause is immediately found and toward people who worry about disfiguring scars. Younger women may worry particularly about this, not only on the beach but, similar to those following mastectomy, at home. I still get upset by patients who cannot trust their medical advisors. I feel this is at the heart of the whole matter. If they do not trust them enough to put their lives into their hands and be guided by them, they are onto a nonstarter. This applies to the choice of operations. A lot has been written in connection with hip replacement, about types of operations, types of prostheses, material used, etc. This must be left entirely to the surgeon and his experience. Indeed, if you voice your opinion, you may influence his judgement with inferior results. This occasionally happens in psychiatry when one bends over backwards to fall in with a medical patient's request, when the best treatment would be to be firm and try to treat him the same as anyone else.

In a country with limited resources, the Health Service should concentrate on those conditions that are not only treatable but in which the quality of life can be so vastly improved.

It is now four years since I had my first hip done and 3½ years since the second. There are few restrictions on my life, apart from being forbidden to run or jump. I tend to get wetter than other people in a shower of rain, perhaps my saucepans boil over more, and people think me "odd" not running to catch a swinging door or a bus. Only on two occasions have I come to a complete impasse. One was when wedged between two fat strangers on a picnic bench with table attached. I could not leave until one of them moved. The other was getting out of a speedboat; I could not take the necessary wide stride over the end and onto the harbour steps. Having a bathing costume on, I sat on the stern and slid over into six feet of water rather to the amazement of onlookers. It is a matter of balancing overprotectiveness with foolhardiness.

Occasionally I feel resentful that I cannot play tennis or even join a jogging marathon like patients with "new" hearts, and I get slightly irritated by people who comment that they thought hip replacements were only for the elderly. When this happens I firmly remind myself that if the situation had arisen 20 years ago, I probably would not be walking now. Each day is a special bonus to be enjoyed to the full, and I am profoundly grateful, as my senior orthopaedic friend suggested, to "God, Mr. Charnley, and the surgeon, in that order."

CHAPTER 12

MULTIPLE SCLEROSIS

MIRIAM C. CHELLINGSWORTH

What is it like to have multiple sclerosis? After five years of MS, I have to say I don't know. Relapsing-remitting MS is an infuriatingly unpredictable and variable illness. What follows is an account of my own MS; others will, I'm sure, have had entirely different experiences.

Summer 1979. I was on top of the world. At the age of 22, I had achieved a lifelong ambition and graduated in medicine. I had spent five years hardly believing my luck at even getting into medical school. Everyone had told me it would be too difficult—I was female, quiet, and shy. No one in my family was a doctor. I was equally good at languages—why didn't I study something "sensible," like French?

Spring 1980. I had enjoyed a very busy six months as a house physician (intern in internal medicine) and had moved to a post in orthopaedics in another city. I looked after many patients with lumbar disc problems so it did not really surprise me when, after lifting a heavy patient, I developed backache and, later, transient numbness in one thigh. I put my symptoms down to hypochondriasis—after all I had suffered from this condition before when, as a student on a gastroenterology firm, I had an "ulcer"!

A few weeks later I moved to a general surgical firm. The work was very hard since the consultant refused to employ locums for our holidays. I ended up doing the work of two house surgeons and being on call two or more nights out of every five. Finally, when my turn came for a holiday, I went home for a rest. By this time both feet were numb, and over the next two weeks, the numbness spread to involve both legs up to the waist and the right side of my trunk. I remember thinking vaguely that I must have a tumour or MS; I rapidly discounted the latter. The only patient with MS I had ever seen was a young man, wheelchair-bound with a catheter—that couldn't be me! I went back to work, ignoring my symptoms; they went away almost completely. At

DR. MIRIAM CHELLINGSWORTH, 30, is a trainee in internal medicine, at present a research fellow in clinical pharmacology at Birmingham University Medical School, UK.

that time I foolishly did not have a doctor of my own. I did not like my boss and would never have told him of my problem.

After this the sequence of my symptoms becomes rather blurred, but they included further paresthesiae in my legs and numbness of the right side of my face. I was again working too hard and also making frantic applications for senior house officer posts in general medicine. Eventually, the thirteenth application proved lucky; I was offered an interview in yet another city. I went along for the experience of the interview although I really wanted a post at my teaching hospital. Much to my amazement I was offered the job, and before I had really thought about it, I accepted.

August 1980. Another move. I packed all my belongings into my little Austin Mini, since I was on call for admissions the next day. I woke with what seemed to be a persistent speck of dust in my left eye, which, 24 hours later, was a fairly large central scotoma. Despite this, I drove 90 miles to my new hospital, fortunately without incident. I now realized that I had MS, and, as soon as I had free time, I went to the library to read about it. I soon found out that my symptoms were typical of MS. I was devastated but told no one—the consultant had gone on holiday and the registrar on his honeymoon. No one appeared to notice that I was effectively blind in one eye, or if they did, they were too polite to say so.

October 1980. Luckily the scotoma had disappeared over a period of three weeks, but I went on to develop further uncomfortable paresthesiae in my legs. Then one night, an emergency call—"Come quickly to casualty! A young child has very bad asthma." I ran downstairs in the dark only to fall head over heels. By morning I was limping badly, not through injury but through weakness.

I realized that I had to tell someone. My consultant, a physician with an interest in neurology and rheumatology, was obviously surprised and upset but was very kind. He agreed with my diagnosis and arranged for me to see the visiting neurologist. The neurologist was also very kind, but what upset me most was his look of pity and sadness. That frightened me more than anything he said—I was very depressed after our meeting. I told my boyfriend (of only a few weeks' standing); he was very understanding and made life worth living for the next few months. I still had to tell my parents. That was, and still is, the most difficult thing of all to cope with. They were on holiday. When they returned I was much better and went home to tell them. Their reaction was predictable—shock and concern. I hated upsetting them, most of all because my elder brother had been seriously ill and had only just recovered.

Throughout this time I had stayed at work but was excused from nights on call. Being busy with a job I enjoyed helped a great deal; I just didn't have time to think about myself. My symptoms settled down without treatment. My boyfriend and I spent a glorious two weeks in Athens. When I got home a letter was waiting telling me that I was to be admitted to the teaching hospital the following week. The neurologist had said that he would admit me for tests and a "rest," but my admission had been delayed because of problems with the opening of the new teaching hospital. He was surprised to see how much I had recovered—I was now walking with barely a limp. I stayed long enough to have my visual evoked responses tested and to have a lumbar puncture, though I now realize that these were not needed for the diagnosis. I survived the lumbar puncture without incident—I think the doctor who performed it was more nervous than I was. Twenty-four hours later I was back at work.

I remained well and passed the first part of the MRCP exam. My ambition had always been to become a paediatrician, but the neurologist refused to hear of it. I must get a "quiet" job and never get tired. My parents had been told the same thing. This had created great friction between us when I had resumed my full duties as medical SHO.

I took my doctor's advice and found a rheumatology post at a teaching hospital in Birmingham. The actual appointment was not without its difficulties. One person on the interview committee wondered why I should want such a job—poorly paid and not popular. He asked me if I had ever been ill, so of course, the whole story came out in the interview—a traumatic experience. He later apologised, and I was given the post, though I suspect no one else wanted it.

March 1982. I was enjoying rheumatology and passed the MRCP. I then had to decide on a career. The professor for whom I worked suggested pathology, but after much thought I realized it was contact with patients that I enjoyed. I decided to continue with rheumatology. To become accredited, I needed more experience in general medicine. I eventually became a registrar at a nearby district hospital. I did not tell them about my illness, mainly through cowardice; I did not know what reaction I would get (I had not been short-listed for another post when I was honest about my problem), and I still hate actually telling people about my MS.

April 1983. I was settled, liked the new hospital, and was buying a house. The work was busy but enjoyable. I spent a marvellous holiday in Canada and the United States. I bought a new car. Then the predictable happened. I began to have more problems. It started with a right hemianaesthesia, followed by weakness of the legs and more retrobulbar neuritis. Each of these episodes recovered only to be followed by the next. They culminated in September 1983, with almost complete loss of proprioception in both arms. This was extremely disabling and frustrating. I could feed myself only with difficulty. I could not write or drive. I took six weeks off work. The most frustrating thing was that the harder I tried, the less I could do. At least with weakness the opposite is true. Also unpleasant were painful dysasthesiae, which made me feel as if I were wearing a corset that was three sizes too small for me and as though I had ten sausages instead of fingers.

Because I had moved, I had a new neurologist. Fortunately I got on extremely well with him. I think he was as frustrated as I was by my frequent relapses and, like me, was not keen on steroids. I started on azathioprine. I would like to have been part of a controlled trial, but my symptoms would not stay stable for long enough. I continued to have minor relapses but managed to get back to work and even surprised myself by learning to insert permanent pacemakers. Again, my consultants and colleagues were extremely kind, though my absence made a great deal of extra work for them.

November 1984. I developed a rash and stopped azathioprine. I moved again—back to the teaching hospital. The government had decided that it could no longer afford planned expansion in rheumatology, so my career had taken yet another turn. I was now a research fellow in clinical pharmacology. Things went well till April 1985, when I lost proprioception in my feet. I restarted azathioprine, unwillingly, since this time it made me vomit. Then I caught flu; over a week I developed diplopia, weakness of both legs and of my right arm. I was admitted to hospital, only to develop a facial palsy and mild dysarthria and dysphagia. For a while I was unable to walk, but fortunately once again, I recovered very quickly. I was back at work within four weeks, although it was two months before I could drive again and my legs are still quite weak. I usually manage to remain reasonably cheerful during relapses, though this one was particularly frightening. It is only when I recover and have to cope with life fully again that I become depressed and realize what might have happened.

Being both a doctor and a patient is difficult. General practitioners and junior doctors tend to be reticent and not treat me as a usual patient. It was refreshing to be admonished by a GP trainee for driving my car when I should not have been, although at the time I was extremely annoyed. I try to be a "good patient," but it's not easy. I must admit that stopping azathioprine was as much due to my dislike of taking tablets, and hence being a "patient" and "sick," as due to my having an itchy rash.

Having an illness like MS has helped me in my work. I now understand what it is like to be on the receiving end of advice like "take a month off." How often do we think before we give such advice to patients? I hope I now stop and think carefully before I give a patient advice that may dramatically alter his or her life-style. I still wonder what would have happened if I had taken up paediatrics. Who knows?

I do not make a secret of my illness, though I've only once told a patient that I have MS. She also had MS and was obsessional about her illness. She kept to a gluten-free diet and would not drink tap water "because it contains too much lead." She was in hospital having given birth to her first child, who was ill in the special care unit. Whenever the paediatrician talked to her, she experienced tingling in her hands in addition to her usual dysasthesiae. She described the latter as "terrible." "I know," I said, "they're awful." "You don't know, you can't know!" "I do know. I have them too; I have MS." I immediately regretted my impulsive remark. Her whole attitude changed to one of pity for me rather than for herself. I find pity difficult to cope with at the best of times; it makes a doctor–patient relationship impossible. I do not see many patients with MS but do not avoid them. I have even told two patients their diagnosis (with the agreement of their consultants); I feel that they have the right to know. I'm not a neurologist, though, and in general, the management of MS is best left to experts.

What of the future? I do not know—no one can tell me what is going to happen, and I would not expect them to. My neurologist seems a lot more optimistic than I am. The fear of losing my independence is much greater to me than the fear of actual disability. My hope now is to do enough work to obtain an M.D., and then to become a geriatrician—about the only growth area in the NHS. Ironic, since I started my career intending to become a paediatrician. Still, I enjoy helping with the rehabilitation of my patients; that aspect of geriatrics appeals to me.

I have been fortunate in never feeling bitter about my illness. I did not think, "Why me?" Why not me? Of my immediate family, I'm sure that I'm the one best able to cope with MS. Of course, I've had a great deal of help from them, especially my younger brother, who lived with me when he was a student. Their support has been invaluable, and I'm grateful for it. Friends and colleagues have also helped greatly, particularly by listening when I wanted to talk. Early in my illness, I came to believe in God, having previously been an atheist. My belief helped a little, though I'm still not a practising Christian. Eventually I would like to marry and perhaps even have children, but that seems a remote possibility at the moment. Today I am just thankful that I am still able to work and enjoy myself. With MS, I've learned to live life one day at a time.

CHAPTER 13

DISC WITH L-5 ROOT COMPRESSION

STEPHEN N. SULLIVAN

It was Friday the 13th! They had taken my glasses, and everything was a blur. There was no pain, but I knew that if I stood up it would start, so I lay on the stretcher outside the operating room. The nurse wrapped my cold feet in a heated blanket. In a few minutes I was going to have an operation.

That was six months ago, but the details remain as if they occurred yesterday. The problem had started a year before. It was an ache in the left anterior hip and buttock, worse in the morning and usually gone by noon. It was annoying because I liked to do my running in the morning. I would get up at 5:45 and jog out to meet two buddies for a ten-mile run. Usually the ache would ease, but gradually it became a pain and then one morning I couldn't finish a run and had to walk home. I thought it was a musculoskeletal problem. After all, I was running over 3000 miles per year. A colleague in the Orthopedic Clinic agreed. I had already ruined my stomach with enteric-coated ASA so he suggested Naprosyn and arranged physiotherapy. He also advised that I stop running for a while. In the middle of winter it isn't much fun running in the snow, so I agreed. Besides, I had become interested in triathlons and thought it would be a good opportunity to improve my swimming, so I stopped running for a month. The pain improved, and so did my swimming, but when I started to run again I found I was completely detrained. It was a blow to go from being one of the best runners in the city to being one who couldn't finish a training run. Then the pain came back! I decided to cut back on my miles and concentrate on the triathlon. I spent more time in the pool and on my bike. Athletically it worked and I won my age category in a few triathlons, but the pain got worse. Not only was it worse and lasting longer, it

DR. STEPHEN SULLIVAN is a 39-year-old gastroenterologist. He lives with his wife and two children in London, Ontario, and works and teaches at Victoria Hospital. For more than two decades, running has been part of his daily life—a form of transportation and a means of dissipating mental stress.

spread. It now involved the left hip, the left buttock, and the lateral aspect of the left lower leg. It still seemed musculoskeletal so I arranged a formal office consultation with a friend in rheumatology at another hospital. She gave me a very thorough going-over and sent me a three-page report. She agreed that it sounded musculoskeletal. She thought that we should make sure I did not have early ankylosing spondylitis or some structural problem with the hip, so I had X-rays of the hip and pelvis—my first investigation—both normal. I also donated 10 cc of blood for a research project she was doing. More physiotherapy was arranged and I was given some samples of a new nonsteroidal. The physiotherapist spent a lot of time trying to figure out which muscle, ligament, or bursa was involved. In the end, we agreed that it seemed to be a problem with abductors of the left hip. Special stretching exercises were prescribed and things seemed to get much better. It was only temporary—a placebo effect? The pain now began to interfere with my work. As long as I was sitting or moving slowly it wasn't too bad, but if I stood for any length of time it got progressively worse. I could get through a routine upper endoscopy, but colonoscopies became impossible. I had to sit down to do the procedure. The marked postural element to the pain made me think that perhaps this was more than just a musculoskeletal problem. I began to read orthopedic journals and rheumatology textbooks. I did a literature search. I convinced myself that I had the pyriformis syndrome. To confirm the diagnosis all I needed was someone to put a finger up my bum and palpate the tender muscle. I found I could not do it myself. Then, the top of my left foot went numb! A pain in the buttock with referral to the lower leg and a numb foot. This wasn't a musculoskeletal problem, this was a neurological problem. Another literature search and then stumbling onto an article in that month's *Annals of Internal Medicine,* Dr. O. Duffy of the Mayo Clinic writing on lumbar spinal stenosis. All the symptoms fit. I wrote him a letter. He replied at length and made some helpful comments, including the suggestion that it might be a disc protrusion.

The problem came to a head in the last triathlon of the season. I came out of the water in good position. The bike ride was incredible. In spite of having to stop for a train I made up over 60 positions and came off the bike in seventh place. As a runner, I looked forward to the run. I had never been passed in the running portion of a triathlon. My leg wouldn't work! Runners were going by. I tried to push the pace, but I couldn't. I lost my age category by 20 seconds. Something had to be done, so back to the rheumatologist to discuss the latest developments. A CT scan of my lumbar spine was arranged. I remember lying in that marvel of modern medicine. It was nearly 7:00 p.m. The only sound in the room was the humming of the air conditioning and the electric whir and clicks of the scanner. Every time it took a slice the red sign above my head flashed "X-RAY ON." I had visions of myelogenous leukemia. The next morning the radiologist reading the films called me. "Steve, you have an L-4–5 disc with compression of the L-5 nerve root."

"But I have never had any back pain!"

We reviewed the films together. There it was in black and white and shades of grey. I went back to my office and called the secretary of the orthopedic surgeon in our hospital who had the best reputation for back problems and the city's largest experience with chemonucleolysis. She told me he was at a conference and wouldn't be back for a week. I told her I would like to make an appointment for a patient. She told me the next appointment was in March (it was now September) and asked me who the appointment was for. I told her it was for me. "Oh," she said. "We might be able to fit you in at the beginning of October."

I told her I would call back. I was outside my field of expertise. What should I do? I asked the hospital librarian to do a Medline search on chemonucleolysis and find me a recent book on back pain. Then I called a friend in the Department of Neurosciences at the University Hospital for advice. He reminded me that some years before, when he and I were doing research in England, he had injured his back. He called home long distance to Dr. G., a neurosurgeon on staff at University Hospital. For his money, Dr. G. was the best. I called his secretary and asked when his next regular appointment was. "January" she said. I thanked her and called the orthopedic surgeon's secretary again and told her I would take the appointment in October. Then I went home to rest in bed. No matter who I saw I knew he would recommend bed rest. As I left the office my secretary said, "Steve, I know Dr. G.'s secretary. Should I talk to her?" I vaguely remember saying, "Okay." On Saturday morning, Dr. G. came around to my home and examined me in my own bed. I felt like a fake. There I lay, feeling no pain, but within 30 seconds of my standing up the pain returned, and Dr. G. pointed out that I clearly had easy fatigability of the dorsiflexors of the left foot. He advised strict bed rest, so for 23½ hours a day I lay in bed surrounded by my books and journals and articles on back pain. I lasted 3½ days. Each time I got up to empty my bladder I timed how long it took for the pain to come. It was getting shorter and shorter, not longer and longer. I phoned Dr. G. and told him of the lack of improvement. He told me I had a surgical temperament—always wanting things to happen in a hurry. I told him that at one time I had planned on being an orthopedic surgeon, until I saw the light. A myelogram was advised. I visited a friend in radiology and asked him who did the best myelogram in the city. "Dr. H. without a doubt. He is really slick." I felt less guilty about "doctor shopping" since Dr. H. had interpreted the CT. Dr. H. arranged the myelogram for 8:00 a.m. the next day. He was slick. It was painless. The only time I jumped was when he washed my back with cold alcohol. There it was again, in black and white and shades of grey—a left L-5 root compression. Dr. H. insisted that I remain upright and under observation until the early afternoon. The radiocontrast medium, metrizamide, is water-soluble and renally excreted, so over the next few hours I sat on a stretcher in our endoscopy room and drank 6 litres of soda water. I found out later that metrizamide can cause seizures if it irritates the cerebral cortex. So much for informed consent, but I really didn't want to know anyway. If it happened, it happened. My secretary took the films up to University Hospital for Dr. G., and I think that Dr. H. called Dr. G. about the myelographic findings, because Dr. G. called a few hours later and asked if I wanted my disc out the next day. I didn't pause to think; I said yes. At 4:00 that afternoon I checked into University Hospital as Mr. Sullivan. I was examined by a medical student. There was no pyriformis tenderness on rectal examination. The resident reviewed the findings with the student and pointed out some classic findings of an "L-5 root." Why weren't they classic before? Then off via wheelchair for a routine preop chest X-ray. A postmyelogram headache had started and I wanted to walk back to the ward and lie down, but that was against the rules. I had to wait for the porter. I waited and waited and the headache got worse and worse. The ECG technician came—sinus bradycardia, incomplete right bundle branch block, and nonspecific ST segment changes. Why an ECG and chest X-ray for a 38-year-old marathoner who on several occasions had gone beyond stage 7 of the Bruce protocol and had a VO_2 max of 72 ml/kg/min? The IV nurse came to do a CBC and cross-match. I thought that this sort of surgery was bloodless. I was overjoyed when the anesthetist arrived. He was a friend who lived across the street from us. We joked about waking me up with the same IQ I went to sleep with. We then talked about blood transfusions and I insisted I could go a hell of a long way on a few litres of saline. He agreed. The chief resident arrived late that night. He confirmed the findings and said that I was booked for 8:00 the next morning. He then embarked on informed consent. I really did not want to hear that I might wake up worse than I went to sleep. A nurse filled me in on the postoperative nursing procedures and informed me that there was a 25% chance of needing a temporary urinary cathether—no way, I thought. I didn't sleep very well that night. My roommate had had a stroke. He spoke only Russian and German and snored like a steam engine. The next morning I requested a private room.

Early in the morning the team made its rounds. There had been some emergencies, so the surgery would be delayed until noon. The history was reviewed and the findings discussed. Dr. G. demonstrated how the left dorsiflexors fatigued. Why hadn't any of the other examiners picked that up? I am 5′ 8″, 135 lbs.; he is at least 6′ and 180 lbs. and towered over the team. He was the only one strong enough to detect the weakness.

Preop procedures, get into a thin gown with ties down the back, shave arm and start IV, lock up valuables and take away glasses. Then the long stretcher ride to the OR. Hospital ceilings are boring and the people were all a blur. A half-hour wait in the cold air-conditioned anteroom. My feet were freezing and the kindness of the nurse who wrapped them in a hot blanket was much appreciated. Transfer to the cold hardness of the OR table and listen to the nurses setting up. It sounded like somebody washing cutlery. The anesthetist said, "Just a shot into the IV, Steve." It stung and then I was floating a foot off the table. What a feeling. All the worry was gone. "Now I want you to take a couple of deep breaths." I made it to one and that's the last I remember. One second I was there, and the next I was gone.

The next sensation was that of warmth. I thought I was lying in the sun by my pool, but I couldn't figure out why a strange lady kept shaking me and saying, "Mr. Sullivan, are you awake?" Then I was awake. There was no pain. For the first time in months the leg felt normal. I felt great. Dr. G. came by before I left the recovery room. The surgery had been uneventful and I had had a sequestered disc that no amount of bed rest would have healed. I was relieved, because I knew that Dr. G. had not been keen to operate on me. By 5:00 p.m. I was famished. The hospital food was great. I talked the staff into taking out the IV and letting me up to urinate. It was slow, but no catheter was needed. The next morning my back hurt—the first time I had had any back pain. It wasn't bad, but it made me irritable, so when the IV nurse came I started to give her a tough time. She wanted to do a CBC and electrolytes. "Why?" I asked. "I am drinking and peeing and the surgery was bloodless." "The doctors ordered it." I shut up and bared my arm.

The team made its rounds and I got permission to go for a walk. I was stiff and sore and slow, but the leg worked perfectly. I was in good spirits. Family and close friends visited. One of the advantages of being treated in a hospital other than the one you work in is that well-meaning colleagues don't keep dropping by, so I had time to relax and read and snooze. The back started to hurt more. I made another walk around the ward. When the evening nurse made her rounds at approximately 9:00 p.m. she asked if I wanted a shot for the pain. "No, maybe just a couple of Tylenol.'' By midnight I was going crazy. Why do things hurt more at night? My hand kept reaching for the call button, but I kept pulling it back. No, I was going to tough this out. Finally, I pushed the button. Heaven is a shot of Demerol when you are in pain.

The next morning the pain in the leg returned. Not very much, but it was there. The resident thought it was probably just some postoperative edema—made sense to me. Another few laps of the ward and I was all set to go home, but it was Sunday and the team wanted Dr. G. to see me before discharge. Besides, my son was having his 13th birthday and things were pretty hectic at home. That night I remembered how well the Demerol had worked, so I asked for another shot. The next morning Dr. G. examined his handiwork. I asked him what things I must not do. ''Do whatever you want, Steve.'' I thanked the nurses and walked out of the hospital under my own steam. Not bad—operation on Friday, home on Monday, two shots of Demerol and about six Tylenol #3. No one could ever accuse this doctor of abusing the system. I didn't even have a prescription for an analgesic. The plan was to have the stitches removed as an outpatient and see Dr. G. for a follow-up in a month's time. I knew that by then I would be back running. But the leg still hurt! Tuesday was warm and sunny and a beautiful day for a bike ride. I got out my ten-speed. The back was stiff and it was difficult getting on and off the bike, but cycling was painless. The next day the ceiling fell in. The preoperative pain was frustrating and annoying, the postoperative pain was at least understandable, but this pain was excruciating. I cursed myself for riding the bike the day before. To get out of bed I had to roll out onto the floor and pull myself up with my arms. Any sudden movement, a cough, a sneeze, a slight bump, and the pain would lance down my leg. To make things worse, it was completely unpredictable. Sometimes a movement would cause the pain, and sometimes it wouldn't. It was as if a gremlin with a cattle prod was following me around. When I wasn't looking he gave me a jab. When I looked for him I couldn't find him. Dr. G. came around and saw me at home. I was a puzzle. Perhaps a sterile discitis. A short course of prednisone was tried and I had the wildest dreams. A friend dropped off some Valium and Tylenol #3, which I washed down with beer, and things became a blur. Anything to blot out pain and consciousness. I asked my wife to buy me a bottle of vodka. She refused. I became an automaton and functioned in a trance. A whole week of my life went missing. The second weekend after leaving hospital I resolved to take control of my life again. Time to get on with things again. I decided to walk over to the home of Marc Roberts, a running buddy. It was only 7 km away. What was 7 km to someone who used to average 100 km a week? I had gone 5 km when a lady pulled over in her car. "I was driving by and saw you so I went around the block and came back to see if you could use some help."

"No, no," I said, "I'm training."

"What are you training for?"

"The human race."

"You sure you don't want a ride?"

"No, I'll be fine."

Who was I kidding? There I was moving as fast as I could, my heart rate was only 62 beats/minute—some training effect. I finally made it to Marc's. I looked at my watch. Sixteen minutes per kilometer. I used to be able to average under 4 minutes a kilometer for 42 kilometers. This was idiocy so I asked Marc for a ride partway home. On the way he and I compared notes. Approximately a year before he had been badly injured in a running accident and it was many months before he could get on the road again. He took up golf and smoking. His wife used to find the cigarettes hidden in his golf bag. We agreed that being injured really did a number on your head. He dropped me off at another friend's place, but nobody was home. I started to walk. On the way I had to cross a four-lane road with a pedestrian crosswalk. I couldn't make it across before the light changed. How must old people feel? When I got home the house was empty. I opened and drank a whole bottle of red wine and sat in a trance in front of the television set. My wife and children came home a few hours later. "How are you feeling dear?" I started to cry and couldn't stop. Now, I've been known to get a moist eye in sad movies and feel choked up at funerals and shed a tear when a patient dies, but this was different. My family had never seen me like this before. I had never been like this before. I sobbed and sobbed and tried to tell myself to stop being stupid. My daughter patted my hand and my wife held me close. My son didn't know what to do. I babbled on and on and on, pouring out all those bottled-up thoughts, dreams, and feelings. It all came spilling out.

The next day I was better—not physically, but psychologically. My head was together. The following day I went back to work. I moved carefully and very slowly. I had difficulty getting in and out of my car. One morning it took me 20 minutes to get out of bed and get dressed. My son had to help me put on my socks. Listening to other people's problems distracted me from my own. My own problem also affected my approach to the problems of others. I had a great deal more sympathy and empathy for those with chronic or recurrent unexplained pain that had failed to respond to the diagnostic and therapeutic touches of the physician or surgeon. One of my more philosophical and introspective colleagues served as a psychological sounding board as I tried to sort out why it had happened to me. Not the physical part, but the mental part.

Once my head was together the pain and disappointment were easier to bear, but I continued to look for explanations and solutions. Nobody knew why the pain had returned—edema, hemorrhage, discitis, retained fragment? Dr. H. offered to repeat the CT scan, but I remembered the red flashing "X-RAY ON" sign. Nonsteroidals gave me a bellyache. A transcutaneous nerve stimulator didn't help. I did pelvic tilts and back stretches twice a day. I could just about touch my knees. I had this feeling that if I could stretch my spine about an inch something would slip back into place and the pain would vanish. I tried hanging by my hands from the pipes in the basement. I tried hanging upside down by my knees from the climbing frame in the local schoolyard. It didn't work. I arranged a back massage. The therapist was very good. It hurt at the time but felt better later. However, the thing that helped the most was the change in my expectations. Walk normally in four weeks, jog in eight weeks, run in 16 weeks. I kept fit by swimming and cycling. I had trouble getting in and out of the pool and on and off the bike. My appetite returned and I gained five extra kilos. I walked pain-free at four weeks and jogged at seven weeks. For the uninitiated, there is a difference between running and jogging. As my daughter says, "It is a bit like pee and poo; pee is fast and poo is slow." I went one mile in nine minutes; it hurt, but I persisted. The weight came off. I ran my first race on Boxing Day. A ten-miler in 61 minutes, only 7 minutes slower than three years before. Then one day I realized that the pain was gone—not always, but usually. Occasionally the ache in the lower leg returns to remind me. I tilt my pelvis and stretch my back every day. I can touch my toes again. Today, as I write this, six months and two days since the surgery, I have just returned from a pain-free 17-mile run. Now that the pain, mental and physical, is gone, I thank my friends and colleagues who helped. For their knowledge, their skills, their patience, and, I am embarrassed to say, for the strings that they pulled.

So why did it happen? Not the disc protrusion or the slow (was I expecting too much?) postoperative recovery, but my emotional reaction to the whole thing. The simple answer would be that I was addicted to running and needed my daily fix. It was a way of leaving my worries by the wayside as I ran home from work. For a while I thought it was something more fundamental, more philosophical (and perhaps it partly is). Our lives are like a river. Sometimes we flow smoothly with the years—walking, talking, toilet training, going to school, reaching puberty, dating, leaving home, getting married, having children, children leaving home, grandchildren, death. Sometimes we challenge the rapids in the river for the excitement—academic and athletic achievement, scholarships, university, medical school, research, grants, publications, promotion. I had reached calm water—a wife who was a friend, kids I was proud of, house paid for, busy practice, lots of publications, and recent promotion to associate professor. The water was as smooth as glass and not very exciting. I knew I would never be a great research scientist; besides, I hated writing grant applications. Teaching was fun, but repetitive. The practice would remain the same, unless I changed directions in midstream. Somebody would have to die before I was promoted again. At that point in my life the excitement seemed to lie outside of my job and my research and my teaching. For over 20 years I had been a runner. During high school I had run well. When I went to university and medical school I devoted myself to my studies but kept myself fit. Over the last few years as that water had become smoother I again started to concentrate on my athletics. The hard work was paying off. I broke 32 minutes for 10 kilometers, ran a sub-2:30 marathon, won the club championship, and had enjoyed more than modest success in triathlons. In a year and a half I would be 40. I was looking foward to it. As a master runner I would be fit and looked forward to the excitement of competition. Suddenly, it was slipping from me. The careful plans, the hard training, the long-term goals were floating away. Looking back on it I feel a little foolish, but I firmly believe that one has to run the rapids, rather than just drift through life.

However, in the end I came to realize that a lot of it was vanity—the erosion of my own self-image. *Mens sana in corpore sano* (''a sound mind and a sound body''). When I think of myself, I think of me as a physical as well as a mental being—running, swimming, cycling, stretching, weights, aerobics. Taking the stairs three at a time. High VO_2 max, slow pulse, trim body, energy to do anything. I had this irrational fear that I was losing it all, that all the hard work was for nought. A bit like a thinker believing he has Alzheimer's. It was crazy.

Perhaps it was the pain, the pills, the booze, the uncertainty, or the unrealistic expectations. Perhaps it was the combination. I will never know for sure, but thank God it is all over (I hope).

CHAPTER 14

HERNIATED DISCS

SAM J. SUGAR

Patients often ask me how to maintain health. I receive quizzical looks when I reply, "Don't get sick." Despite the circumlocution, it is the best advice I can give anyone, and especially good for physicians. By not getting sick, a physician can avoid a host of unpleasant experiences with which he is uniquely *unqualified* to deal. Unfortunately, my body would not listen to my own advice, and I had a serious illness that affected me deeply at a productive point in my career.

The firstborn son of Holocaust survivor refugees to America, I fulfilled my parents' dream by becoming a physician, despite (or because of) having to work from age 11 to help defray expenses. While my college career was fairly distinguished, my medical school experience was mediocre. By graduation, I was married with a family, and my work ethic, rather than any extraordinary talent, landed me a position as a chief resident. The year of chief residency was exciting, stimulating, and a terrific career builder. Yet that year also proved to be a year of recurrent severe back pains and sciatica, which had plagued me occasionally until that time but which eventually led to a series of problems and operations that devastated me.

My earliest recollection of sciatica and back pain came at age 11, when suddenly, while playing baseball, I was afflicted with pain in my back radiating into my scrotum and legs. Our general practitioner placed me at bed rest. After a couple of days, I felt pretty good and returned to my usual activities. I noted that I would occasionally have stiffness, even to the point where it prevented me from playing baseball. Nonetheless, since the problem was only episodic and not very severe, I chose to ignore it. In high school, having been active in

DR. SAM SUGAR is a 39-year-old practicing specialist in internal medicine and primary care in Evanston and Glenview, Illinois. He is a member of the faculty of the Department of Internal Medicine at Northwestern University and the Evanston/Glenbrook Hospitals. His special interests include hypertension and medical administration.

sports, I noticed severe stiffness in my back and occasional shooting pains down my leg sometimes after athletic competition, but never to the point where it kept me out of competition. I had had little exposure to family illness since all my relatives had been killed in the war. My own illnesses included recurrent strep throat treated in the hospital with gentian violet. I had undergone a cardiac cath for a ventricular septal defect at age 14, but since the cath took only a day or two out of my life and the results were good, I never really played the sick patient or even knew anyone who had.

In college I had no back trouble at all, but during my first year in medical school I began to have difficulties. These were acutely made worse when, picking up shower gifts for my fiancee, I noticed a sharp, persistent pain radiating into my leg. The pain was severe and did not resolve with a couple of days of bed rest, but it did eventually get better after I took some over-the-counter pain medication. However, the pain recurred and flared at the worse possible time—during our honeymoon in September 1969. I was so afflicted with back pain and sciatic radiation that I could not even carry our bags to our hotel and had to be admitted immediately to the hospital when we returned home, for ten days of traction, physiotherapy, and diathermy. At this time, the first set of X-rays ever taken of my back revealed severe spondylolisthesis and slippage of L-5 on S-1, causing impingement on a nerve root. I was told to lose weight and to exercise, and I would get better. Needless to say, in medical school it was impossible for any of those things to happen. My back pain was controlled with Extra-Strength Tylenol or Excedrin, but there would be stretches—especially after sitting in lectures for hours—when I would be in excruciating pain from extremely severe sciatica. However, because I was young and strong and resilient, I made up my mind that my medical school career came first, and that I would overcome most of the pain simply by blocking it out of my mind, resting, and staying off my feet as much as possible. During medical school I chose clerkships, depending upon the status of my back, and I opted for the medical clerkships that were the least demanding because standing on my feet for long periods of time was simply not possible. This was not a hardship because I preferred medical clerkships to surgical ones anyhow, and in medical clerkships I was better able to control the amount of time I spent on my feet. Nights on call were difficult and involved sleeping on bad mattresses in poorly furnished call rooms. With care, the use of a back brace, and the avoidance of any lifting, I managed to stay out of difficulty until my chief residency in internal medicine. During that strenuous year, long days were *de rigeur*, and I found myself sporting an impressive sciatic scoliosis by the end of the year.

By the time I entered practice, I had made it my business to have several more sets of X-rays and some physical therapy, and at the advice of an osteopathic friend, I had even been to an osteopathic physician for an injection of some God-awful substance that was supposed to stabilize my back. It didn't work, but I was amazed at all the popping noises this man could produce from within me by moving my leg around! During these early attempts at becoming a patient, I remained aloof and superior to my pain, figuring all the while that doctors can't get sick and that my ailment was only trivial and would eventually require some kind of treatment, but this treatment could be postponed indefinitely. My level of activity outside of work was shrinking, though. Whereas I had loved competitive sports, they now were out of reach. The absence of pain was recreation enough for me. My attendings supported this view by advising me to "tough it out." To this day, I don't know how they expected me to do that. I was big and appeared strong, but my pain was melting my strength.

In my first years of practice, a certain physician gained some notoriety for his injections of chymopapain into a star third baseman, and because I thought his procedure might be helpful to me, I traveled to Elgin one day to speak to the physician, observe his technique, and discuss my case with him. X-rays in hand, I presented to his office. He examined me briefly and invited me to his hospital, where he performed procedures during the day. He introduced me to his OR nurse, a 350-pound male. In those days, patients undergoing chemonucleolysis were under general anesthesia, and it allowed the doctor to rely very heavily on his male nurse for the performance of the procedure. After viewing the procedure and the expertise of his staff, I felt somewhat relieved until he gave me a list of patients on whom he had performed the procedure and recommended that I call them to determine their outcomes. Nothing was mentioned as to my suitability for the procedure and I never did call any of those people, preferring not to become a patient at that point, but storing the information about chymopapain for future reference. I became intimately familiar with the literature, and when it became clear that most of the experimental work leading to the use of chymopapain and chemonucleolysis was then on rabbit ear cartilage, I demurred. I was further dissuaded from this technique when I asked what the eventual metabolic disposition of the disc and chymyopapain were, and no suitable answers were available.

By the time my back pain became unbearable, I had been in practice six years and had accumulated one wife, three children, three partners, three offices, seven employees, and all the responsibilities and anxieties and tribulations that go along with the accumulation of these things and people.

The last siege started on the third visit to the health club "to get into shape" on the machine for the abdominal muscles. The sciatica began first in one leg and then in another, the back spasms followed, and I vividly recall seeing patients in my office the next morning while I was in great pain, even though I had taken two or three Tylenol with codeine to suppress the pain. I was in such agony that I had to leave in the middle of a physical and inform my office staff that I was going home to lie down, and I collapsed in a heap as I arrived home, just barely able to crawl into bed.

The frustrating part about sciatica and back pain is that it doesn't hurt very much when you're on your back and lying still. It's just that when you try to walk, breathe, eat, urinate, sit, or any of the other normal functions of daily living, the pain is almost unbearable. At this point, my corset wasn't much help and none of the medications I took made any difference. I discussed the matter with my partners, my wife, and my family and decided that I would see an orthopedist, who advised me that, yes indeed, I had some back problems and that after a few days or weeks of bed rest I would be just fine.

I always felt uneasy when seeing the orthopedist. I wondered whether all patients with back pain provoked the kind of response that I felt I saw in him—namely, that of doubt and the question of malingering. I, too, had been taught about the malingering patient with back pain but was insulted when the orthopedist asked me if I was really having that much pain. This was one of the first real negative experiences that I incurred after having officially become a patient.

Becoming a patient is a process. It starts with having to give up certain rights and privileges. Among the first to go is privacy. Once your ailment is divulged, it seems that everyone knows about it in every detail. I felt somewhat uncomfortable having to disrobe in front of nurses and assistants with whom I had only enough familiarity to cause distress. I suppose that the pain of shedding my outer garments was really that of shedding my shield of invulnerability and leaving the domain of physician and entering that of patient. The patient is a very dependent person. The physician is not. The patient depends on the kindness of those around him. The physician does not. I found myself constantly having to demand that I pay for any services rendered—not because I really wanted to pay for them but to justify my position of demanding information and prompt response to my questions. I did not want to be treated like any common patient, because I was a doctor who just happened to be a patient. I found it also unsettling that I was given information about my illness as though I was an expert in back problems, when, as an internist, I clearly was less than an expert. I was expected to prescribe medications for myself, which I found puzzling. I found myself frequently wishing that I could be treated for a few moments like any other patient—to get the sympathy that I tried to provide my patients when they were ill—and at other times to be treated with respect and reverence due my position. It was a frustrating business.

In an effort to avoid the major surgery apparently required to correct my problem, I was given the option of going to a certain hospital in Toronto for an injection of chymopapain. At this time, papain was not legal in the United States and only one doctor in Toronto was in the business of providing this treatment. I was advised to come to Toronto, check into a hotel, and present myself on a Tuesday morning at this physician's clinic in the hospital—anything to avoid surgery! It was in Toronto that I learned the true meaning of terror. In their system of medicine there is no personalization, and I felt as though I was treated very shabbily and had an extremely poor result, with the complication of arachnoiditis from the injection and no follow-up whatsoever. Consequently, after returning to the United States on a stretcher, I was at bed rest again for another month before anything could even be considered with regard to therapy. It was during that time that I began to sense the loneliness that had gradually begun to supplant the feeling of overwork that most physicians feel. In our daily encounters with colleagues and patients, we are frequently flooded with "good morning"s and "hello"s and casual "how are you"s. I quickly found that with regard to the colleagues that I had developed on a casual basis and to whom I had referred hundreds of cases, "out of sight, out of mind" appeared to be in operation. Though I'm sure it wasn't intentional, I was surprised and stunned by the lack of sensitivity my colleagues showed in not at least *sending* their regards to a colleague who was ill. This was in stark contrast to my patients, who sent hundreds of cards and letters and gifts and flowers during the entire length of my illness, which only made my physician colleagues' poor manners more obvious.

When it became obvious that surgery would be necessary to correct the severe problem, I consulted my orthopedist again. It appeared he did not believe the severity of my illness and said that he would need to see the results of a myelogram that was done. I was pleasantly surprised by the skill and compassion shown by the radiologist at my own institution who deftly performed the dreaded procedure with precision. I had made the decision to seek care in my own institution, a teaching hospital affiliated with a major university. I believe in retrospect that that was an error. Being in my own hospital increased my feelings of insecurity and, because I was neither a doctor nor a patient, I was greeted by the familiar "hello"s of the people working in the hospital who were confused to see me lying on a cart rather than walking through the hall. Their compassion was welcome. But my colleagues simply didn't know what to say. I can recall vividly being wheeled into the myelography room and running into one of the surgeons at the hospital, to whom I had sent many cases. He just looked at me and waved as if it were perfectly normal for me to be on a stretcher. This incongruity has confused me to this day. What was even more frightening and confusing was the reaction of my orthopedist when he saw the myelogram, indicating the extreme severity of my disease and the multiple discs involved. He came to my bedside, sat next to me, and said, "Sam, I can't tell you how surprised I am. I really didn't think you were sick. You certainly weren't fooling." This may, of course, have been his attempt at humor. However, it struck me as being very crass of him even to mention it.

During my hospitalization many tests were performed, including a CAT scan. To those of you who have never personally experienced the tests that you frequently prescribe for your patients, I recommend that you take the time to investigate these tests thoroughly and personally. For those of you who have never had a procto or a lower GI or an IVP or a CT with infusion or arterial blood gases or myelogram—and for those of you who order these tests with alarming frequency—I would suggest that if you knew the brute force of these tests, you would think twice before ordering another one.

The CT machine is a good example of how a patient can be consumed by hospital technology. To have a CT scan done, one must be literally engulfed by the machine. You lie there quietly in a room devoid of other human beings, dependent on whirring motors guided by unseen hands, probing deep inside you without feeling. It is an eerie, other-worldly feeling that one hopes is justified by the lack of physical pain it causes.

Now a full-fledged patient, I realized that I would have a period of disability, and I'm grateful to my partners for accepting the responsibilities of my practice while I was laid up. They dutifully showed up in my room as often as they could, but I know they were uncomfortable visiting me for the same reason that I'm uncomfortable visiting colleagues in the hospital now. We are never really sure whether our medical colleagues are patients or doctors. We don't know whether their shields of invulnerability have been pierced or not. We don't know how to act in front of them because we don't know what they need. If they were patients, it would be easy. They would need our support and understanding and skill and attention. But as physician to physician, we know so little about each other, owing to the cursory nature of our intercourse with one another, that it can be a struggle sometimes just to enter the room. For the rare physician who has the ability to see his colleague as a patient in pain, I offer the advice to come often and stay for a while.

Since surgery was the only solution to my problem, I opted for a neurosurgeon to perform the complicated operation. Neurosurgeons are the real surgeons, for real patients with real illnesses.

I recall very clearly being admitted to the hospital and asked to wear a hospital gown, at which point all the funny jokes about the backside of those gowns no longer seemed funny. I remember my subdued irritation at how cursory I thought the history and physical performed by the resident was. My irritation at the nurses was less subdued when I felt that the care they rendered was less than adequate. Even my wife, an R.N., was confused and shocked at the level of care I got and responded by doing some private-duty nursing for me. Somehow, it seemed more appropriate to vent hostility at nurses than at physicians. Perhaps this fraternalism is what will always keep doctors and nurses on different levels. I found myself arguing with laboratory technicians who demanded to take blood more than once from me and forbade this duplication of procedure. I felt no remorse or compunction about complaining since I had fully come to accept my role as no longer a provider of health care but a consumer, and it is amazing how different things look from one side of the bed to the other. Especially at our own institution as physicians, we are constantly looking for ways to take care of problems after they have arisen with our patients in the hospital. In general, we tend to react to medical problems rather than predict them. When you are a patient, it is very clear that if a problem strikes, you want a solution right then and there, and a physician is available only for a short time during the day, whether house staff or attending. The nursing staff and nurses aides are the ones who handle your immediate problems, and there is no remorse about letting them know about your unhappiness with regard to any particular problem. Whether they solve it or not is not as important sometimes as having complained.

Because I was vocal in my complaints, I was assigned a special nurse, who proceeded to ignore me with even greater vigor. I specifically remember an instance after surgery in which the intravenous solution I was receiving contained nafcillin and was clearly causing burning, pain, and swelling—obvious signs of phlebitis. I informed the nurse of it and she said the IV should stay in for another couple of hours. I clearly recall, through the haze of the postanesthetic state, that I told her she would have exactly 30 seconds to get the IV out of my arm or I would pull it out myself. The conversation was via the intercom, and I began to count. When I reached 30, I pulled the IV out of my arm and proceeded to let my arm bleed all over the floor on purpose. After that incident, nurses did respond when I called. Additionally, I learned new respect for the drug nafcillin and since then have given it with great caution and strict IV phlebitis precautions with a diluted solution. My colleagues in infectious disease say this is ridiculous, but they've never had nafcillin phlebitis. As a doctor, I have also learned to listen to my patients' complaints about nursing services. This is not meant to be a knock on the nurses because they do the best they can, but it is clear that in every hospital I've ever been in, nurses are tremendously overworked, undercompensated, and burned out long before their time. This is unfortunate, but I was absolutely convinced that I, as a patient, did not need to pay the price for it.

Being a patient brought forth in me, in a magnified fashion, the fears that most people have upon becoming a patient: helplessness and the feeling of aloneness, compounded by the feeling of being a stranger in my own hospital. There is such an inescapable feeling of dread for physicians as patients. Perhaps it comes from the fact that we know better than anyone else what goes on in hospitals, if only anecdotally. We recognize our shortcomings both as doctors and as human beings, and fear the worst for ourselves. Normally, a patient would have some of those fears allayed by his physician, but as a physician myself, I found the small amount of comforting that was given to me by my attendings and the complete lack of it afforded to me by the house staff to be disquieting and quite detrimental. On the other hand, my vantage point as a patient allowed me to appreciate with clarity, for the first time, the absolutely critical role that personnel whom we casually refer to as "ancillary" have to play in the recuperation and eventual recovery of a patient. Student nurses, whom I always viewed with sarcasm because they were always hoarding the charts I needed, visited my room once or twice during their training and their cheerfulness and attentiveness brightened my day. The volunteers whom I would greet cursorily and without really knowing names appeared in my room regularly to deliver cards or flowers or just to say hello, and they brightened my days considerably.

The orderlies and transportation service workers within the hospital who dutifully shuffled me from X-ray to surgery, to the room, to physical therapy were always pleasant and managed to have a smile and a "get well soon" on their lips. I was flabbergasted by the number of cards and telephone calls I received from my patients. Their attentiveness and outright love were the most pleasant surprise of all. All of these niceties were in stark contrast to the reactions from my colleagues. I could not understand why my patients could find the time in their busy days to make phone calls or send cards or flowers or candy, while people who spent half their lives in the hospital didn't find time to stop by and wave, even though my room was on a major thoroughfare in the hospital. I deduced some of the reason for this when one or two of my colleagues did show up and had no idea of how to act in my presence. Before my illness and since, it has been easy to meet and discuss things with these very same persons, but it is clear to me now that they and many of our colleagues have no idea how to pay a sick call. We know how to make rounds; we know how to write orders and make progress notes, do consultations, and read various graphs and charts; but it is a truly rare physician—at least in my experience—who can visit the sick, give comfort, and be comfortable doing it. Perhaps we are all too familiar with illness, too calloused from multiple encounters with illness, to recognize that our patients and especially our colleagues need a special kind of love and comfort that can only come from the knowing smile of a trusted colleague. That smile, that visit, can never be replaced by flowers, candy, fruits, or cards. A personal visit is mandated; nothing else will do.

After an article of mine on the isolation of the ill physician appeared in the *New England Journal of Medicine* (describing my feelings of anger about how few of my colleagues responded in what I thought would be an appropriate fashion to my illness), many of these very same colleagues came up to me after my return to practice to say, "I know you weren't talking about me in that article because I did send a card and I *was* thinking of you but I never had a chance to come visit or call." These people were well-intentioned, but I can translate their sentiments into "I didn't know what to say and I didn't feel comfortable coming into your room, didn't want to look at your chart, and I didn't want to know about your illness." This type of avoidance behavior tends to allow the well physician the luxury of maintaining the mirage of his immortality. It allows him to avoid social contacts that could become embarrassing for him, and, most important, it allows him to remain aloof from the personal nature of illness by maintaining his status as a caregiver rather than a care-receiver. I believe that for these reasons, most physicians who become ill will experience the isolation and frustration that I and many of my colleagues have faced when we were ill.

The hospital is a scary place. Patients who come in ignorant of what goes on in hospitals are probably far luckier than physicians who know a little bit about everything in the hospital. In my own case, I had an experience that demonstrated the rote manner in which the hospital can work to the potential danger of the patient.

I am a nonsmoker, but one day while lying in bed five or six days postop, I noticed what I thought was a burning rubber smell in my room. I called my nurse and naturally no one responded. I was not in a position to get up and investigate, but I could see from the corner of my eye without twisting too far that the electrical connection to my bed had been frayed and had begun to melt. While I didn't think it was a terrible emergency, I asked the nurse to come in right away to disconnect my bed. When she responded that she was busy, I told her that she had better hurry because I thought there was the possibility of my bed catching fire. This was a terrible mistake.

Three nurses rushed into my room and found a smoking electrical cord. I thought this was fine and asked them to disconnect it, which they promptly did, and I said, "Boy, I'm glad that's over." Before I could get the words out of my mouth, they had telephoned a fire code directly to the operator, who called a "99" with my room number on it. When this announcement was made over the hospital speaker, chaos erupted. Apparently the operator, knowing my room number after having received many calls from me, announced that the patient in room 4136 was having a cardiac arrest or some other emergency. As a result, dozens of nurses, doctors, technicians, firemen, EKG personnel, and people I had never even heard of came rushing into my room. I shooed them away with the cane that I had acquired and told them I was fine and to get out of my room, but they kept coming. I sensed immediately that I was in danger. I crawled out of my bed, onto the floor, out into the hallway. I figured I was safer out there than getting cardioverted by accident. Interestingly, the response from the cardiac arrest team was one of disdain, saying, "Boy, you really scared us." I had no intention of doing anything of the kind and felt fortunate to be alive after such a scare myself. Two hours later when I was finally allowed back in my room and a new bed had been acquired, the nurse scolded me for telling her there had been an emergency. I was incredulous but thankful to God that I was alive and that the hospital system had not overtaken itself and done me harm.

In another instance of the hospital system, a renal mass appeared on a CT scan of my lumbar spine. The CT doctor showed me the films and said he didn't know what the mass was but he would get back to me as soon as he could. The next five hours were tension-filled and I was convinced that my back surgery had led to the discovery of renal cell carcinoma. The ultrasound examination later that day cleared my mind a bit, but I wonder if I would have been better off not knowing why the ultrasound was ordered. There has been no follow-up of that renal cyst and I'm not sure that my primary care doctor even knew that the ultrasound was performed, again indicating a sort of abdication of responsibility when physicians become patients. For some reason it's assumed that we will follow up on our own abnormalities or that someone else will.

Aside from my bed almost catching on fire, my postoperative course was relatively unremarkable until I developed mild arachnoiditis, the one dreaded complication of neurosurgery of the back, and as a result, I was placed on prednisone therapy. As an internist, I had used prednisone hundreds of times in my practice, and I had always been careful to warn patients of the psychological effects of the drug and how it could cause euphoria, ulcer, brittle bones, and diabetes. But nothing can prepare you for an appreciation of prednisone's stunning power and side effects better than taking the medication yourself. I took prednisone for a couple of weeks only, but my mood swings, as judged by my family and friends, were incredible. I had crying jags, spells of uncontrollable laughter, sleep disturbances, a voracious appetite, and gastritis treated with Tagamet. Doctors would do well to familiarize themselves intimately with every drug they prescribe to appreciate better and respond to their patients' pleas for help when the drugs cause side effects that the patient is clearly aware of but the physician might miss.

I had to wear a steel-ribbed back corset and use a cane for several months. I viewed these medical appliances with ambivalence and sometimes exhibited them as a badge of courage but other times hid them to avoid dealing with the implications of my need to use them.

At home I noticed what I considered to be unusual behavior on my wife's part. After struggling with me for so many months to finally achieve what we hoped would be a cure, my wife began to leave home early and stay out late, leaving me alone for hours during the early part of my home convalescence. At first I thought she was disgusted with having to be the wife of a temporary invalid, but slowly came to realize that she was simply living her normal life-style—shopping and doing all the things required of a wife: managing her children, household, and life. My life had been so geared to being out of the house that it was unusual for me to be at home and alone. After my daily ritual of bathing, showering, and taking my whirlpool and stretching out, I found myself with hours of nothing to do. In speaking to patients about this phenomenon, I learned that this happens not only to physicians but to all work-oriented heads of household. We all find it very difficult to sit home and not do the things we're used to doing.

One thing I found helpful was the large number of books that friends had sent, and I immersed myself in reading long novels. I appreciated the opportunity to reintroduce myself to literature. The reading, however, could occupy only so much time, and when I was feeling up to it, I went out and bought a computer system and learned to program the computer and develop some small simple programs for future use in the office. I was convinced that this was a skill that would stand me in good stead and that, by becoming computer-literate, I was doing myself a wonderful favor, but in truth, since my illness, I use my computer only to balance my checkbook.

During my convalescence, I was reintroduced to an understanding that generations of physicians had reached before technology took over medicine—the importance of rest. Not only was my spine in need of rest so that it might mend, but I began to understand the need for restoration of the psyche and soul from the wounds of being sick, and I appreciated the opportunity to take it for all it was worth. At the same time I also became aware of my innate need to be busy. These two conflicting forces in my life were easy to reconcile in that I would rest until I got tired of resting, and then be busy until I got tired of being busy so I could rest again. This repetitive pattern was broken by periods of visits from friends and telephone calls, some minor book work, and meals. I found it a soothing existence that lent itself to the healing process. In fact, it was so restful that I began to sense resentment in my partners, who were diligently working to carry their own practices and mine, and I began to get sly remarks about how easy I was taking it and wasn't I ready to come back to work. I was sufficiently circumspect about this to let it pass and recognize the primal importance of my recovery, because if I didn't get better completely they'd have a practice of mine to take care of for a much longer time.

At the time of my illness I had three boys, aged 10, 8, and 1. My older boys were completely convinced that after Daddy recovered from this nasty surgery, he'd be able to do everything he ever did before, except he'd be able to do it better. A major source of comfort for me was the innocence of my youngest boy, who knew nothing more than love itself, and we gladly shared our love in a leisurely fashion that was not available to my first boys because of my time commitments and career. To this day I feel an extra special attachment to my youngest son, Bradley, who is the last brilliant jewel in my crown.

My mother and father are of European descent, so when I was in the hospital they found it absolutely critical for me to be fed in a manner that confounded my nurses and doctors but gave comfort to my parents. Although I was limited to nourishing liquids, my parents would show up daily with two rib steaks and a baked potato, which I wolfed down with abandon, happy to keep their secret from my doctors. It was this type of gastronomic nurturing that made patient and parents feel wanted, needed, and cared for. It may have been wrong medically but was right spiritually.

During my hospitalization, I lost a great deal of weight, and one day while I was being wheeled from my room to physical therapy in a polo shirt and shorts, one of my medical house staff saw me and asked if I were related to Dr. Sugar, whom he knew but remembered as being much heavier. I still don't know whether he was joking, being kind, or being stupid.

An activity that occupied happy moments for me during my recovery was filling out insurance applications to collect on the disability insurance policies whose premiums I had been paying for years. It made me feel smug that I had had the foresight to be fully covered for medical disabilities, and each check I received brought me great elation. What was even more fun was fighting with one particular insurance company that refused to pay a claim and winning the case without having to resort to lawyers. Knowledge of the intricate workings of insurance companies and their arcane and illogical ways of paying their legitimate debts has stood me in good stead as I argue with them for my patients. Without disability insurance my illness would have been a tremendous financial burden. Making these policies available to us is one of the great services provided by our medical societies.

My reentry to the real world took place gradually in an orderly fashion. My follow-up care was routine and my recovery uncomplicated after a few stormy days and weeks. Ultimately, four weeks after surgery, I was readmitted to the hospital with an acute episode of severe back spasms and underwent emergency CT scanning and other testing. This was resolved so quickly that I'm not sure what happened, but the day and a half in the hospital reconfirmed how uncomfortable I was at being there. Since I and my doctor had had more than enough of my illness, we both decided that I should continue to recuperate at home as if nothing terrible had happened.

My follow-up since then has been sporadic, with only occasional chats in the hall with my surgeon. No specific office visits or tests have been ordered, but my surgeon has advised me that I must lose weight. Additionally, he has given me curbstone advice on swimming, jogging, and tennis, none of which I have ever done or intend to do.

I returned to the office part time several months postop and was stunned by the outpouring of love and affection by my patients at my return. Many of them had waited for months to be seen, insisting that I was the only one who could take care of their illnesses. I was extremely flattered and touched by their sincerity and devotion. My office staff had kept everything going, my partners had kept the practice going, and they were more than anxious for me to get back in the saddle. After a period of several weeks, I felt I was in the groove, thinking clearly and acting with facility. In the beginning, I was a little clumsy with the instruments of daily practice. It took me a little longer to do reflex testing, a little longer to pump up the blood pressure cuff. But I was enjoying being a doctor again and relishing the fact that being a patient was quickly becoming part of my past.

Returning to the hospital was interesting also. I had a meeting with my chief of service and officially notified him that I was coming back to work. Although I am sure he was sincere in his welcome back to the department, somehow I felt as though he had never been a patient at his own hospital and that he had never experienced what I had experienced. I found myself wishing to explain to him what I had gone through, but decided it was inappropriate.

My story does have a relatively happy ending in that I am now back in full-time practice and have been for some time. I still list 10 to 15 degrees to starboard because there isn't much left of the left side of my lumbar spine. I am back playing sports to a small degree, and I don't lift things anymore unless I absolutely have to. Though my quadricep muscles are a fraction of the size they used to be, they're symmetrical now. They don't hurt very much or very often, and although I have an occasional twinge of numbness and occasional pain, life is a great deal more bearable now. My illness has helped me understand some things that only my patients understood before. It has helped me to develop an attitude toward patients, and especially patients who are in pain. I now feel I can understand all the grief, the anguish of the patient, and pain, and can relate to the patient who is hopeless and afraid of hospitalization. I can understand the apprehension of the preoperative patient. I can empathize with the patient who is afraid of an invasive test. In fact, my experiences with many of these tests have allowed me, with a great deal of confidence, to tell my patients that "I've had this particular test; it isn't any fun but it's not as bad as you think it is. I survived and so will you." For some reason, patients find this far more comforting than bland reassurance based on statistical probability and evaluation of the medical literature. Our shared human pathos as physicians who have had significant life experiences, both personally and professionally, with the sick, the pain-ridden, and the dying is an extremely valuable commodity. I view my illness with mixed emotions, but certainly it has been a process that has allowed me to gain insight and had made me a more compassionate physician. More importantly, it has made me a far more compassionate man. I now go out of my way to find friends or colleagues who are ill. I make it my business to see them. It is my responsibility to ask them if there is anything that I can do for them. A stumbling block in this endeavor has been, however, the secretiveness of physicians about their illnesses. I suspect that this is fairly widespread and makes it difficult for me even to know when there is a physician in the hospital to visit. It is also difficult for me to know whether I am breaching confidentiality by my knowledge of my colleague's illness, but given my own experience, I feel comfortable sacrificing confidentiality for the greater reward of visiting the sick.

If I were to distill out the most important and overwhelming emotion or attitude that I experienced during the unnatural time of my illness, it would be displacement. For those of us who are highly trained, highly motivated, successful caregivers, it is a shock and an enormous displacement to divest ourselves of the robes of superiority we wear as physicians and don the patient robe that exposes our fannies. Learning to cope with that displacement can mean the difference between successful recovery with serene convalescence and a stormy, unhappy, disgruntled recuperation, leaving permanent emotional as well as physical scars. In the end, however, my original advice to a potential patient still gets top billing—"Don't get sick."

CHAPTER 15

PARKINSON'S DISEASE

DONALD B. HACKEL

My feelings about writing this essay on my life with Parkinson's disease are mixed. On the one hand I am afraid that there is nothing especially important or unique in what I have experienced. On the other hand, I feel some enthusiasm in using this opportunity to review my situation, perhaps because of a feeling that in so doing I might discover something about myself.

I had never really been sick until March 1972, when I developed a mild to moderately severe case of infectious hepatitis. I felt lucky, however, that I wasn't as sick as the prosector of the autopsy from which we both probably caught the disease. She was unable to return to work for more than six months while I was better after only one month. In September of that year I noticed some awkwardness in writing which disturbed me since I was in the habit of writing the first drafts of my reports and manuscripts in longhand. This "writer's cramp," as I thought of it, was noticed by the secretary, who had become used to my old handwriting and was bothered by its deterioration. The letters tended to fade off into smaller and smaller sizes, which is typical of Parkinson's disease and even has a name, "micrographia," so that if I had been alert enough—or interested enough—I would have been able to make a diagnosis at that point. Shortly after this I became aware that my facial muscles were tense, that I had trouble smiling, and that I was bothered by frequent eye blinking. I had not yet put the two sets of symptoms together and did not worry about them since they had come on so gradually. Furthermore, they did not significantly affect my ability to do my daily work, and I passed them off as merely changes that might be expected with aging.

The symptoms did progress, however, and I began to have some real difficulty in sitting through an hour's lecture (although not in giving one) because of the eye blinking, which was exaggerated by the ex-

DR. DONALD HACKEL is a 65-year-old professor of pathology at Duke University who is active in teaching and research. His major interest is in cardiovascular disease.

perience. The eye blinking really got to be embarrassing when it interfered with my ability to talk freely on a one-to-one basis with others, especially since it was made worse by emotional stimulation. When, for example, a problem was brought to me for action or advice, I found that my muscles became more rigid, the eye blinking got worse, and it was difficult to concentrate on the problem at hand. This was so even when I had no real personal involvement or any stake in the problem and would not ordinarily have had any reason to be nervous about the situation. Still, it was embarrassing and it brought out another symptom that I had, until then, pretty much ignored, a slight tremor of my right hand. It started with difficulty using my hand in quick repetitive movements such as brushing my teeth or shaving. I recall it first appeared about a year after the onset of the "writer's cramp." The tremor came on only once in a while, and I remember the first time when I was no longer able to ignore it. This occurred while I was a guest speaker in the pathology department at Yale. I was having lunch before the talk and rattled my spoon, but I was able to eat lunch without actually spilling any soup and to present my talk without undue difficulty.

By this time I had, of course, begun to think of the possibility of Parkinson's disease—although I hoped that it might be almost anything else. My dislike of this disease was particularly strong because of my experience with the helplessness it produced in people I knew who had had it, and I certainly did not want to be dependent and a burden to my family. However, the slow course of the symptoms and the minor interference with my professional activities until then encouraged me, and I finally went to see a neurologist. He recommended that I try L-dopa as a diagnostic test, and, with some trepidation, I started taking the drug. I wasn't sure whether I wanted the drug to work—which would confirm my fears that I had this bad disease—or whether it would be better for it to fail—which would mean that I had something that could be worse but might be better! In any case, I was surprised and pleased at how dramatically it relieved my symptoms so that I began to "feel human" again for a change. Ever since this experience I will admit that I have been less of a therapeutic nihilist and recognize the value of drug treatment when it is specifically indicated.

My reaction to the trial therapy with L-dopa surprised me. It was one of relief! I was partly relieved, of course, at having an answer to the cause of the bothersome symptoms and a drug that would help alleviate those symptoms. However, in retrospect, it seems to me that there were some other considerations which influenced me and which are difficult to describe clearly: (1) I felt some relief at finally hearing that I had Parkinson's disease. (2) This was explained by me at the time as the natural result of finally having an answer to the troublesome symptoms. (3) I did not want to tell my colleagues or even my family (except for my wife) about the diagnosis until the symptoms became so bad that I could not avoid it. (4) I can now see another reason for the feeling of relief as being due to the fact that I would now be released from the expectation (mainly from myself) that I continue to achieve and move upward rather than to keep on with my present work, which was clearly what I most enjoyed doing. (5) My reason for not wanting to talk about the diagnosis—I told myself at the time—was a desire not to be "labeled," but it was probably also due to a reluctance to use the disease as an excuse to avoid the pressure which I felt was a good and desirable stimulus, and which had served me well in the past.

It is now about 13 years since I first noticed the symptoms of Parkinson's disease, and I really cannot complain very much. I have been able to continue most of my activities, including teaching the pathology course to first-year medical students, continuing as director of the course with responsibility for organizing and overseeing it, and participating actively in teaching a laboratory section of 20 students. In addition, I am the department "professional advisor," which means that I am responsible for the 17 or so elective courses that we give to third-year medical students, and in addition to which I give an elective on cardiovascular pathology each year. I have been able to continue my experimental research work as before, and my other medical school responsibilities are not much different from what they had been—although I have somewhat curtailed my involvement in committee work. My national consulting activities have been almost completely eliminated. I especially miss the project site visits and study section meetings that I used to participate in frequently for the NIH. I enjoyed them because I made so many good friends through them and felt that they were my one best learning experience.

I end with two comments:

1. The fact that my symptoms were preceded by a bout of infectious hepatitis makes me wonder whether there is a causal relationship beween that illness and the subsequent development of Parkinson's disease. As a scientist and a physician, I am alert to sequential phonemena looking for a relationship. Is what I experienced coincidental? After all, neither infectious hepatitis nor Parkinson's disease is rare. Is it causal? There is no scientific evidence for such a relationship. However, I can't help wondering.

2. I would think that my experience with Parkinson's disease should be comforting to other newcomers to the club, since the disease varies greatly in its speed of progression and can respond well to drug therapy. Thus, the only reasonable attitude is one of optimism that your affair with the disease will be as slowly developing as mine has been.

CHAPTER 16

PARKINSON'S DISEASE

LOUIS B. GUSS

I learned I had Parkinson's disease when I had a daughter in college and two other children preparing to follow her—quite a blow. My family was my first concern, and then there was the realization of all the manifestations of the illness well remembered from my medical texts.

A painful left knee was my first symptom in 1972 when I was 58 years old. I used some simple analgesics and bought an exercise bicycle. Since I stood many hours a day in my office practice, I thought exercise might be beneficial.

In September 1972 my wife and I went to Yugoslavia, where I attended sessions for my CME credits. It was here that I first fell. At the time, I thought I had merely lost my balance and tripped. A few months later I went to Atlanta, where I took a course in infectious diseases. In the hotel bathroom I noticed that my bare feet stuck to the tile floor. Getting in and out of a car was getting more difficult. Also, my handwriting became smaller and almost illegible.

When my symptoms increased I consulted my friend and internist, Dr. M., who thought I had Parkinson's disease and suggested I consult a neurologist for verification. This must have been difficult for my colleague and friend to tell me.

Dr. P. of the Department of Neurology confirmed the diagnosis. I was disappointed because I felt I had so much that I wanted to do. He was most supportive and encouraging, and I needed that so much. He thought that I would be able to carry on my practice for an indefinite time and do what I had to do (or at least that was what he told me).

Artane mg 2 t.i.d. was my initial medication. After a few doses I was elated because I felt stronger and was able to walk without diffi-

DR. LOUIS GUSS, 71 years old, retired after 30 years of pediatric practice. First, last, and always he has a keen interest in pediatrics and the welfare of children. Since his affliction he has been interested in the current findings and research of Parkinson's disease. He is eager for a new effective medication that will eliminate the "off" moments of the present "on-and-off" syndrome.

culty. Two days later, however, I developed nausea, and this was a great disappointment. This was badly timed because I was looking forward to driving to Vermont to pick up my daughter, who was attending a summer session at Middlebury College.

The dose of Artane was decreased to mg 1, and this in combination with Symmetrel kept me going. I was able to function fairly well and carry on a practice for another 11 years. My stamina was greatly diminished, however, and I tired easily. It was difficult for me to project my voice, and because of my instability I fell several times. How to get up was something that my wife and I had to figure out. I would have to roll over and get on my knees, place one foot flat on the ground, and have someone pull me by my belt. Something stationary in front of me to hold onto was most helpful.

An area of great concern to me was how my patients would react to having a pediatrician with a condition such as Parkinson's disease care for their children. Would they think that I was incapable? My mind and judgment certainly weren't impaired but I'm sure that there were those who felt that their physician should be not less than perfect. Nevertheless, many still trusted me implicitly and this was rewarding. I'm sure this trust gave me strength.

I did not feel like my old self, and I definitely could feel a change. My wife and I were so disappointed. It was difficult to accept and we could not even call my condition by name. And—most of all—we didn't even want to speak to others about it. At the same time my colleagues and co-workers were considerate and sensitive to my condition. How often the girls in the nursery helped me tie the strings of my gown! The first things I gave up were attending cesarean sections and taking care of newborns.

Even though I would have liked to have felt more limber, Dr. D., the neurologist to whom I was assigned, felt that at this early stage of illness my medication was appropriate. Fortunately, I was, and still am, practically tremor-free. As he explained to me, "More medication or L-dopa would be like shooting a bird with a cannon." This philosophy has stayed with me through the years—"Use the least to be the most effective."

So for another period of time I managed to plod along the best that I could. As a result of the Symmetrel my feet and ankles became edematous and I had to wear larger shoes. I also developed an ulcer on my right foot that was extremely difficult to heal.

Until June 1983 I managed to carry on an office practice on a limited basis. At this time the medications were no longer effective and I was stiff, weak, and unable to walk. I thought that "the day" had come.

Then I consulted with Dr. R., a local neurologist who had much knowledge and experience with Parkinson's disease. I found him to be compassionate, brilliant, and interested in me not because I was a physician with Parkinson's disease but because I was a patient in distress who needed medical attention. My wife and I were already making adjustment to the almost complete disability when he advised hospitalization. This was to monitor and regulate new medication and to begin physical therapy for me to be ambulatory once again. Needless to say, my wife and I felt that this was a gift of rebirth. He gave us great faith and encouragement. All our negative feelings were dismissed, and we were imbued with the spirit of hope. I will always be grateful to him for his sincere interest. The sparkle of his eyes and facial expression denote the reward he derives when I am functioning well. He is a dedicated physician and a very special person.

The EMT who accompanied me to the hospital in the ambulance was one of my former "little patients." He said that it was about time that he did something for me since I had attended him on several occasions for asthmatic attacks. It is comforting to know people, especially in times of distress. Even though it seems strange to be on the receiving end, I have readily accepted the role of being a patient. When one is "down and out," there certainly is no choice. I recall that I felt very helpless and weak.

In the course of about two weeks I was stabilized on a combination of Artane, Sinemet, and bromocriptine. Physical therapy was used, beginning with passive leg exercises when I was in bed. The therapists helped me to walk again. Never did I think that I would have to learn with a walker. I was apprehensive about getting into the car to be discharged. The therapist accompanied me to our car and showed me what to do with my body and legs. I lacked confidence, and I was fearful of falling. It really takes time to learn how to balance oneself.

For a few months I continued with physical therapy. The rehabilitation staff were interested and supportive. They also used massage for my neck, back, and chest. I enjoyed the massage very much because it relaxed my tight muscles, but unfortunately the effect was only temporary. Nevertheless, the entire therapeutic team is so delightful that visiting them in itself would be therapeutic.

I experienced nausea, probably from the Sinemet, mostly in the early morning. Saltines and cracked ice helped. Flushing and frequent hot flashes from the Sinemet were almost unbearable. Faintness, headache, and lateral numbness of the head came from the bromocriptine. I was functioning, but it was a big price to pay. Tagamet was prescribed for symptoms of hyperacidity. This worked fairly well but I had an intense headache. When I eliminated the Tagamet and changed to Zantac, the headache diminished and the acid control was effective.

Constipation is another drug-related problem. Because of the anticholinergic effect the stool is large in diameter and dry. As a result of passing "cement," I developed an inguinal hernia. Increased fluid intake, figs, and a Fleet enema every other day really are helpful. Hard peppermint candy helps with the dryness of the mouth.

To complicate the management of my illness, I have a fairly good size hiatus hernia. The anticholinergic drugs used for Parkinson's disease increased the symptoms of the hiatus hernia. The most distressing is abdominal distention. At one time there was absolutely no peristalsis and I must have had an ileus. Nothing was moving and I felt as if I were going to blow up. Reglan was ordered. What a marvelous "Roto-Rooter"! My GI tract was relieved and I was more comfortable. However, it completely canceled the Parkinson drugs and I was stiff and practically unable to walk.

Bromocriptine also presented other problems. I developed ergotism with hemorrhagic areas on my toes. The thought of gangrene is not a pleasant one. When the medication was eliminated my toes became warm and pink again.

So my present medications are at a minimum. The regime is Artane mg 1 t.i.d., Sinemet 25/100 1 every two hours during the day (this had diminished the hot flashes somewhat), and Zantac b.i.d. I still am able to walk, eat by myself, and get along fairly well, but, of course, my performance is not as good as when I was on the bromocriptine. However, it is best to be able to function fairly well at the least. It's like a balance. For a while I was wearing out the pages of the PDR checking out all my symptoms.

Special commendation is to be given to the staff of the surgical supply company for the many comforts that were given to me. Just to mention a few: straightening out the kinks in the motorized bed, solving the problem with the wheelchair, and suggesting the special mattress for my sore and aching back. The Thermophore moist heat pack was also very helpful for my stiff neck. They made several adjustments to meet my needs and were always courteous and caring. When we moved to our town house apartment a chair lift was promptly installed.

In retrospect I do feel that having the responsibility of my office practice gave me the strength to carry on and a purpose to life. It would have been very easy to have "given in."

As you can see, it has not been any one person that has contributed to my functioning *status quo* but a group working as a team. I now have been retired for two years, and I am trying my best to enjoy it.

I am not happy to be dependent upon others, especially my wife, who anticipates my every need. But I believe that I am now resigned to this fact, and I accept it as graciously as it is offered. To my family, friends, and colleagues I will be ever grateful.

Another one of my disappointments is that I am unable to read as much as I would like because of the atropine effect of the medications.

So my day's physical activities are often limited to a walk about 10:00 a.m., when my medication (which I refer to as "my fix") enables me to take off. I enjoy visiting friends as well as having them visit us. Movies and television have been helpful.

Traveling is not the easiest because there are many adjustments for me to make and a great deal of planning for my wife. This past December we flew to California and visited with our daughter, son-in-law, and two grandchildren, but I am more comfortable at home. I certainly did have the royal treatment—we were given the master bedroom and they had rented a motorized bed for me. No doubt I am insecure being away from my physicians, but it is necessary that I be more courageous.

Since I lose my balance easily and find it difficult to walk in close areas or behind another person in close range, I have a lot of mental programming to perform.

Just the other day my carpenter and friend, Richard, put some ball casters on my chair at the dining room table. This enables me to be comfortably seated. We are still learning to be innovative to make life easier.

I do think that I would prefer having syphilis. At least I would have deserved the risk taken, and the treatment is specific and effective. However, my faithful wife of 41 years might have some reservation in this regard. So, inasmuch as I had no choice in being afflicted as such, I am making the best of it.

PART III

NEUROPSYCHIATRIC DISORDERS

CHAPTER 17

CEREBRAL CONCUSSION

LAWRENCE R. FREEDMAN

A little over two years ago I set off for a usual day at the hospital. After breakfast I put on my bicycle helmet and gloves and started off for my five-minute refreshing ride in the cool morning air. About 200 yards from my home, passing a construction site, I noticed a small truck emerging from an alley...

I learned much later that someone had called the paramedics, who found me on the ground and brought me to the hospital where I was admitted with the diagnosis of cerebral concussion. I have no memory of the event or of the subsequent six-day hospitalization. I am told that I was confused and disoriented, but not unconscious. It was not until three days later that I easily recognized my family. I am told that I complained of considerable headache during the first days after the accident, that my appetite was poor, and that I suffered from severe shoulder pains. Since there were no fractures, the pains were attributed to the fall.

A CT scan of the brain upon admission to the hospital revealed a small amount of intracerebral blood, which resolved by the time I was discharged. Yet, since there was no reliable information about how my accident had occurred, a cerebral angiogram was performed to rule out aneurysm as the precipitating cause. The angiogram was negative. I have no recollection of any of the procedures or of any of the events in the hospital, even though I am told by my family that I seemed to participate appropriately in the consideration of what was done and signed the required permission forms. I probably looked better than I actually was since I also recognized visitors by name but had no recollection of their visits even a few minutes after they left.

I was on a neurosurgical service where my management consisted of close observation and two prophylactic medications—one to assure

DR. LAWRENCE FREEDMAN is Associate Chief of Staff for Education, West Los Angeles Veterans Administration Medical Center, and professor of medicine, UCLA School of Medicine.

the stability of my blood pressure and the other to prevent the possibility of convulsions.

It is hard to be precise about when I began to realize that I had a bicycle accident and had been hospitalized for a week.

The first clear memory I have, and treasure, dates to the early days at home when my daughter talked me into going for a walk around the block. I was anxious about the walk—I wondered if I would be able to maintain my balance walking down the front steps. I wondered whether it was as safe outside as I felt it was indoors, at home. Going down the steps turned out to be quite easy, and it felt wonderful to be outdoors. The weather was good, the air was delicious. Still, I was very pleased when we arrived back home. Exhausted, I went directly to bed.

My daughter told me later that when we had gotten halfway around the block, I wanted to turn in a direction that, she explained to me, was the wrong way. She seemed so sure! I told her that exceptionally I would go her way, but that I would bet her a million dollars that we wouldn't arrive home that way. I still owe her the money!

An early memory is of the worrisome fatigue that had me spending a good part of the day in bed. Taking a shower was particularly tiring; doing anything was, in fact, exhausting. Even food had lost its attraction.

Another early memory dates to about three weeks after the accident when I awoke with generalized teeth-chattering shaking chills that lasted over an hour. My wife, worried, called my internist, who came over as soon as he could. He and I both concluded that I was probably having a reaction to the blood pressure medication. My other medication, an anticonvulsant, had already been discontinued before I left the hospital because of my developing a generalized skin rash. I was now medication-free. Within 24 hours my shoulder pains disappeared, my appetite improved, and I was no longer enveloped by the cloud that contributed so much to my fatigue. I continued to feel very good being at home. I became aware of a resting, recuperating process within me to which I abandoned myself completely.

There was one thing I noticed in the early days at home that disturbed me greatly—I was no longer interested in listening to music. I heard the music, I knew it was music, and I also knew how much I used to enjoy listening to music. It had always been the primary unfailing source that nourished my spirit. Now it just didn't *mean* anything to me. I was indifferent to it. I knew something was very wrong.*

*I have since spoken with two people, both musicians, who had the same experience after a head injury. They were greatly reassured by hearing of the complete restoration of my "musical connection."

The realization that something was wrong was the major issue I had to struggle with during the months that followed. I felt that I had been far, far away and had now "returned," that I was now doing and experiencing things that I knew and understood from a distant past but had not done for a very long time. The sight of trees and flowers was spectacular—colors were delicious and exciting.

Along with the excitement of discovery there was the fear and anxiety of what seemed uncertain or unknown. After not having driven an automobile for a month, I was suddenly not sure that I knew how to drive or how to deal with traffic and was not sure that I was capable of doing any sport. I was uncertain of my ability to move quickly and appropriately.

I was pleased to have visitors, but I didn't mind when they left, and I wondered when I would regain the full pleasure of being with people.

Professionally, I had similar anxieties when I returned to work part time after six weeks at home. I was concerned about seeing patients, making rounds, and working with students and residents. I felt the need to be particularly attentive in the hospital to even routine matters. This must have contributed significantly to my fatigue.

The first talk I had to give, about three months after the accident, was accompanied by a lot of anxiety. I took a long time in preparing it and worried about the most unlikely aspects of it. When the talk went easily and well, I realized that my main difficulty at this point was most likely due to the uncertainty and anxiety related to the thought of doing something, rather than an inability to actually do what I contemplated doing.

Guessing the probable source of my difficulties did little to help resolve them. I realized that my physicians had not addressed the psychological consequences of my injury, nor had they prepared or advised my family of the inevitable anxiety that would accompany recovery. I felt intensely alone with my worries, too frightened, too protective, and too insecure to do anything but worry more. A potential vicious circle was at hand that made our family life gloomy and tense. My wife and my daughter helped me to decide to consult a psychiatrist in an effort to bring some relief and attend to the escalating doubts and anxieties. In retrospect I realize that the more I recovered, the more frightening and shaking the whole event seemed and the more I worried. My meetings with the psychiatrist were fascinating but, more importantly, were immensely helpful and, in fact, constitute one of the important gains that this accident carried with it.

The early period of recovery at home was, in a sense, reexperiencing childhood. I was told what I could and could not attempt, I was cared for, I slept a lot, and there were few demands put on me; I had no responsibilities other than to "emerge." I can best characterize this as a time of infantilization.

Coincident with feeling infantilized, I was gradually naggingly aware of having passed a period of time when I had existed but about which I had no memory. The thought that there was a time when I might have been dead occurred often.

The image that I still retain of this early time after my accident is that of being enveloped by combined feelings of uncertainty and constraint—as in childhood, coming immediately up against the anticipated uncertainties and constraints of aging and the void that may be death. It was as if the inner devices, which normally kept my early experiences separated from concerns of future dependence by a "healthy" distance, weren't working properly. Life events, fears, and memories seemed linked when, in fact, they were far apart. I searched to find my proper place in my present three-dimensional landscape, which, although familiar, needed a readjustment of scale. I felt as if I were looking through a powerful telescope that brought vaguely perceived objects too near. In one's "normal" adult state, the memories of childhood and the unknowns of aging are generally perceived through the wrong end of a telescope—both extremes of life are vague and seem a long way off. The accident had somehow turned the telescope around.

Professionally, these experiences gave me a vivid insight into the complex human issues that loom so large in caring for the aged, to whom childhood seems near and who, at the same time, struggle with feelings of loss of competence and increasingly dependent needs.

On still another personal level, feelings of this early period after the accident required that I focus attention on my relationships with my wife of over 30 years and my children. For me to have become "the child" in a setting where I had been the parent and husband and then to return to the latter status required devoting considerable thought and feeling to my place within the family. This effort was, of course, essential to my personal sense of identity but was even more rewarding on an inner level for all of us.

What did I miss most as a patient recovering from a cerebral concussion? I wanted my physicians to talk to me; I needed them to talk to me, particularly as I improved and knew what I wanted to discuss and was able to retain more of what was being said. As I look back, I know that I was unaware of this need at the time and was, therefore, incapable of expressing it. Yet I believe I would have benefited enormously from regular meetings with my physician, especially during the first few months after being discharged from the hospital.

I would have wanted to hear about the experiences to be anticipated after such an injury, about their evolution, about their impact on me personally and professionally. I would have benefited from the identification of any signs of progress and encouragement as to the probability of full recovery.

In this regard, it had been particularly satisfying for me to see the relief of the two musicians (described earlier) with whom I spoke after their cerebral injuries, when I described my difficulty in "connecting" with music and the recovery from it after my accident. This was an experience that was troubling to both of them—indeed, so troubling that they did not/could not bring it up in conversation with me.

I would have benefited from the opportunity to express concerns and ask questions. It is clear to me, however, that I would not have gotten to personal issues without having first developed a relationship of trust with my physician, and such relationships take time to develop.

I realize, as I write, that I sound like the army of patients who have expressed and continue to express these sentiments. But why is this dimension of care so lacking? Several reasons come to mind. Perhaps one important reason is that physicians are poorly compensated for their time unless they carry out well-codified, remunerative procedures.

Another reason is that the human aspects of illness and medical care are not infused with the attention and emphasis that they deserve. In the physician, human understanding and involvement is presumed to be inborn and then enhanced by experience—and sometimes it is. But "sometimes" is not enough and, most important, is unpredictable. The reality is that such care requires instruction and guidance—elements that are conspicuously absent from our traditional formal medical teaching. I hope the current effort of the American Board of Internal Medicine to focus on "humanism" will require that attention be directed to this vital dimension of medical care.

However, it is not at all certain that identifying the need to consider the human aspects of illness and addressing them in the curriculum will be sufficient. After all, Dr. Kübler-Ross began her pioneering work on death and dying about 20 years ago, and, despite her accomplishments and the development of hospice as a care unit, the usual professional response to terminal illness, still today, is withdrawal. The human aspects of the care of patients with nonterminal illness also have broad implications. The subject matter will require definition, and medical student and house staff instruction will require that both faculty and students explore personal feelings and attitudes about not only death, but also about illness in general, and personal vulnerability. These issues are, perhaps, brought into particular focus in caring for a colleague.

It is surely the human aspects of care that patients are looking for when they search for practitioners of "holistic" medicine. I suspect that patients are driven to practitioners of a variety of "paramedical" practices because traditional physicians seem so unavailable to attend to nonbiological aspects of illness.

In my experience and for my family, it was the nurses who were most alert and sensitive to our needs for both human and biological dimensions of medical care. The nurse was the major conveyor of information and feelings, the translator, the interpreter of questions and answers between the patient, his family, and the physicians—in all directions. This is a major component of care that does not receive the acknowledgment and respect it so richly deserves. The role of the nurse should be accorded the most careful attention and nurture, particularly at this time of rapid change in the organization of medical care.

As I reread my discussion of the human aspects of medical care, I feel that it is incomplete because I know that these issues have been raised many times in the past and yet the general dissatisfaction with care continues. Indeed, there are many who believe that we physicians are less effective in providing this human dimension of care today than we were in the past, when we could do little to influence the biology of disease but when we could at least talk, listen, reassure, and comfort.

Recent comments by Oliver Sacks pertain directly to that aspect of care which is lacking today.[1] Sacks has called attention to the reaction of an individual affected by illness "to restore, to replace, to compensate for and preserve his identity." He suggests that it is "an essential part of our role as physicians" to study or influence the means by which individuals react, no less than it is our responsibility to direct attention to the primary illness or injury.

Somehow, coincident with the spectacular advances in science and medicine in recent years, the physician is perceived as being less aware of/competent to manage the human aspects of medical care. We can perhaps be aided in our efforts to incorporate this responsibility into our general understanding of medical care by referring to the means by which mankind has responded generally to change.

Arthur Schlesinger, Jr. has estimated recently that more change has taken place in the past two lifetimes of man than occurred in the first 498. He went on to observe that whereas "science and technology revolutionize our lives, memory, tradition and myth determine our responses."

I would like to suggest that this idea is transposable to what I have been referring to as the biological and human aspects of medical care. The biological dimension of care is easily seen in terms of the science and technology that revolutionize our lives, and I believe that the human aspect of care is inseparably intertwined with the memory, tradition, and myth of the patient and the society in which he lives.

Schlesinger's use of the word *response* to characterize the relation of memory, tradition, and myth to science and technology brings to mind the principle established by Newton's third law of motion, that "for every force acting on a body, the body exerts a force having equal magnitude in the opposite direction along the same line of action as the original force."

Applying Newton's law, memory, tradition, and myth become the means by which the individual exerts a force of equal magnitude and in the opposite direction along the same line of action as the original force, science, and technology. In medical care terms, the human responses to illness generate an equal force in a direction opposite to the force of the biological consequences of illness.

In other words, what traditionally has been referred to as the dissociation between the attention directed to the biological and that directed to the human consequences of illness is, perhaps, more easily understandable as conflict, since the human aspect of care would address powerful forces that have arisen in opposition to the biological forces requiring attention and care. The physician, in directing his attention primarily to the biological forces responsible for illness, becomes inevitably linked to these forces. It is not surprising, therefore, that he would be viewed as inadequate to deal with the patient's human needs. In order to address the human aspects of care and illness, he would also have to direct his efforts in opposition to the biological aspects of illness with which he has become identified.

There is another dimension to the dissociation/conflict between the biological and human aspects of medical care. Perhaps the youth of science and technology generates a pressure to struggle against the power of memory, tradition, and myth, which, after all, have been around for a long time and which have a firm hold on the attitudes and behavior of mankind. Perhaps science has understood, as did Robert Pirsig,[2] that "there are human forces stronger than logic." In other words, perhaps scientists and technologists, with all of their spectacular achievements, feel that they must struggle to achieve dominance over those powerful archaic forces—forces that are still stronger than logic—which continue to maintain their power.

It is not difficult to understand the profound personal conflicts generated in patients by scientific triumphs such as blood transfusions, artificial organs, organ transplantation, artificial insemination, surrogate motherhood, and still others. Yet the meaning of these advances is rarely considered in the light of memory, tradition, and myth. If my hypothesis offers a valid explanation for the conflict between the biological and human aspects of illness and care, we are not likely to reduce this conflict until we start learning how to talk about it. I suggest that the first step would be to encourage physicians to begin questioning themselves about their personal views and then to encourage their talking about them with each other. Ultimately, it will require skill and sensitivity to learn how to incorporate this understanding of human aspects of illness and care into the traditional educational programs of students and physicians.

I remember when, during the recovery from my concussion, I realized that I no longer understood or felt music. It was then that I knew something was wrong with me. As I reflect upon the emphasis in medicine today and the forces pushing it in the direction in which it is evolving, I no longer understand the music; I know something is wrong.

REFERENCES

1. Oliver Sacks, *The Man Who Mistook His Wife for a Hat* (New York: Summit Books, 1985), p. 4.
2. Robert M. Persig, *Zen and the Art of Motorcycle Maintenance* (New York: Bantam, 1974), p. 17.

CHAPTER 18

ALCOHOLISM

"DR. MAGOO"

I became ill without ever recognizing that I had a disease, and began my recovery when I had major medical, social, legal, economic, emotional, and spiritual problems that were overwhelming me. My illness progressed for 25 years, during which time it moved imperceptibly at first and extremely rapidly at last.

Although I was well trained at a prestigious eastern college and medical school, and had completed rotating internships and specialty and subspecialty training, I had never been given any training in the recognition and treatment of my disease. In fact, I did not even learn I had a disease until treatment was in progress. A further paradox was that my treatment was not by doctors but by ordinary lay people to whom I am eternally grateful for saving my life.

I had always considered myself a social drinker, and the people I socialized with seemed to drink as much as I did. In college I found that I drank at parties and football games but always drank for the effect that it gave me—escape, euphoria, and the chance to be uninhibited. It did cause embarrassments such as public intoxication, vomiting at times, and passing out, but since it was periodic drinking, I never had any difficulty until the last few days before graduation, when I was told that I was going to be expunged from the records—as if I had never attended college. This was directly related to drinking and a prank pulled off as a lark. Fortunately, the dean recanted and I was graduated to go on to medical school.

Because I knew that the challenge of medical school would be a big undertaking, I decided to do everything in my power to attend to my studies without competing problems. I decided, therefore, to give up my girlfriend. She had often been embarrassed by my drinking, disapproved of it, and, I felt, lorded it over my head—controlling me to a certain degree. I also severely curtailed my drinking, limiting it to a few

"DR. MAGOO" is a former navy physician who now has a private practice in the northeastern part of the United States.

noontime beers and a sandwich at a bar so that I could face the cadaver after lunch in anatomy lab. The lady instructor told me to stop going to the local liquid lunch when I came stumbling into the lab and fell down. She suggested that if I wanted to pass the course I would have to change my ways. She made sense, so I used only the weekends to party, as I had done in college.

After graduation from medical school, I entered the U.S. Navy to fulfill my military obligation, which I completed 20 years later at retirement. My first duty was at Pensacola, Florida, where I learned to fly and studied to become a naval flight surgeon. In California, at my first duty station, I was informed by my commanding officer that my job basically concerned itself with the three A's—Airplanes, Alcohol, and Ass, which are the three things most pilots are particularly interested in—in that order. I was happily married, now had my wings, and felt the only important thing to do was to work on the third A. Fifteen years later my drinking had progressed from binges to daily social, and finally to a fifth of vodka or more daily as maintenance drinking.

At this time a series of events occurred that made me consider that I might have a drinking problem. On reporting aboard a carrier for a Mediterranean cruise, I decided to limit my drinking and determined that I would go "cold turkey"—stop drinking altogether since I would not be able to get booze at sea. My only concession was to smuggle a bottle of vodka aboard for medicinal purposes. I awoke the next morning covered with my own vomitus, lying in my stateroom and missing my cover (cap), which I never found and presume went overboard! Here for the first time I realized that I might have either asphyxiated or drowned and concluded that from now on I would control my intake of alcohol.

On return from the cruise, my life went from bad to miserable. The harder I tried not to drink, the more I thought about it, tried not to, but again and again awoke inebriated with an empty bottle beside me. I tried total abstinence—over and over—never getting more than a few days or weeks before prolonged binges. I tried Antabuse and nearly died because I drank while taking it! I made promises to God, my spouse, my friends, my priest, my boss, and I think even to the garbage collector and broke them all. I went to court to face drunk driving and hit-and-run charges. I answered a letter to the chief of naval operations why I, a "four-striper," was singing and dancing on the same stage as the Sea Chanters of the Navy Band before the D.A.R. at a Washington, D.C., hotel. The final act of insanity happened three years after the near death on the carrier.

My sister had come down to visit us in Maryland, and on a spring Saturday afternoon while I was in my "cups," I started chasing a dog around my backyard with an axe, with intent to kill the pet who had tipped over my garbage cans. *My wife threatened to call the police and my sister fled the house with the children to protect them against the madman, their father.*

At this point, I had reached my "low" and determined that not only had my "cure" not worked but my alcoholism was so progressive that I was dangerous to self, others, and loved ones. At my wife's urging, I decided to attend an AA meeting. Here I met a very dear medical friend with whom I had spent many an hour drinking when we were both stationed at Naples, Italy. He told me, embarrassed as I was to see him there, that I was in the right place and that he had begun to attend meetings only six months before. He told me that the navy had an excellent course on alcoholism for senior officers at Long Beach Naval Hospital and recommended that I attend it, admitting that I was an alcoholic when I arrived there. He said that the education and treatment were immensely sped up by going to what is affectionately known as the navy's "School for Surrender." I agreed to do so and a week later was in "drydock."

After meeting the director of the program, a truly great professional in the treatment of alcoholism, I was sent for therapy to my doctor, who is and was a marine corps gunnery sergeant. What a change of roles—the doctor is the patient; the therapist, a layman. My next therapist, when I returned from Long Beach Naval Hospital to my own hospital, was a black second-class navy cook. These two men were remarkably knowledgeable about alcoholism because they were also recovering from the disease and taught me a way of life—how to live without alcohol, one day at a time. They made suggestions as to how to deal with the obsession and compulsion to drink. They provided me with the tools to deal with my daily problems without a chemical answer to them. They showed me true love, compassion, and understanding, and made me believe in my self-worth and led me to recovery. I had to give up the role of healer and accept the fact that I was vulnerable to a disease so insidious that it almost killed me before I accepted the fact that I had it. I entered daily AA meetings with joy and enthusiasm. I was introduced into a local doctors' AA group and was told that I would have to begin helping other sick alcoholic doctors for me to get better. "You can't keep it unless you give it away" is the axiom. I was learning a new language, a new way of living, and I was beginning to enjoy each and every day—without alcohol. I was told that my recovery depended in great part on attendance at ordinary AA meetings and that the doctors' group was only a portal into the much greater fellowship of recovering brothers from every walk of life.

I abandoned the illusion that I was the director of my recovery. I saw that it lay in the hands of others, nonprofessionals who could give me good-quality sobriety if I would only let them show me the way. In turn, I vowed to help others just as I had been helped by strangers. No longer would I direct therapy, but would offer my hand and heart to anyone who might listen to me. I offered myself to help those still sick and still do so in many capacities.

I have eight and one-half years of sobriety now and am immensely proud of my greatest achievement—sobriety. It has brought me a life of unique friends. It has strengthened my love for my family. I practice medicine as a solo practitioner and have offices in two towns. I have weathered the death of a child and a parent without having to resort to alcohol or pills. I realize that every day is not so great, but it's 100% better than any day while I was still drinking. I feel good about myself. I have regained my self-confidence. I am not ashamed of my actions. I am respected in the community as a valuable and conscientious physician. My wife and my family can trust me. My actions are predictable. I'm fun to be with and enjoy many recreational activities.

Most of all, I work hard in my spare time, helping people discover how to recover from ethanolism. I have made known to all my colleagues that I am a recovering alcoholic and welcome any referrals of physicians or patients of theirs to introduce into AA. The reward for doing this is enormous. Although I cannot predict whether they will recover, I am astonished how many "make it" when someone cares about their problem and holds out a helping hand. The simple faith in God, a sharing of my spirituality with others, and a firm belief in allowing God to enter my life has been the most important force in my own personal recovery.

Finally, I no longer feel like a patient. Instead, I feel like a person with a disease in remission. I know that if I take my medicine—AA—as much as possible, don't take the first drink, and live my life fully and daily with what I always wanted to do anyway—help people get better—I have been given a gift given to only a few—sobriety. I know that there are many out there still drinking and drugging who will never recover, and I grieve for them. I will still try to help them if they will let me. Finally, I've come the full circle—from patient to layman helping others, teaching them a way of life that is unparalleled in joy and love—and I don't have to be a doctor to treat this disease, the strangest paradox of all.

CHAPTER 19

DEPRESSION

"LOUISE REDMOND"

This is a hard thing to talk about. I suppose that it is why it is important for me to talk. It is also a hard thing to think about. It becomes very fuzzy, trying to catalog the beginnings of it all. When did I first have problems with depression? If I could state that clearly, I suppose there would be no need for me to write it all down.

Perhaps first I should look at me from the outside a little. Depression is such an inside sort of disease, and, I think, depressed people think so much inside themselves that it may be important to look from outside to get a sense of perspective. So who am I, from the outside? Such definitions always seem to start from one's occupation. I am a pediatrician, nearly 40 years old, married to a surgeon, the mother of three children. We have lived in this small southern town for four years, having spent the first 11 years of our marriage in the military. My husband and I both were reared in northeastern cities, and this move to the country has suited us well. He is in private practice; I am in public health. We are blessed with a good marriage, plenty of creature comforts, good health, and good children. So far, so good.

Still looking from the outside, I probably represent a fairly typical woman in medicine of my generation. I was able to finish pediatric training before beginning a family and completed a fellowship after the children were born, never interrupting my medical career. I've published a little, taught a little, practiced a little, and, until the energy crisis of middle age hit, considered myself a superwoman along with so many of my contemporaries. I suppose many people in this community still consider me such a person. But they only see me from the outside.

The inside parts go back a long way, at least one or two generations. My father, of whom I must be nearly a clone, committed suicide

"DR. LOUISE REDMOND" is a pediatrician employed by a public health district in a small southeastern community. She is trained in adolescent medicine and has a special interest in behavioral pediatrics.

when I was in medical school, two weeks after my marriage. His depression went back many years and appeared refractory to the interventions available 20 years ago. I remember so vividly, in the dark days, Dad sitting in his chair in the living room, staring into space, for long hours at night. I remember our confusion about his silent periods. He was a good father to all of us, a good husband to my mother, but seemed incapable of purging himself of the demon that finally claimed him that January morning so many years ago. "Why?" we asked over and over, for years and years. "Why?" asked his friends. "Why?" asked his psychiatrist, whose intervention and medicine were unable to change the end of the story. And "Why?" I asked, for such a long time afterward. I no longer ask why. I finally understand.

As we asked all those questions, for all those years, we seemed to uncover some partial answers. There may have been other suicides in my father's family, although such things were rarely discussed. My younger sister had an acute depressive break eight years after my father died. At first it appeared to be related to life circumstances and to some delayed grieving over Dad's death. But gradually we began to understand the biochemistry of unipolar depression, and our family began to accept the fact that some of us were prone to this disease. Somewhere during all of that questioning, the extent of my own illness began to define itself.

The first well-defined episode of depression I can remember occurred when I was in my late 20s. I had been given clomiphene to induce ovulation after one successful pregnancy, two miscarriages, and some difficulty with reestablishing a normal menstrual cycle. My biologic clock was ticking away, or so I felt, and the risks of clomiphene seemed worth the benefits of a successful pregnancy. Neither I nor my obstetrician had any real appreciation of what this hormonal preparation could do to a person with biochemical depression. I found out, three months into the regimen.

Because of lack of ovulatory response, my dose had been doubled for five days that month. I remember some vague discomfort during the first two cycles, but the depression that month, after 48 hours of clomiphene, caught me totally off guard. I remember coming home from work, dismissing the baby-sitter, and falling apart. My husband, a surgical resident, would not be home from work for several hours. I began to cry uncontrollably. I spent an hour or so huddled on the floor, sobbing, holding my confused young son. What was happening to me? I was sure I was going crazy but was not sure why. My head hurt. I think my brain must have hurt. Over and over again, my thoughts returned to my husband's gun collection. Where, oh where, did he keep the ammunition? But what would I do with my child if I decided to shoot myself? There must be someone I could call. Musn't disturb my husband during evening rounds. Can't call my family, 2000 miles away. They'd only worry. All my friends are physicians, and I can't let them know I've gone crazy. But it hurts so terribly bad. The gun would make my head stop hurting. What good is a crazy mother to a child, anyway?

A long time passed. Somehow I got up from the floor, fed my son, and got him ready for bed. I paced around the house, not really looking for the ammunition but bothered by the obsessive thoughts. When my husband arrived, at nearly nine o'clock, I was pale and exhausted. "What's wrong?" he asked. The tears began again. This time there was someone to give some of the pain to. That's always the way, it seems. Giving some of the pain and the fear away takes some of the power out of this thing that happens to me. The inside thinking, so terrifying when faced alone, becomes less so when it is examined from the outside. I think it is the inside thinking that causes that awful pain in my brain.

We talked and talked, attempting to make some sense out of what had happened to me that day. The clomiphene connection became apparent, and once I stopped taking the drug, the depression lifted, like sun coming out after a terrible storm. We were both frightened, though we tried to make light of the whole episode. It was many months before I realized that all of the ammunition left the house that night. We decided that the time had come for me to seek professonal help to sort out both this episode and its relation to my father's illness.

My first attempt at seeking professional help was short-lived. As a military physician, I had free access to a large health care system. The psychiatric end of that system, however, was a great mystery to those of us who practiced "real" medicine. I didn't trust many physicians and was not at all sure I wanted to have the words *Mental Hygiene* stamped on my all-too-public military health record. I saw a psychiatrist twice, was as unimpressed with his expertise as I'm sure he was with my level of trust. I decided I could handle this problem without psychiatrists. And for quite some time I did.

It would be a long time before I again had a frightening depressive episode. A pattern began to emerge, very gradually, which I began to understand some years later. Somewhere around October, I would begin to have trouble with sleep. Shortly after that the myalgias and arthralgias would begin. By later December I would be well into an "inside thinking" mode. Sometime in early January I would say to my husband, "I think I'm depressed again." And with that admission would come the beginnings of relief. By the end of February I would feel well.

There were variables that would influence this general pattern, I discovered. Fatigue, particularly a hectic night call schedule, would make it very much worse. In retrospect, I had always had some minor difficulties with depression during my residency rotations in the nursery. I'm sure now that was less from trouble dealing with the type of work in the nursery than it was from lack of sleep. Job stress made the level of depression much deeper. Conflict on the job, difficult supervisors or co-workers, unpleasant assignments, especially in the autumn or winter, would precipitate significant problems. I learned, when in an inside thinking mode, that it was best not to overextend myself in any way. Giving a dinner party could be overwhelming during bad times and a source of great pleasure when I was feeling well.

It is a strange thing to look at all of this from the outside. So many things seem obvious from a distance that simply have not been clear up close. Perhaps it is the old principle of denial of illness. It has been very difficult for me to admit that this illness exists. And it is, after all, very simple, with a little bit of medical training and no objectivity, to give oneself almost any disease but a mental one. For one thing, the symptoms are so vague.

I speak of early morning awakening as the harbinger of this disease. It surely does not come labeled that way. It begins as a nagging problem, just trouble getting to sleep after a trip to the bathroom or awakening to comfort a child in the middle of the night. One starts by thinking of the most recent job stress and ruminating on it perhaps a little too long. The next night and the next it happens and one finds oneself thinking about old job stresses and reliving past mistakes, real or imaginary. These problems keep one awake for 30 to 90 minutes and often preclude sleep until 5:00 or 5:30 a.m. The worries stretch into the future. One worries about a spouse or a parent or a child dying. One thinks about all of the terrible things one has done during a lifetime. Why would anyone put up with being married to me? What right do I have to pretend to raise children? Everything I've accomplished in life is a joke! If they only knew how little I knew, they never would have given me a medical degree, a license, board certification, a job. The thoughts move faster and faster. It reminds me sometimes of one of those lamps they used to have in bars, where the beer advertisement hovers over a rippling waterfall, constantly in motion. My brain won't stay still. The thoughts are moving too fast. I'm spinning around. I'm doing it again. I'm going crazy. It's that awful pain, the inside thinking.

I mention arthralgias and myalgias. I have never seen this described except in the vaguest of terms, but there is a strange kind of physical pain that accompanies depression. Joints start to ache but never swell. Muscles ache. I'm embarrassed at the number of sed rate and rheumatoid factor slips and CBC reports (all normal) that fill my military medical record. The pains are very real. I think back to the times we would laugh at my father for complaining about sore skin, or sore hair. I now understand that skin and hair can hurt, in the absence of viremia or a collagen disease. Looking from the outside, the possible explanations are fascinating. Maybe brain serotonin is low because it is misplaced to muscle or joint, or even hair follicles! Looking from the inside, it simply hurts and confuses.

The fatigue of depression can also be confusing. Partly related, no doubt, to the sleep loss at night, the lack of energy can call to mind all manner of hormonal dysfunctions and physical ailments. One's legs ache and simply feel too heavy to carry one's weight. There are terrible episodes of sleepiness, occurring in the afternoon and early evening hours. If one yields and goes to bed early, it seems as if the early morning awakening and its attendant terrors come sooner and are much more intense.

And then there's inside thinking. *Inside thinking* is a term I use to describe a kind of paranoia in which one can almost hear one's own thoughts. I wonder what they're saying in the next office. I bet they're talking about me and how awful I look. They probably suspect that I'm a little crazy right now. It must show on my ugly face. And my boss, why did he give me that assignment at this particular time? He must know I'm not doing well. Probably wants to keep me locked up in the office for a while so no one will figure it out. He must be sorry he hired me. And my husband—I'm sure he wishes we had never met. Who would marry such a person as me? Probably stays with me because of some crazy loyalty, some antiquated ideas about wedding vows. He'd be so much better off if I weren't around and he could find the right kind of wife and mother for these poor children.

It becomes, then, a very short step from inside thinking to suicidal thoughts. "Better off without me," coupled with that awful pain in my head, logically becomes a wish to eradicate the pain. The thoughts are at first passive, and they sort of play games with my mind. They flit in and out—I wonder how it would feel if. . .—and I can at first dismiss them fairly easily. But they get more persistent. They begin during the long night hours but soon intrude in my thinking during the day. And there comes a time when they make the transition into active planning. How could I do it so the kids wouldn't know? Don't want them to go through what we went through with Dad. How could I do it so no one could find me and stop it? I'd never want to do it halfway. The thoughts start to hurt and the lamp in my head starts to spin around faster. I find myself literally holding onto my sleeping husband at night, trying to make it all stop and stand still.

So how close am I to really being crazy? I have to think that as long as I *can* hold onto someone, that I *can* keep the thoughts under control, that I *can* find a time when I feel better—as long as all that still happens, I'm okay. I am convinced, however, that the patients I see professionally who have mental illness are in pain and that their pain is as real as the pain from a surgical abdomen or from a growing tumor. Psychic pain *hurts*, and seeing oneself as mentally ill hurts. It is infinitely more respectable to ascribe that pain to a physical ailment, however terrible, than to a mental illness. And so the denial. Who's crazy?

There comes a time in every illness when the denial is no longer enough and one must seek accurate diagnosis and treatment. I'm reminded of the occasional patient who comes out of the woods with a fungating cancer that has been present for years. Am I not just as shortsighted? My cancer grew a long time, hit some kind of critical mass, and became a source of pain year round, before I finally crawled out of my hole and sought help. I suppose there's some rationalization called for here, and my cancer analogy may help. "I don't trust doctors," says my patient from the woods. "I thought it would go away by itself." "I'm afraid of pain." "I can't take the time off." "I can't afford it." Add to that concerns about professional reputation, insurability, status in the community, and, quite simply, a fear of the truth, and you have my reasons for denial.

At any rate, I arrived at the psychiatrist's door after many false starts. I'd tried to put myself on medication a couple of times in the past, without success. My autonomic nervous system goes into overdrive with imipramine, and a minuscule dose at bedtime causes gastrointestinal symptoms severe enough to wake me three hours later. So added to my distrust of the medical and psychiatric professions came distrust of pharmaceuticals. I was fortunate in having a younger sister who served as a role model in this regard. Her response to medication, her excellent rapport with and trust of her own psychiatrist, and her willingness to have all sorts of hormonal testing done in search of an accurate diagnosis made my transition into care fairly smooth, at least in my own eyes. We already knew this was a familial unipolar depression, that it could respond to certain antidepressant medications, that it did not appear to be related to abnormal adrenal functioning. Our original seasonal variations had extinguished over the years, so we assumed this was not a light-responsive illness. Pity the poor psychiatrist upon whom I laid this barrage of facts at my first visit! Apart from the usual difficulties of treating a physician, he was faced with an agenda of preformed assumptions and possible therapies, as well as a list of things that hadn't helped, along with "insight" that bordered on rumination. Much to my relief, he took me on, despite all my baggage. We are manipulating medication more or less together, he is soundly slapping my hand when I abuse the role confusion beyond his tremendous tolerance, and I am alive and thinking clearly enough to recount this tale.

It does bring me back to the issue of trust, however. I have always believed that trust and confidence are the most potent tools in the healer's armamentarium. Surely that is even more true in the relationship between patient and psychiatrist. It is difficult to quantitate that trust. When I say the things I've written here to another professional, I lay bare a good part of my soul. I have a remnant of the layman's fear of psychiatry: Can he really read my mind? Does he see underneath what I'm saying to some part of me I cannot see? Would it even help me if he could see that far? Or would it simply leave me more vulnerable? It is difficult to find someone with whom I am willing to take that risk. On the other hand, the idea of giving the pain away has driven me on. Find someone to share it with. Take some of the power from the pain. Then it becomes livable.

Under some circumstances, one might be able to accomplish this with help from religious faith. I was brought up Catholic. In my early years, depression ("despair") and suicide were considered mortal sin, and a Catholic who took his own life was denied Christian burial. With more enlightened thinking, the illness associated with suicide has become apparent to the Church, and the rules are less rigid. My family found tremendous consolation in the rituals of my father's Catholic funeral. How dreadful it would have been had that comfort been denied the survivors!

There are many stories of depression and despair in the Judaeo-Christian tradition. I have found solace in studying the stories of Job and Judas and Peter and Gethsemane. If I could not find solutions to my illness in study and prayer, I believe, it is less a problem with the source material than it is with my distorted thinking and perceptions. Again, inside thinking makes outside help difficult to grasp.

I often wonder if my illness has helped or harmed me in my dealings with patients. I believe depressed people find each other and often seek help from providers who themselves have been depressed. I find treating depressed people very difficult. Perhaps it stems from feelings of inadequacy—if I could fix this disease, I wouldn't have it myself—or perhaps it brings painful thoughts too close to the surface. For whatever reason, I do not feel I am an effective therapist for a depressed patient, although I do believe I can diagnose the condition accurately. It is always with a sense of relief that I suggest a more competent therapist than I to deal with these problems. I'm not always sure that I'm being fair to that therapist.

With that exception, however, I believe that experiencing this illness has heightened my sensitivity to many other problems. It is very difficult to project an impersonal image when one is so acutely aware of one's own vulnerability. My dealings with patients must be more personal; I simply cannot take myself too seriously. And understanding my own illness and my reluctance to use or trust health care providers gives me, I believe, an advantage over my less vulnerable colleagues. The human condition afflicts us all in one way or another. If I have this weakness, I also have some talent, and I will use it to help my patients as my therapist has helped me. With all of our sophisticated technology, the medical profession is effective insofar as we, its practitioners, inspire trust and confidence. In that sense, we are not very far removed from our horse-and-buggy colleagues of another generation. To listen, to empathize, to walk in my patients' shoes, weak though I be—these are the measures of my worth as physician and healer.

A postscript to this account: I have chosen to remain anonymous as I write all of this, although any who know me will recognize my story. I have not changed facts or descriptions of events. It is a sad commentary on the state of our professional understanding of mental illness that I am afraid of the consequences of telling my story openly. I wonder how many of us would really refer patients to a colleague who openly seeks psychiatric help and openly takes prescribed psychotropic medications. My residual layman's fear of the psychiatrist extends, I am ashamed to say, to his patients. Surely it is for us in the profession to attempt to allay those fears. But until we can deal with each other's illnesses with empathy and understanding, there will be no way for us to accomplish this with our patients. I hope that somehow my story may contribute to understanding of depressive illness. And I hope that someday I might be comfortable in signing my name to an essay such as this.

CHAPTER 20

DEPRESSION

A. ROSEMARY MACKENZIE

A proper description of what happened to me requires some brief autobiographical details. At the time the story begins, I was in my mid-30s, married, with no children. I am a general practitioner. This is a peculiarly British occupation by which I contract myself to the Health Service to provide primary health care to all who register with me as patients. I am totally responsible for these people—nearly 2000 of them—24 hours a day, 7 days a week, 52 weeks a year. Unlike most general practitioners, I am not in a partnership, although I share on-call with another doctor for nights and weekends. When I took on my practice I had been working in hospital medicine for several years but had had only one year's experience of general practice. There had been several changes of doctor in the previous few years and the practice was a mess—records badly kept, patients dissatisfied. Apart from the other doctor with whom I shared cover, there were three other general practitioners in town. There was a long tradition of rivalry between the practices, not improved by irregularities in my practice that had occasionally given my colleagues extra—and unpaid for—work. All four of my colleagues were men, and I felt they did not look kindly on an inexperienced woman taking the post. My practice is in a seaside town in west central Scotland, an area of dying heavy industry, urban decay, and high unemployment. It is also home—where I wanted to live and work. It takes about an hour and a half to get to Glasgow, the nearest city.

I know that when I first took on the practice I felt fine. It was extremely hard work, and I was reduced at times to extremes of rage or frustration or exhaustion, but I was not unhappy. When I first began to feel unwell I thought it was just a sense of anticlimax after a year and a half of getting things into some sort of order. I first formulated the

DR. ROSEMARY MACKENZIE is a single-handed general practitioner working on the island of Bute, a holiday resort in west central Scotland. She is married with no children. The little time she has to spare from general practice is spent gardening and writing.

idea that I was depressed in December 1980. I was in London, having a short holiday, and I felt I simply could not bear to go back home. It was just after John Lennon was shot. I found that event very distressing—no doubt, many people of my age group did—with feelings that youth and hope were gone. There was no way I was going to tell anyone how I felt.

Having decided I was depressed, I treated myself with antidepressants, in fairly modest doses, and I felt a bit better. For over a year and a half I did this, varying the drug or the dose from time to time, though within fairly conservative limits, more or less depending on what free samples I happened to have around. My own general practitioner was the doctor with whom I shared a rota. Once I said to him something like "I've been feeling a bit down recently," to which he replied, very quickly, "I hope you're not going to be one of these people who go through life taking drugs." I rapidly translated my complaint into the idea that my migraine had been bothering me a lot and ended up with a prescription for analgesics. He was a person who was rather switched off anyway about psychiatric complaints—later I heard him describe someone for whom he was writing a reference, "She's got a psychiatric history, you know"—and also I think he felt threatened that I was not going to be able to do my work and would leave him with additional responsibilities.

In the autumn of 1982, I went on holiday, came back, and thought, "I can't face going to work." Of course, I did manage to work, but I finally asked for help—by letter! A friend in town, a doctor, but not in practice, found me a psychiatrist. In turn, he demanded that I have someone local to attend to me. I agreed, largely because I felt that otherwise I was putting an undue burden of responsibility on my friend, and with intervention, I found myself with one of my other colleagues. He and my psychiatrist together put me on a less homeopathic dose of tricyclics and I very rapidly became very much better. For months, I complained that the dry mouth due to the drugs was affecting my voice. Then one day, my doctor said, "What's that scar on your neck?" That scar was from my thyroidectomy, and I was, of course, quite myxoedematous. After thyroid replacement therapy, I felt amazingly so much better physically that I only then appreciated the degree of physical discomfort I had been in. Four months later I looked at the bottle of amitriptyline, thought, "I don't need this," and took no more. I was cured. Occasionally, when I have had minor viral illnesses, I have felt for a few days as I did before. When I wrote about it afterwards, I didn't write about the myxoedema, because the object of the article was to say: It's all right to have a psychiatric illness, it's all right to ask for help—and I felt to raise the issue of having been physically ill would be a cop-out, a way of saying I didn't really have a psychiatric illness.

The symptoms I had are all documented in the textbooks, but no textbook can describe the kind of despair I felt. What I noticed first was a feeling of "I can't cope" about things that ordinarily would not bother me at all. In the mornings I would wonder how on earth I would manage to get through consultations. The day's work seemed unbearably long and difficult. The prospect of unplanned visits, unexpected calls, worried me, yet the essence of my kind of work is its unpredictability. I dreaded "difficult" patients, and more and more patients seemed difficult. I could not concentrate; indeed, I could not think. I stopped reading or listening to music. Instead of driving around as I usually do with the car radio on, I went around in silence and in my mind recited quotations about death. I cannot now even recall correctly the poetry that reeled through my mind; then I was word-perfect. Most of all I felt guilty and ashamed and worthless, and this was one of the things that made it impossible for me to tell anyone or get help.

The diurnal variation was quite marked. By evening I felt almost myself, I didn't have the sensation of dread, and I didn't think about death, but my concentration and interest were still very poor. In the evenings sometimes I would be frightened that I would kill myself early one morning. I knew I didn't really want to die, that I had a remediable disorder. I knew quite clearly all the time that it was me that was ill, not the world that was wrong. As a doctor, I have experienced patients suiciding and I knew well that it would be a terrible thing to do to my family, but I would invent the scenarios for credible accidents. Fortunately, perhaps, they were all incredibly complicated, and I had far too much inertia to begin to perform them.

It was only when I started getting better that I realised how impoverished my life had been for over two years. Recovery, in fact, proved quite expensive since every time I went to town to see my psychiatrist, I came back loaded with books and records and clothes. When I was well again, I realised that I had coped by progressively narrowing down my vision of life. I dealt with patients by being uptight and authoritarian and censorious. This is quite easy in Britain, where the medical profession is still very paternalistic, and by most people's standards, I was probably easygoing, but when I look back on my attitudes in the light of how I see things now, I think I was very rigid and judgemental. On the other hand, I learned a lot of how it feels to be a patient, and that may have altered my attitudes a lot. If I hadn't been ill, I might still be as paternalistic as anybody else. I dealt with life outside the practice by just not doing anything. I accepted social invitations only where I could not avoid them. I invited no one to my home. Whether I had sleep disturbance I don't know. An insomniac with a telephone liable to ring at any time, I always sleep so badly that I doubt it could have become much worse.

It was extremely difficult to ask for help. Partly this was the illness itself. The effect of depression probably depends to an extent on the character of the sufferer. I felt a great deal of guilt and unworthiness. I believed that if anybody knew how inadequate I was, he or she would be appalled and disgusted. I felt no one knew what I was really like, that it was necessary to conceal myself because otherwise no one would like me. I was brought up on the Scottish virtues of independence and self-reliance. I was a woman in a male-dominated profession. I had never failed to get where I wanted, and I had never felt unfairly treated, but I had always felt I had to prove I could do the job as well as my male colleagues, with no concessions. More than all this, I saw my role as a doctor to be someone who cared for others, and it was very difficult to step out of that role into that of supplicant.

There were three doctors to choose from. I didn't know any of them very well. I chose to consult the person I did because, although almost our only communication had been arguments at meetings, I had always thought we would get along if we got to know each other. At the same time I was able to say to myself that he couldn't think much worse of me than he already did. I expected him to be fairly horrified at having to treat me, but I relied on the fact that I knew him to be an extremely conscientious person to give me a fair hearing. I thought I would get five minutes now and then in the surgery and instructions to keep on taking the tablets. In the event, he was incredibly supportive, far beyond what I thought was necessary, though he may have estimated my suicide risk higher than I did myself. He saw me in his own home, and after a formal consultation in his office I spent the rest of the evening socially with his family. I assume this was basically a courtesy extended to a colleague, but the social part of the consultation did a lot to retrieve my self-esteem. I had presented myself to him with what I felt were dreadful weaknesses and faults, and I very much wanted reassurance that he did not think me a terrible person. The fact that he had me meet his family and appeared to enjoy my conversation and company made me feel very much better about myself and about the fact that I was imposing on him for care. If I had been in his situation, I would have been flattered and concerned. It is perhaps reasonable to think that that is how he felt (once he knew he wasn't going to have to do my work for me). Being asked for help is what turns people like us on, after all. I knew I could quite easily feel very angry with him once I felt a bit better because he had seen me like this, and I had, as it were, warned myself of this reaction. He knew that too; he said to me that one day when I was better I might wish not to see any more of him. I never did feel that; I like him too much to get angry.

Over the last four years I think we have become friends. I still visit his home regularly. He still puts aside a time for a formal interview from time to time. This is important to me. If our relationship now were purely social, it would be difficult for me to tell him if anything was wrong. This level of care is way beyond what either of us would give an "ordinary" patient. It did carry home to me how very destructive of self-image serious illness can be; how, as doctors, we see people stripped of their public persona. I had felt it was a fault of mine—time-wasting, self-indulgent curiosity—that I tended to chat with patients, ask them about things not related to their illness. I came to understand that this was not necessarily so, that conversation was one way of saying—in spite of what I have seen and heard—you're all right, worth getting to know. I also saw how easy it could be to manipulate people into the role of invalid. For a brief moment I wondered if I would go on producing complaints after I had really recovered to retain the gratification of my doctor's interest. In fact, the day I decided I was recovered I could not refrain from telling him so, I was so delighted with myself. However, I could see that it is very easy to manipulate people into the role of invalids because it is mutually gratifying, because they become hooked on the attention and we become hooked on being needed. Because we became friends, with a lot of interests in common, I never had to say to my doctor, "I don't need you anymore." If we hadn't developed this friendship, I don't know how I would have coped when that day came, knowing that it can be quite a hard experience for the doctor.

I don't know quite what I expected from a psychiatrist. In Britain, the medical profession, in general, still thinks of psychiatry as something slightly weird and disreputable. On the other hand, I had this fantasy figure, like the character played by Montgomery Clift in *Suddenly Last Summer,* who with a few well chosen words would unravel my whole life. In the event, I did not find my psychiatrist important to me, and I looked on my visits to him largely as an excuse for a day out in the city. However, I think the fact that he was there did take some of the burden of responsibility off my general practitioner. He did suggest I have ECT, and from the depths of ignorance, I refused. If it happened again, I would agree; indeed, I would like ECT early in the illness so that I can make a rapid recovery without enduring the side effects of tricyclics. I have taken pains to become a bit better informed about psychiatry in general and this aspect of it in particular.

I did not at any time consider going for help to anyone but a doctor. My closest friends were going through a crisis in their own lives; otherwise, I might have confided in them, but they live at the other end of the country. I find it quite easy to mix socially in the town, but all my friends are either patients or friends or relations of patients, and I find it necessary to be basically "all right." I decided years ago I was an atheist and have not given religion more than a passing thought since. It simply did not occur to me to go to a minister or priest; nor could I ever—the gulf between their belief and my disbelief makes me feel that on important matters we are not speaking at all the same language.

The effect of tricyclics was to make me feel very much better but still not quite myself. I compared it with walking on a tightrope: all right so long as I didn't stop and look down. The medication prevented my looking down. I never once missed a dose. I knew I wasn't cured and said so when my doctors said I was well and tried to reduce the dose. The day I knew I was better, I knew it with absolute certainty and stopped the medication there and then with no ill effects; I felt I could not even wait till my next consultation, I had such an urgent need to stop it.

Both my general practitioner and my psychiatrist from time to time tried to get me to talk about "myself"—about my relationships with my family and my husband, about how I felt about not having children. I just could not talk about these things, not because I felt I was hung up about them, but because I thought they were of minor importance and irrelevant. My general practitioner then suggested that I should write about myself instead, and I tried to do this. I wrote endlessly, mostly at two o'clock in the morning. I tried to write about myself, but what appeared on paper were essays on medical practice and ethics, on politics and nuclear disarmament, on world peace and conservation. At the end of it all I came to the conclusion that perhaps these were the things that really did concern me, and that being the case, I had better get on with it and do something about it. To date, I have bought a lot of labour-saving machinery for the home and hired a domestic help, since I have decided to give up on the idea that I have a duty to be a perfect homemaker as well as following my professional interests.

I have now joined Greenpeace and the Medical Campaign Against Nuclear Weapons. I have written several articles for different journals and magazines, I have appeared (briefly) on national television, and I have got involved with the teaching program at the local medical school. My illness gave me a period of introspection during which I sorted out my priorities. It also gave me a sense of mortality and time passing, which has given me the impetus to do things I had formerly only thought about.

One thing I was aware of as a patient was a terrible need to express my gratitude to my general practitioner. This was something I had not thought of formerly. It's always gratifying when patients say, "Thank you." It's pleasant but a bit embarrassing when they give you gifts, especially when the gift may be more than we feel they can afford. All the time I was receiving so much help and support I was thinking,

"Please—let me give you something." I found a way to do this, but I thought patients must feel like this. It must be dreadful to be always receiving and not be able to give anything in return. Indeed, it is a kind of insult to say to someone that they must take but there is nothing they have worth giving. An impersonal gift would not have answered my need. It is perhaps easier for my patients to give things to me because it is easier to find something to give to a woman than to a man. Perhaps what we should let people give us is their concern for us; let them express sympathy with our joys or sorrows.

My parents and my brother live in another town, and they know nothing at all about my illness. We are not a very close family, and it is 20 years or more since I confided in them. What my husband thinks about it I know not. All the time I was ill, I said nothing to him. I eventually told him a little when I wrote about it, because he was likely to read the article. He has not asked me anything, for which I am thankful, and I assume he does not want to know the answers. I might not have been able to go on living with him if he had seen me with my self-respect in shreds. I suspect he may have found me easier to live with when I was depressed, when I sat quietly at home and didn't argue. Now I am very much more busy with things that do not involve him, much more self-determining and independent.

It is difficult to look at those four years as anything more than a waste of my life. Possibly, my attitudes have changed because of it, but I suspect all the ideas and projects I have now would have happened anyway, that my illness just meant a four-year interruption. In retrospect, I became quite frightened. I lost four years largely because I would not or could not ask for help. I think I was at considerable risk of dying; I am quite appalled when I think of that. I hope I wouldn't do that again. I don't think I'll get the chance to; I am being looked after as never before in my life. I am extraordinarily lucky to have found a physician who cares that much. I wrote an article about it afterwards; I hope that by talking about it and writing about it, I may make somebody somewhere pick up the telephone rather than a bottle of pills. I know that the worst thing a patient can do to me is come to grief rather than ask me for help. It would be a terrible thing to die of pride.

There were two pieces of verse that circled relentlessly round and round in my brain:

> Darkling I listen; and for many a time
> I have been half in love with easeful death,
> Called him soft names in many a mused line
> To take into the air my quiet breath.
> Now more than ever it seems rich to die,
> To cease upon the midnight with no pain.
>
> –Keats, "Ode to a Nightingale"

and

But at my back I always hear,
Times winged chariot drawing near
And yonder all before us lie
Deserts of vast eternity.
Thy beauty shall no more be found,
Nor, in thy marble vaults, shall sound
My echoing song; then worms shall try
That long preserved virginity,
And your quaint honour turn to dust,
And into ashes all my lust;
The grave's a fine and private place,
But none, I think, do there embrace.

-Marvell, "To His Coy Mistress"

CHAPTER 21

MANIC-DEPRESSIVE PSYCHOSIS

MICHAEL ROSE

A dog that shot past me, a yellow rose in someone's lapel, could set my thoughts in motion and obsess me for hours. What was the matter with me? Had the hand of the Lord reached out and pointed at me? Well then, why me? Why not just as well at some man in South America? When I pondered these things, it seemed more and more incomprehensible why precisely I should have been chosen as a guinea pig for a whim of God's favour. It was an extremely odd way of going about things, to leap over the whole human race in order to arrive at me; for example there was Pascha, the rare book dealer and Hennechen, the steamship clerk.

—Knut Hamsun, *Hunger*, 1890

It felt as though I had somehow logged into the spirit of the age. Clouds gathered in great vortices, blizzards swept in from the blue in late April, and the winds rocked buildings as solid as Oxford. I thought and believed I might be Judah Maccabaeus riding my gorgeous old motorcycle Bucephalus around London, England, and Northern Europe to the Gates of Hell. In fact more like Don Quixote upon Rocinante, inspired by visions of Dulcinea serving in a sandwich bar, to take on the world in expiation for some obscure sin I had committed but could no longer recollect. Or Spartacus maybe, with Doc Holliday at the OK Corral. The confused details as a matter of fact are quite funny but perhaps out of place in a text intended for serious academic colleagues. So I will herein limit myself mainly to the aftermath and thoughts of recovery, though I am now back more or less in the condition in which I started—in a locked psychiatric ward with access to a

DR. MICHAEL ROSE is 49 years old and currently live in Findhorn, Scotland. He was prematurely retired from medical practice in haematology at St. George's and St. James' Hospitals in South London as a consequence of his mental disturbance. He hopes to retrain as a teacher, as it seems unlikely that he will be able to return to medical practice. He is married with two children.

word processor. Hence, it it clear that whatever hesitating credit I give to the beneficial effects of lithium carbonate in the management of manic–depressive psychosis (or whatever we choose to call it), I remain intermittently as crazy as I ever was. Though the place is congenial, I don't want to convey the impression that I like it or am prepared to subside into a prolonged state of quiescence, or settle for a mess of pottage. I want more, much more. To be free to run and play tennis, for a start.

> He was insane. And when you look directly at an insane man all you see is a reflection of your own knowledge that he's insane, which is not to see him at all. To see him you must see what he saw.[1]

The incipient notion of what had happened, a recognition that something had been the matter, marked the onset of mental recovery. It was the key to that recovery, the internal beginning to a process that has taken many months to percolate to the surface. Writing about it has demonstrated, at least to me, that I could, after a fashion, recognise the authority of Robert Lowell's descriptions of states of being into which I had also ventured.

I did not believe fully in the authenticity of the manic–depressive syndrome until I had read Ian Hamilton's biography of Robert Lowell,[2] by then myself recovering from an acute manic episode in a locked ward for the third time in two years. The poet's life had been bedevilled by a succession of manic illnesses that had urgently required hospital admission in the United States and later in the United Kingdom. These had undermined his many marriages, friendships, and relationships, though much survived. He was established amongst the foremost poets of the age before his death in 1977.

"Walking in the Blue" from *Life Studies* describes the internal institutional experience amongst his psychotic companions in the locked ward:

> before the metal shaving mirrors...
> we are all old timers,
> each of us holds a locked razor.

The experience of madness is at first barely retrievable, merely some residual details:

> I lie secured there, but for my skipping mind.
> They keep bustling.
> Where you are going, Professor,
> You won't need your Dante.
> What will I need there?
> Is that a handcuff rattling in a pocket?

Curious objects peculiar to the environment remain memorable and "the pinched indigenous faces of these thoroughbred mental cases," fragmented, bewildered mentalities making pitiful and futile pleas against the odds, whilst those of us fortunate enough to reach recovery, however transitory, just watch and listen, witnessing barely recognisable vestiges of our own insane experience performed before us, surpassing any theatrical avant-garde. In due course graduated privileges consign the time that insanity is over and recovery begins. The carefully landmarked days proceed still with a painful languour.

My illness has lasted now for about two years, and I have been in a number of institutions, some indifferently staffed, others by remarkably compassionate and understanding individuals who tolerated insults and fearsome assaults without vindictiveness. Two years is a long time out of professional circulation—things forgotten, things not learnt or heard of—but the most daunting problem is the prospect of further episodes of mania. Depression, if it occurs, is a more private feature of the syndrome. Mania is very public, with a multitude of interested parties. Some patients are said to respond well to lithium carbonate and to have their lives changed if they avoid other precipitating agents. Others, like Lowell, have fewer and less severe attacks after they have had lithium. Yet others are less fortunate.

Before I had appreciated the destructive force of the manic attack, I remained attracted by the "tropical terrain of the affliction," and certainly the depression that followed my first episode of mania was partly mourning for a Paradise Lost. Now eventually I feel more satisfied with what I can make of ordinary opportunities and do not search for transcendental powers from signs in the sky. Though hopefully "cured, I am frizzled, stale and small," recalling the "majestic lunacies of the pre-lithium days."

Questions remain: Will there be further episodes? How frequently? Will they be as debilitating? No one can offer guarantees or even reliable answers yet. Meanwhile, what about my capacity to work, to earn a living, to occupy myself and fulfill my responsibilities? The qualities required of a doctor are vastly different from those of a poet. A hospital consultant is nothing if not reliable. My unreliability is already manifest. Rehabilitation should be, if possible, a dire uphill struggle. It seems as though the illness was more of a problem in Lowell's life than for his creative work; perhaps it even amplified the range of his imagination. Hamilton offers no opinion. Of course it did.

Fashioning a new career will be an uphill struggle too, but the mid-40s may be a good time for a change, and I, too, have a yearning to become a poet of a kind. Perhaps in my case that is what the syndrome was partly about, "a measure of my essential discontent."

We feel the machine slipping from our hand
as if someone else were steering...[3]

Now I am not certain what the message was; perhaps that I had survived, could read and write, and needed a little help from friends. In the interim, music occupied my senses, familiar classical and romantic pieces resonant with memories of adolescence and its heroic delusions, contemporary rock with conspiratorial lyric and beat. As well as Lowell and Hamilton,[2] I read William James and warmed to the tranquillity of such illustrious company and the inspiring modest optimism:

> I have swum in clear sweet waters all my days; and if sometimes they were a little cold, and the stream ran adverse and something rough, it was never too strong to be breasted and swum through. From the days of my earliest boyhood, when I went stumbling through the grass,... up to the gray-bearded manhood of this time, there is none but has left me honey in the hive of memory that I now feed on for present delight. When I recall the years...I am filled with a sense of sweetness and wonder that such little things can make a mortal so exceedingly rich.[4]

Ten of us were confined in more or less luxurious conditions, from time to time moving in unobtrusively on one another. Occasionally there were violations, though in spite of our being nominally the most disturbed assembly in the hospital, the environment was remarkably civilized and good-humoured.

Looking back, it seemed as though I had behaved like "a buffoon maddened with a vision of the Apocalypse." However, to write about it now is no longer to risk entry into whirling incoherence but to witness metaphors and intention, to rearrange the content in cerebral safety, and to deal with the details as I wish for my current fancy.

To do this, however, I had first to recover. The psychiatrist supervising my case had claimed shortly after I was overtly sane that I was fit to resume work. Fortunately, in the event, my employing authority took many months to conclude that it was prepared to have me back. During that time I was able to recover vestigial synthetic mental activities: perception, attention, memory, thinking, action, reading, and writing. This recovery seemed to take place abruptly after months in neutral. For instance, it took me about five months to be able to count my change after a simple transaction in a tobacconist shop. More surprisingly, I observed that my physical capacity to run a four-mile road circuit in South Wales was compromised by torn ligaments and contused joints, as I aspired to speeds I could not attain. Then, over cross-country circuits of similar distance, I ran gently, satisfied with deteriorating times for about three months, when suddenly, without making any conscious decision, I cut minutes off the best times I had ever run, as if some blockage had been released; I could also run farther than ever before. That also coincided with an abrupt return of social competence. "The birds of fortuity had alighted once more on [my] shoulders."[5]

Whilst awaiting this emancipation, which I had no confident grounds to expect since I had been advised I was already fit, I occupied myself with scraping paint off the woodwork, replacing broken and cracked panes of glass, and prising crumbled cement from between the bricks of our home, which I repointed throughout a rather solitary autumn. The mailman passed by our house each day without letters, apart from those most welcome documents dispatched by the Department of Social Security.

My family and a few friends were unconditional with their support. Without them I would have submitted to hopelessness, vagrancy, or worse. My employers preserved me on full salary though they had no statutory obligation to do so. That was extremely benevolent and made a critical difference to our domestic stability.

Nevertheless, by the time I was able to celebrate what Oliver Sacks describes as the Rabelaisian gusto of convalescence,[6] there seemed precious few to celebrate with. It seemed disturbingly and, I suppose, uncharitably as though

> ...the real poignancy of the story is that there is no longer any Zion: he cannot say, but what he is going back to has no zest and no promise. He returns to the city, "to outworn friends who kept one talking in the dead jargon on one's past," to face the bare necessity of making his own soul, creating his own culture, without help from environment or institutions.[7]

But no; it transpired quite differently. I had months face to face with the crumbling walls and cracked peeling paint, often without conversation from daybreak to sunset, though with friendly greetings from neighbours and tradespeople, wondering what had happened. It seemed 20 years after I had graduated, as if my scientific knowledge and comprehension had become irretrievably unequal to the representations of medical disorder upon which I was assumed and had assumed myself to have some insight. I felt also that I had become estranged from the bedrock of clinical activity and had elaborated smokescreens of evasion. In the event, these were facilities I was soon able to recover, granted access to libraries, lectures, patients, and colleagues. It was, however, a morbid hiatus.

On the other side of the smoke I had observed another culture, an apparently glowing world of spruce-covered hills, tropical coastlines, and dancing orange people at full moon, living magic and romance, crime and danger. I wanted to be of their number and compose vivid episodes, incessant beginnings, each swept aside by the next, holding time back by the scruff. I was impatient to "caress the light." Still now, beneath cobwebs and fingerprinted dust, deep within cupboards amongst old photographs and the verbal detritus of a life run riot, remarkable wreckage remains. My view had then seemed attractively kaleidoscopic, with configurations pointing first this way, then that, then all ways at once, dictating action that I sought to follow without hesitation, confident I was bound for the Promised Land, "riding my mind at a gallop across country in pursuit of an idea," at the head of a column of policemen and psychiatrists.

And thus:

> I plunged without a clue into a labyrinthe of images that we are warned against in those Oracles which antiquity has attributed to Zoroaster.... "Stoop not down to the darkly splendid world wherein lieth continually a faithless depth and Hades wrapped in cloud, delighting in unintelligible images."[8]

At first there seemed to be plot and form, a coherent action, more coherence even than "real life"; the coherence of fiction. To be insane is to live fiction, to assume a star role in your own life as author and player. The statements and actions of others are apprehended outside schemes of social and institutional convention, as if they, too, were scripted by the same idiosyncratic author. But the imaginative overlay of fiction cannot be lived because, loaded with metaphorical charge, it violates too many practical conventions and breaks with the restraints of social possibility. "Those blessed structures, plot and rhyme..."[9] break down on the first page, in the first paragraph. And I was hopelessly adrift amongst "The disintegration of images into a whirling incoherence [which] is more than impotence: it is damnation."[10]

In the second hospital I was shown how to make plates and mugs, I built a scooter for my nephews with expert guidance, drilled manually for hours through steel bars, worked with weights, played table tennis (the sexiest game in the world), tennis, and badminton. This bevy of activity for a formidable preparation for discharge. Later there were fortnightly joint sessions with my wife and children too, and in due course we were seen safely out of the harbour, once more into open seas.

As a doctor I was perhaps an unusually truculent patient, reluctant to relinquish my autonomy to attendants whom I considered inferior, ignorant, and superficial, who sought to administer treatment before reaching a diagnosis, before even addressing me, as if there was but one possibility and hence no need to talk. They would discuss my diagnosis, they said, "When you are better..." "Better than what?" I protested. I had never felt better in my life. My manifest contempt may have had some bearing on the punitive dosages from the pharmacopoeia that I received, and there is little doubt in my mind that the dereliction which followed my initial mania (described as depression, as if an integral part of a well-recognised syndrome, rather than an iatrogenic consequence) was drug-related and the "manic relapse" part of the same improperly treated process. That is to say, I believe the condition was amenable to much earlier resolution by subtle means, moderate medication, and thoughtful enquiry rather than the sledgehammer blows that were dealt with such abandon. Upon recovering a measure of sanity I encountered many problems that at first I could not contemplate at all. I felt that in certain respects my life was already over and I would, at the age of 47, have to reconcile myself to declining mental and physical capabilities. My thinking was dull, monotonous, and painfully slow. This cerebral "numbness" seems to correspond with the features that Luria described in association with massive frontal lesions.[11] The disorder seemed as reproducible and persistent as if, like Kazetsky, I had been shot through the cranium with shrapnel.[12] Merely the haemorrhage was spared and there was no pain. Without the shrapnel it all seems less explicable and, of course, less honourable.

The sporadic frames of mind in which coincidence and the relationships between things produced arresting images and ideas seemed at the time to veer too closely to the vivid characteristics of insanity. It was almost six months before I could look up from my feet once more and recognise Orion and Sirius without fear of uncontrollable primitive convictions, overwhelming inspiration, and deluded expectations.

The transactional basis of my relationships with people—relatives, friends, and colleagues—seemed depleted and doubtful. I did what I could, which was at first little enough, and then, for no obvious reason, coincident with being able to run well again and being able to count my change, I was able to engage in more complex intellectual and social processes without apprehension or self-doubt.

There was, of course, marked discontinuity between my own thread of exclusive personal experience and the general current of affairs, which at first seemed difficult, if not impossible, to bridge. If, in the event, it had been in practice impossible, it would have been less directly due to the underlying facts themselves than to consequent attitudes, my own or those of my contemporaries. My reception at work was initially somewhat cool, though I was pretty cool myself—"nowise cool for being curbed."

Perhaps, however, the illness—the experience itself—is viewed as a lifelong condition (which it may well be), if not a life sentence:

> These gloved hands I look at now, steering the motorcycle down the road, were once his! And if you can understand the feeling that comes from that, then you can understand real fear—the fear that comes from knowing there is nowhere you can possibly run.[1]

But I look over my shoulder and there is nothing to run from.

Depression as I have experienced it on and off over the years now seems dissipated, as if from necessity building from the ground I have been able to discover what was required, to identify what I had to do, and to find out how to do it—then do it. It seemed important to acquire at least a modest degree of confidence and versatility to negotiate the inevitable succession of problems and to identify the proprieties ("It is much more important to dig a half-buried crow out of the ground. . .than to send petitions to a president"[5]).

> Failure to solve problems—for example a crossword puzzle—can lead to a state of trivial misery that we may call a "minidepression." The solution found, the "minidepression" disappears. Depression during a time of loss (of a job, friends, prestige, etc.) may be a period during which the brain is looking (searching) for a solution to the problems that cannot be solved, at least in a relatively brief period of time. Eventually, we may find a way of accepting a substitute for the person we have lost, but this may require a considerable reevaluation of what we may desire in our personal relationships with others. Whether by conscious effort or unconscious mechanisms, the information stored in our brains may have to be reorganised. We may eventually piece together a solution to our being unemployed or our friends' misrepresentation of our worth. A loss of self-esteem, for example, may motivate us to "outdo" a former friend and to change our mental image of him.[13]

And hence of oneself.

The raw material of my delirium bleeds still in chaos, expressed in abortive essays and fleetingly observed in a multitude of curious snapshots, fading towards the final sequence in darkness and mist. But by then neither words nor pictures could contain the cataclysmic blaze of anger and I smashed the door with a pickaxe, rampaging onto the street quite capable of massacre.

Now,

> Now all my lies are proven untrue,
> And I must face the men I slew.
> What tale shall serve me here among
> Mine angry and defrauded young?[14]

Slowly the metaphorical possibilities of my deranged experience reveal themselves:

> Understanding a metaphor is as much a creative endeavor as making a metaphor, and as little guided by rules. . . .No doubt metaphors make us notice aspects of things we did not notice before;. . .[15]

And if, as Nietzsche put it, "We have art, in order that we may not perish from the truth," then that may perhaps be "A New Option," as the Dice Man concludes.[16]

> I tell myself I have reached an age, the age of unreliable menace. The world is full of abandoned meanings. In the commonplace I find unexpected themes and intensities.[17]

Yes, it is simply a fact and I hope that I have managed to salvage some modest synthesis from this illness, if that is what we choose to call it, perhaps to lay before whatsoever interested parties might prematurely have concluded it to have been a terminal condition.

I have quoted frequently and from many sources. Where I have done so, the pieces were observed like signposts through thoughts in which, for obvious reasons, I could not fully trust the authority of my own impressions. I needed the weight and brilliance of other minds to follow and with which to blend. It is difficult not to end with Robert Lowell, who, more than lithium carbonate, I suspect, offers the possibility of a new beginning:

> Fertility is not to the forward,
> or beauty to the precipitous—
> things gone wrong
> clothe summer
> with gold leaf.[18]

And now it is summer.

It was, however, a long and savage winter, with a brief and beautiful spring.

The path that I trod was strange to me and even stranger to my companions, who left me one by one. In this chapter, I pick out landmarks left by others declaring their views. Now I must describe it as I saw it; it was a matter of survival:

> I kick-started and rode astride Wolfgang, polaris metallic like an Arctic Wolf, purring slowly down through Camberwell with menace towards the grey chilling river, furious and hungry for the land...[19]

Which, for what it is worth, is more or less how my own story begins.

ACKNOWLEDGMENTS

To the editor of the *Lancet* for permission to reproduce the passage adapted from "Manic Depressive Illness." To the physicians, nurses, and ancillary Staff of MH, who will know who they are without being named. To my father for reading preliminary drafts and for his helpful comments. To my wife for delightful conversations in extremely difficult circumstances and for standing by me through thick and thin. To our close friends and colleagues. To our families, without whom I would have nothing left.

REFERENCES

1. Robert Pirsig, *Zen and the Art of Motorcycle Maintenance* (London: The Bodley Head, 1974), p. 82.
2. Ian Hamilton, *Robert Lowell: A Biography* (London: Faber & Faber, 1983).
3. Anonymous, "Manic Depressive Illness," *Lancet* 2 (1984), p. 1268.
4. William James, quoting Theodore Parker in *The Varieties of Religious Experience* (London: Penguin Books, 1982), p. 82.
5. Milan Kundera, *The Unbearable Lightness of Being* (London: Faber & Faber, 1984), p. 78.
6. Oliver Sacks, *A Leg to Stand On* (London: Duckworth, 1984).
7. Graham Hough, "Culture and Sincerity," *London Review of Books* (6–16 May 1982), pp.6–7.
8. W. B. Yeats, "Hodos Chameliontos" (1922), quoted in "The Magician," Daniel Albright, *New York Review of Books* (January 31, 1985), pp. 29–32.
9. Robert Lowell, *Epilogue: Day by Day* (London: Faber & Faber, 1977).
10. Daniel Albright, "The Magician," *New York Review of Books* (January 31, 1985), pp. 29–32.
11. A. R. Luria, *The Working Brain* (London: Penguin Books, 1973), p. 210.
12. A. R. Luria, (1973) *The Man with a Shattered World* (London: Cape, 1973).
13. Israel Rosenfield, "The New Brain," *New York Review of Books* (March 14, 1985), p. 34–38.
14. Rudyard Kipling, unknown source.
15. Donald Davidson, *What Metaphors Mean. Inquiries into Truth and Interpretation* (Oxford: Oxford University Press, 1984).
16. Luke Rhinehart, *The Dice Man* (St. Albans: Panther Books, 1972).
17. Don De Lillo, *White Noise* (New York: Viking, 1985).
18. Robert Lowell, "Homecoming," *Day by Day* (London: Faber & Faber, 1977).
19. Michael Rose, *The Capua Gate* (unpublished novel).

PART IV

GASTROINTESTINAL DISEASES

CHAPTER 22

ULCERATIVE COLITIS AND AVASCULAR NECROSIS OF HIPS

JUDITH ALEXANDER BRICE

I

"Well, Judy, you've got what you've been working on." With that cryptic statement my gastroenterologist, aware of my dread of ulcerative colitis, walked out of the room. He'd known of my fears because of our discussions centering on my extensive family history. My mother had needed a colectomy after becoming critically ill with ulcerative colitis during my adolescence. My brother had struggled with two severe bouts of Crohn's disease. Symptoms of irritable bowel plagued me from childhood. Clearly I was no stranger to gastrointestinal distress or disease. Yet, suddenly, with my doctor's stark pronouncement, it seemed my fate had been sealed.

When my gastroenterologist returned a few minutes later to prescribe Azulfidine, he lectured me out of my tears, leaving me to struggle alone through my own worries of smelliness, uncontrollable diarrhea, and possible body mutilation. His hostile, seemingly critical attitude conveyed to me that my illness was somehow my own doing. Guilty, anxious, only marginally aware of my own fury, I returned home. If it was my own doing, how could I undo it? My overwhelmed state could find no reply. Nonetheless, before my health would improve to this premorbid state of functioning, a search for this answer would take center stage and undergo numerous transformations. Kindled that day by a doctor just a little too busy to concern himself with the impact of a few words upon a single patient, the search was continually fueled by my own personal makeup, my medical training, and

DR. JUDITH ALEXANDER BRICE, age 43, is a general psychiatrist in Pittsburgh. She has a private practice in adult and adolescent psychiatry and is the medical director for a partial psychiatric hospital program for children and adolescents at St. Francis Medical Center. She is a clinical instructor in psychiatry at the University of Pittsburgh Medical School. She is particularly interested in psychological issues of patients struggling with chronic disease or handicaps.

all of the uncertainties of etiology inherent in a "psychosomatic" disease.

As inflammatory bowel disease goes, I was fortunate to have seven years with only two disabling, though brief, flare-ups. But within a year of the diagnosis, I became steroid-dependent and every time my prednisone was reduced below 20 mg I paid the price. My body knew the difference; try as I might, I couldn't fool it with lower steroid doses. I searched for other magic cures. Usually, just as I would give up, a friend or a colleague would say, "I had a friend who drank chamomile tea every day and hasn't had a symptom of colitis," "I know someone who gave up roughage and...no colitis since," or "I know someone who...." The list was endless. It was hard to stare down that last glimmer of hope and say, "No, I've tried enough." Psychoanalysis, special diets, quack blood tests supplemented a routine complement of steroids and Azulfidine.

One of the unspoken tenets of my medical training was the belief that there is an answer out there; if you only knew more, if you were a little smarter, you could find it. This attitude resonated with my background. My father, as a research hematologist, had known the joys of discovering unexpected connections and curing disease through careful, meticuluous, undaunted scrutiny of facts. I kept feeling that if I only knew enough, if only I were smarter, I could find the way out. I discovered the hard way that I could only come up with some of the answers some of the time.

The stigma of ulcerative colitis as a "psychosomatic disease" (despite the renunciation of that etiology today by most gastroenterologists) was ever present. This made coping very difficult and heightened my primitive guilt and a pervasive feeling of being different and estranged. When I dared expose myself to close friends and relate distress over worsening symptoms, I felt vulnerable to statements like "Well, it does sound like your job has been stressful lately" or "I'm sure being pregnant has gotten you anxious." It seemed as if many friends felt they could be helpful by pointing out what they considered to be a likely life stressor. They seemed to be in search of an acknowledgment on my part; if I agreed with them that an event was distressing, then this, in itself, would be curative.

These interpretations became, for me, corrosive indictments. I began to feel that mine was tainted anxiety, open for easy critique. Indeed, eight years after the diagnosis was made, on the day before I finally went to surgery, my surgeon informed me that I did not strike him as being "like most ulcerative colitis patients" who were "compulsive" and "insistent on dotting all the *i*'s and crossing all the *t*'s." At first I took this as a complement when he said it, but then, as time passed, I realized that this too was an expression of his and others' underlying sentiments: Ulcerative colitis patients were psychiatrically disturbed in a particular way and their disease manifested this physiologically.

The insecurity engendered by carrying the psychosomatic label was greatly exacerbated by the symptoms of the disease itself and others' reactions to them. In our society we quickly learn the taboo against speaking of our toilet habits in public. Bowel movements, diarrhea, flatulence, bodily odors are all considered personal and private. I felt embarrassed to tell my friends about my "unmentionable" habits. When I did tell them, I both sensed and imagined their discomfort. Their unease and my sensitivity caused painful reverberations. As my time living with the disease wore on, I increasingly felt lonely and I became ashamed of my embarrassing symptoms and disease.

Fortunately, for the seven years following the initial diagnosis, my life was not very disrupted. The intense emotional painfulness of my two monthlong flare-ups receded in my mind as I moved along through each day's events. However, fear of what I then considered might be my ultimate worse prognosis, namely an ileostomy, was never far from my mind. I dreaded such a fate, perhaps because my mother had needed one precisely when I was undergoing the metamorphosis of puberty. My second gastroenterologist, alert to my concerns, yet also aware of the dangers of steroids, kept trying to wean me off. Every two or three months we would need to reassess. As my appointment time approached I became increasingly anxious. I was always frightened lest this would be the time that an ileostomy would be recommended.

My doctor was usually quite calm and matter-of-fact. Unlike my friends, he was willing to hear about my symptoms without embarrassment. This and his respect for my thoughts and impressions were invaluable in mitigating the embarrassment, insecurities, and fear that shadowed me. Psychoanalysis, too, was very helpful. I never could pinpoint specific emotional factors as the cause of aggravated symptoms. However, careful self-scrutiny did help me understand how my own unresolved childhood problems were impeding an optimal adjustment to the stresses of my illness.

In January 1982, my ability to cope faltered, however, after the seven years of moderately good health. My illness became suddenly worse, apparently triggered by a severe gastroenteritis that hit everyone in the household. They recovered; I did not. Overnight my life became an unpredictable roller coaster. One day I was up, both physically and psychologically. The next day I was down. My colitis and my responsiveness to steroids no longer made even a modicum of sense. Not only was the course of my flare-ups unpredictable but also the intensity of my symptoms on an hourly and daily basis was unpredictable. It felt like a nightmare. I might have four and a half good days and then suddenly find myself needing to run to the bathroom six times at the end of the fifth day. My inability to be reliable and steady in all areas of my life, especially in my profession, was devastating to me. Because of the stigma of ulcerative colitis, I was reluctant to let other professionals dependent on my services know of my illness. Yet I had no choice but to cancel out unpredictably and frequently at the last minute. Had I known that my illness would ultimately take its toll for one and a half years before I could once again function consistently at work, I would have terminated my commitments for that period of time. But clearly I was blind to this retrospective view and so I kept trying to anticipate, and failing.

The sicker I got, the more unreliable I became and the more angry others got as their lives and plans and work became disrupted. Like most physicians, I had taken much pride in my work and had derived much of my self-esteem from my commitment to others. Suddenly, I was having to renege on my family, friends, patients, and colleagues. When I did not renege, I was often preoccupied by my symptoms and my concerns about whether I would get through the day without an embarrassing, urgent interruption. As my functioning became compromised in this way, I began to hate my body. I joked about trade-ins, but beneath the levity was an increasing shame, guilt, and dislike for myself. I felt betrayed. It was as if my body had suddenly and unpredictably turned on me; my most trusted friend had transformed itself into my biggest adversary. I felt dirty, smelly, and unfeminine. My self-esteem, so inextricably linked to an integral image of myself, eroded further.

In February and March I was twice admitted to hospital in an effort to control the ravages of my illness. If anything, these admissions were countertherapeutic. The insensitivity of some medical personnel greatly exacerbated my struggle to maintain self-respect when my functioning was disintegrating. One time, for example, between X-rays for an upper GI series, when I explained to a technician that I was too weak to walk very far to the bathroom and I would need ready access to one, she grumped at me, "Well, make up your mind if you need to go or not." Shortly thereafter she left me unattended in a hallway, hooked up to an IV with no bathroom at all accessible. Even as I write now, five years later, I wish to scream back, "If I could make up my mind, I wouldn't be here at all." Then the vindictive thought continues. "And I suppose you have never had diarrhea?" I imagine myself saying in a most sarcastic way. At the time I was too sick and too desperate to realize how angry I was. I needed help and I was helpless. I tried to be more compliant.

During these hospitalizations and then another one in June, I found it very difficult to switch gears. As a doctor, I was functioning in a profession of strength, of intellectual activity, of control, and of independence. These qualities did not easily mesh with those of a passive, compliant patient. One minute I was the psychiatric consultant, heading up case conferences, seeing private patients, and supervising residents. In my personal life I was running the routine of a household, relating to the needs of my husband, and taking care of a 2-year-old son. The next moment I was in the hospital with everyone from maintenance crew and janitorial staff to medical staff feeling entitled to enter my room without knocking. Within hours of being in charge of many aspects of my life, I suddenly found myself surrendering control over almost every aspect of a daily routine. Social boundaries, professional boundaries, personal boundaries were repeatedly subject to thoughtless violation. Doctors walked into the bathroom to examine me on the commode. Well-intentioned and unthinking volunteer staff walked into my room unannounced and interrupted very personal phone conversations to deliver my mail. Maintenance staff were there to greet me when I walked out of the shower. Nursing staff entered my room at night, clanging ice pitchers and laying out new linen. I didn't want clean pajamas; I was a light sleeper and wanted rest. I wanted a modicum of privacy, respect, and control.

During my second hospitalization in March 1982, I felt as if I'd found the answer. I put a sign on the door requesting politely that people knock and wait for an answer before entering. I am convinced that this wish for a normal quantum of privacy branded me as a kook among the nursing staff. I was to pay dearly for it during my subsequent hospitalization. The routine, I found out, was bigger than I.

The unwritten rules of the hospital were corrosive to my increasingly fragile identity. Already alienated from my body, I felt more and more fragmented as the staff's concept of my identity diverged from the person I felt I was. To them I was Judy, the ulcerative colitis patient in bed 612, who was uncooperative and irritable when they walked into her room without knocking. Ignored were my professional identity as a physician and my personal identity as a mother, a wife, and a competent and feminine woman who was not used to being treated as a passive, sexless infant. In March, I was discharged on high-dose steroids, grateful to be at home and at least in charge of such mundane matters as who saw me naked and where, and who entered my living space and when. I was still terrified, however, because my body was not getting better and remained out of control.

Two months later I was asymptomatic but very cushingoid. My gastroenterologist tentatively brought up the subject of an ileostomy and I balked. My self-esteem was at rock bottom and it was virtually impossible for me to imagine living a satisfying life so disfigured. We agreed on another opinion. The person I sought out had an excellent reputation. He conducted a cursory history with a sharp tongue and I was ill at ease throughout the sigmoidoscopy and physical exam. I was so ill at ease, in fact, that I dismissed his recommendation for an ileostomy, a recommendation based on his concern about long-term steroids. I moved on.

My conviction that there must be an answer out there if only I were smart enough or wise enough to find it was goaded on by my own prejudice in favor of the big teaching hospitals. I learned of the Koch procedure (a nondisfiguring surgical procedure resulting in an internal ileostomy), and in June I decided to go to the experts in New York City to have it done. A well-respected internist and family friend helped make the arrangements. The plan was for me to be admitted to a medical service, reevaluated by a well-known gastroenterologist, and then (if he agreed with the recommendation for surgery) transferrred to a surgical service for surgery. After six days in hospital, I had seen my gastroentrologist only three times (including once for a colonoscopy) when he whisked into the room. "It would be madness," he expounded to me and my husband, "for you to get a colectomy." He dismissed, summarily, the long history of steroid use and dependence and the fact that he'd seen me only when I was taking a daily dose of 60 mg of prednisone. And he insinuated that my turmoil of the last month around having an ileostomy had been needless and senseless. His answer to my dilemma was 6-mercaptopurine. He made light of my concerns about side effects and the excessive use of steroids for several more months while the 6-mercaptopurine would be taking effect. The risks, he stressed, were minimal. My husband was outraged: How could he say it was madness when two doctors in Pittsburgh had recommended an ileostomy? My gastroenterologist did not say that he felt he was smarter and more informed than the roughnecks in Pittsburgh who had been treating me. He only implied it.

But I was looking for magic and I wanted to believe I'd found it. Sadly, the price for my magic would prove to be high. I returned to Pittsburgh, 6-mercaptopurine in hand, suffering intermittently from a steroid-induced lethargy that came on suddenly and left me feeling weak and exhausted. For several months I took my new medicine, gradually trying to lower the steroid dose. My symptoms did improve somewhat. However, I teetered on the brink of terror, worried to the point of intermittent panic about agranulocytosis. My white count and hematocrit dropped. I was so preoccupied with this known side effect of 6-mercaptopurine that I did not pay much attention to mild hip pain. "Arthritis," I told myself, and the pain seemed to go away. My colitis improved, my steroid dose was "lowered" to 45 mg per day, and I began to relax. For the third time in nine months I went back to work, and I became more physically active with my family.

I recall one particular fall weekend, wandering around a tiny West Virginia town, the orange leaves crisp against a brilliant blue sky. The hip pain returned. It seemed so illogical, so stupid, so irreconcilable. I felt psychologically together, happier, better. Once again I attributed the discomfort to mild arthritis. My siege of illness, I told myself, was coming to an end. But the pain continued, and in a few days, at my internist's recommendation, I had an X-ray. It was negative. I convinced myself that the problem was only minor; perhaps I needed arch supports. I desperately wanted to be well and so, for a couple of days, I put off my gastroenterologist's recommendation to call an orthopedic surgeon. Vaguely, I knew something could go wrong with my hips. My brusque consultant had mentioned avascular necrosis and my memory was rekindled whenever my hips ached. However, I had accustomed myself to trying to ignore the myriad side effects of all of the drugs my condition required. For me, in fact, one of the many struggles of being a doctor living with a chronic disease was trying, on the one hand, to use all my medical knowledge to master the disease and, on the other, to let go of excessive worry and concern. I experienced constant tension in the process of sorting out. In this case, I had sorted out my hip pain and placed it in a back cupboard, out of sight and mostly out of mind.

As our supply of Tylenol dwindled, however, and codeine got added to the armamentarium of drugs I was daily ingesting, I decided to telephone an orthopedic surgeon. In no way was I prepared for the degree of alarm on the other end of the phone. The orthopedic surgeon asked me how soon I could come in. Within 12 hours I was getting a bone scan. That night, *over the phone,* I learned the results. "My dear, your hips are being supported by dead bone. At any moment they might collapse. From here on you must act as if you are paralyzed. You must bear no weight on your hips at all. Come into the hospital tomorrow; I will meet with you and discuss what should be done first. This is a very serious matter."

When my husband and I went in, we had to discuss my future *in the cafeteria,* because the hospital had no rooms set aside for doctor-patient conferences. The facts, I was told, were simple: My femoral heads were dangerously close to collapse. I might not walk again normally; there was no definite course to the osteonecrosis. It was caused by steroids. I needed to get off my hips as fast as possible. Only after a colectomy could I even consider surgery on them. My doctor hastily outlined some of the options but emphasized that he put credence only in his own procedure, the live bone graft. He stressed that it was only

40% successful and would require extensive time in hospital and in rehabilitation. I hated crying in the cafeteria, but there was nowhere to go, and nowhere to run to.

Suddenly, within 26 hours, my focus had shifted. I had traded in one chronic, debilitating, and embarrassing disease for two. Not only would I need to have an ileostomy, I was now being told I'd need to be in a wheelchair for an extensive period of time and might never walk again normally. I felt devastated, angry, guilty, and terrified. Time, magic, and choice had vanished. I needed a colectomy immediately to avoid any more bone destruction. My gastroenterologist picked the surgeon and I was scheduled for surgery three days hence.

My guilt and despair surfaced in an unimaginable intensity. I had felt increasingly saddened each time I'd had to leave my son and go into the hospital. I was devoted to him and I knew he could not comprehend what was happening. I felt tremendously sad that he was having to go through this immense upheaval. Unfortunately, my emotional conviction that if I'd been smarter I could have avoided this mess resulted in my feeling overwhelmed by guilt. Cognitively I knew it was not true. Emotionally, however, I felt it was my fault that my son was having to endure such pain and emotional trauma at such a young age. I was mercilessly hard on myself, especially in those days before surgery.

II

The colectomy, in November 1982, was awful but the postop course was worse still. I did not recover. Each time the nasogastric tube was pulled, I became nauseated, developed back pain, and vomited within 36 hours. The nasogastric tube was then reinserted, left in for a few days, and then once again the picture repeated itself. My pain was atypical, my course was atypical, and in addition I was more helpless than a typical postop patient because I couldn't walk. Perhaps for these reasons, perhaps because I was known to the hospital as someone who had bucked the system by asking for some privacy, perhaps because I was a doctor who was able to assess the quality of medical care, the nursing and medical staff began to dismiss and overlook my needs. For example, after my urinary catheter was removed, I developed an atonic bladder and I was unable to void for over 14 hours. I begged the nurses to call the doctor for a straight cath order. They began to bicker with me: Maybe I didn't really have to void, maybe I just felt like I had to. "It's been 14 hours," I told them. They couldn't palpate a bladder; maybe I just had not received that much liquid. "Check my I+O's," I politely requested. No order was written for a straight cath, they countered; the doctor must not have wanted to do it. "Does he know I haven't voided in 14 hours?" I asked. In desperation I stupidly agreed to take a Valium (prescribed for sleep) while they called the doctor and got an order. An hour later, I became adamant. They told me they had assumed, when I agreed to the Valium, that the problem was solved. They had not called the doctor. One more hour later, to my relief, they got the order and to their chagrin, my bladder had indeed been full.

Over the next week terror eclipsed my frustration, as the hospital staff's passive neglect evolved into aggressive abuse. It seemed as if my continued illness was a thorn in everybody's side. When I did not get better on schedule, ready explanations were offered. Clearly, in the nursing staff's mind, I did not *want* to get better. Their attitudes reflected this. Some tried to cajole, some became hostile, the majority became condescending. Their expressions of disgust were thinly disguised. Their intent was acutely clear. One nurse told me that I just needed to learn to adjust and live with the pain I was experiencing. I replied that if things were as they should be, I shouldn't be experiencing this pain. This statement fell on deaf ears. Fewer and fewer people believed that I had a "real" problem or "real" pain. When a UGI series was read as negative, that clinched it as far as my doctor was concerned. Convinced, despite my complaints of anorexia and back pain, that I was clearly on the road to recovery and should not need anything else, my doctor discontinued all orders for pain medication. In front of the nurses he lectured me about the hazards of excessive use of opiates for pain control when the pain was not enough to warrant it. The stage was set for the worst nightmare of my life. Unfortunately, the nightmare was not a dream.

Within a few hours after my surgeon's visit, my pain gradually increased. At my request, my private-duty nurse asked the charge nurse to call the doctor. For over two hours the charge nurse put her off, convinced that I was a "crock." I was in severe pain and I began moaning. She continued to ignore it. I rang my call bell. No one answered. Finally, my husband went out to the hall pleading with the charge nurse to attend to me. She ignored him. I became desperate, crying and screaming, since the pain had become excruciating. My husband went out and pleaded again. Finally she barrelled into the room. "Doctor Brice," she exhorted, "I want you to quit moaning and quit manipulating. I have another patient in the next room moaning, and if you think you are going to get me to give you morphine or call your doctor, you are wrong." With that, she stomped out of my room.

Life had seemed bleak before, but never as bleak as at that hour. I knew I was obstructed but I couldn't get anyone in charge to listen to me, let alone believe me. My doctor had all but forbidden me to call him directly when I telephoned him during my first postop obstructive episode. I was desperately ill, helpless, and in an instant my most important helpers had become accusers.

The wrenching terror of that night and that hour has remained as vivid as if it happened yesterday. Others had been my hope. The personal smile, the human touch, had come to mean everything. In that instant, my world shattered. Cruel neglect had become a reality as I had never known it before. Unfortunately, I knew it then and I know it now. I know the terror of its recurring and I fear that terror will loom with me forever. "What if. . . again?" I ask myself at the oddest times. And I work and rework it again and again in my mind, trying to prepare myself for another assault of inhumanity when I am sick and vulnerable. The solutions I see are not admirable. I do think that if ever that occurred again I would threaten to sue, muster witnesses, and call my lawyer day or night. At the time I felt too helpless. I was unprepared, acutely ill, and could think of nothing but relief from pain. I wished I was dead.

After about a half hour of my husband's continued pleading, the charge nurse returned only to exclaim, "Oh, shit!" when she observed the 1000 cc of biliary vomitus that I'd vomited since her last visit. She knew then that she'd made a mistake in her assessment. She scurried about, helped to clean up the vomit, did call the doctor, but did not speak to me.

Two days later and one month after my initial surgery, a laparotomy revealed massive intestinal adhesions. The surgery that was to take one hour ("at the most," my doctor predicted) extended into four and a half hours. My husband and my mother paced in my hospital room. With no word of my condition or the reasons for the delay, they could only imagine the worst; a cardiac arrest was in both of their minds. When I finally went to the recovery room, they were summoned to a hallway that ran outside of one of the operating rooms. There, *standing up,* with other patients being wheeled by on guerneys, my surgeon told them that he had really had a rough time operating on me. He told them that I was "riddled with adhesions" and that they would come back for the rest of my life. My husband could have none other than visions of unending surgical procedures. Never had he or my mother encountered such a breach of empathy. My husband still becomes enraged when he remembers the terror of that four-hour wait and then the shattering news implying that I would go on being severely sick like that throughout my life. It seems to him and my mother now that my surgeon was more concerned for his own exhausting morning than for the impact of his words as they *stood* in the *hall.*

As for me, when I was wheeled into the recovery room, I was to encounter one of the most sadistic nurses imaginable. My first memory is of waking up in severe pain and being extremely cold. A nurse came and took my pulse, and I asked, "Could I have another blanket?" That was enough to antagonize her. "I just brought you one; I'm not going to bring you another," she barked at me and disappeared. When she came back to check my pulse, I pleaded with her. "Please be nice, please be nice," I recall saying. "I'm freezing." Angrily, she brought over a sheet, threw it on me, and again walked away.

It seemed like an eternity until change of shift, when to my relief a responsible nurse came on duty. The other nurse had been so cruel that when this new one brought me blankets and asked me how I was feeling, she seemed to me like an angel.

Unfortunately, she was a recovery room nurse, and once being wheeled into the ICU I was to lose sight of her and again be at the hands of some severely and pathologically sadistic nurses. I was already imprisoned in my body. It began to feel, though, that I was imprisoned as well in a Nazi concentration camp. In probably the best private hospital in Pittsburgh, I was continually terrorized and tortured psychologically.

After three days I was marginally stabilized and I returned to a regular room. My condition worsened, however, and there were many more grim times. I developed gastritis and bled through my nasogastric tube. My surgeon came in, watching the blood drain, and lectured me. "The problem with you, Judy, is that you are too anxious," he expounded. All the while he was talking I was hooked up to an IV line, a hyperalimentation line, and a Jackson Pratt tube, and I had a nonfunctional ileostomy bag strapped to my waist. To this day I wonder how he might feel if he were in such a situation. I also wonder why, knowing I was anxious, and telling me that my hematocrit was stable, he ordered two units of blood in the middle of the night without ever saying a word to me about it. I wonder what he thought that might do to my "excessive" anxiety or to my trust.

The more sick I became, the more my world diverged from the world that had been mine before my illness. Every day was a struggle to accommodate each to the other, to bring them to a single focal point and keep them in a single image. My world was now the world of tubes and drains and repeated stabs and punctures and pushes and shoves. The "real" world was somewhere else again: my son, two years old and motherless; my husband, struggling to shelter him, support me, and continue his own life; and my mother, fighting her own nightmares of a similar illness. The world full of other people and places, the world that saw the first snowflake of winter drift peacefully to the ground—that world had vanished. I felt driven, however, to move toward it. As the last burnished leaf clings to the oak tree before Thanksgiving departs and winter sets in, I clung to the life in others. I knew I had to reel it in, to touch it. I consciously forced myself every day to grasp toward it. I was so physically weak and uncomfortable and so emotionally depleted that even this effort felt excruciating. Word by word, sentence by sentence, I deliberately tried to inch myself outward, engaging the staff, my family, my private-duty nurses, my friends to talk about their lives, their families, their battles with the snow or whatever. They were my link with life; reaching out became my salvation.

My surgeon's soul could not reach back. Frequently, when he came to see me, he would not look at me. His gaze would often avoid mine to wander toward the window or the television. I yearned for him to sit for a minute, hold my hand, give me some reassurance. He never did. He checked the NG tube and noted it was draining copious amounts of fluid. He checked out my ileostomy bag and noted the absence of any output. We both knew these were not good signs. The sicker I became, the colder he became, and the more death loomed in our minds.

My husband and I knew that he was taking my failure to recover as a personal failure. Our hints at another opinion were either ignored or summarily pushed aside. Seeing the concern in my husband's eyes, my surgeon protested his innocence. "I can't imagine that I did anything wrong," he exclaimed to my husband on more than one occasion. He seemed more and more irritable the more I did not get better. My husband and I were very frightened of being forthright in requesting a second opinion, for fear he would take offense and take out his feelings against me and my care. My care was too critical to be jeopardized. My life hung precariously in the balance.

The wish to get out of this predicament propelled me and my husband onward. My gastroenterologist had continued to follow my progress, although it was our impression that my surgeon was upset when the gastroenterologist visited me and conveyed his impressions about the best treatment. Casually, in an aside to my husband, my gastroenterologist suggested that perhaps my recovery was impeded because I was unable to walk. My husband then lauched a crusade. For several days he tried to get my orthopedic surgeon to discuss my immobility with my surgeon and gastroenterologist. Finally, after several unanswered phone calls, my husband again telephoned my orthopedic surgeon's office, this time irate. Up against his anger, the secretaries obliged and arranged a meeting. When my husband finally succeeded (after a full week) in meeting with the orthopedist, the answer came swiftly. "If they think her immobility is causing the problem, for God's sake get her up to walk." Frustrated beyond belief, my husband complained of the lack of coordination of medical care. "Medical care *is never* coordinated!" was the doctor's only reply. Indeed, it was not, at least among these doctors. My husband then refused to leave the orthopedist's office until he called the floor and relayed the message to rescind the order for complete bed rest.

I got up and walked, but still after several days there was no evidence of improved gastrointestinal function. As my condition worsened and I became weaker, I had more than one meeting with my husband and a friend trying to decide if it was worth the risk of alienating my surgeon in order to get in a consultant. I spent hours talking to my private-duty nurses about when and how to make the choice. Planning, even if it was just planning a meeting to plan a strategy, became one more way of coping with the hours of being so very sick and helpless. I finally decided to wait until after Christmas before approaching my surgeon about a consultant.

My surgeon decided on Christmas eve to pull out the nasogastric tube one last time. He told me then that if this effort failed he foresaw several months of hyperalimentation. Miraculously, that proved to be the right time. In delighted amazement, I returned home only five days after the tube was pulled.

III

When I left the hospital I could only sit up for a maximum of 15 minutes without becoming totally exhausted. Even with crutches, I could not walk for more than a few steps without experiencing moderate pain. I was delighted to be alive and at home but I was very scared and depressed. I was returning to a home that I had known as an independent, albeit sick, woman, wife, and mother. But now I was disfigured, dependent, and crippled. The adjustment was mammoth. I felt like a shipwrecked survivor treading water in a stormy sea. As hard as I tried, I felt ominously close to drowning. My family, a few friends, and a very special private-duty nurse buoyed me and my spirits. Had it not been for them and a few others I think I would have given up. As it was, they kept me afloat, encouraging me with their warmth, acceptance, and optimism. My husband and I tried desperately to hold onto the miracle of my survival to give us confidence in approaching the next hurdles. My 3-year-old son's joy in my return home was a shining star. Without it, the battle seemed endless, hopeless, an inglorious struggle for an inglorious end. But the beacon of his happiness gave clear direction. I had no choice. I had a job to do and that was to get better. My recovery became a mission.

I began to search for the next answers: how to get over my hip disease and how to get around with it. I sought out a second opinion and got a radically different recommendation. Concurring with the diagnosis, this second orthopedic surgeon suggested core decompression ("burr holes") of the femoral heads. He felt that there was no good evidence that live bone grafts were at all beneficial and he had known several patients who recovered full hip function from the burr holes. The quandary I was in was enormous: how to decide between two well-recommended doctors suggesting radically different procedures and each acknowledging about a 50% failure rate. I was too weak and too crippled to get around easily enough to make a library search feasible, and even then, how would I learn enough fast enough to make an intelligent decision? Being interested in psychiatry I'd managed to "avoid" orthopedics in medical school and now needed to make a crucial orthopedic decision. To the chagrin of my husband, I coped with this problem not unlike the way I coped with my uncertainty about handling my ulcerative colitis. I began to collect additional opinions.

The problem became confounded, however, when the additional opinions differed substantially from the first two. Still believing in a magic "right" answer and still holding Harvard in highest esteem, I called two different physicians there. One, convinced that he would have to see my X-rays and scans to make a definitive recommendation, was adamant that if the diagnosis of avascular necrosis was correct, then I needed a bone graft of a different kind than had been recommended. He encouraged me to travel to Boston, emphasizing how difficult it is to diagnose avascular necrosis. The second Harvard physician I called recommended a core decompression. Yet another eminent Harvard specialist told my orthopedic consultant in Pittsburgh that this procedure was a waste of time. His practice was to wait until the hips fractured and then replace them.

Each of the physicians I talked to was very convincing. For a couple of weeks I tried on their recommendations the way a well-dressed woman might try on several spring coats. It frequently took me a day or two to take the latest person, or opinion, off a pedestal. For several days my husband would come home from work only to find out that I'd completely changed my mind about what direction to take. Untrained in medicine and hearing only second- or thirdhand about yet one more opinion, he couldn't help but be one step behind me at the least. I was desperate for a right or magical answer. He was resolute about moving ahead in a sensible way. The tension was great as we each struggled with the uncertainty and controversy.

In the end, I placed my bet with the only recommendation made by more than one of the six physicians I eventually consulted: a bilateral core decompression. As I look back, I see that my choice to go with this procedure was as much determined by the character of the physicians as by the "majority" opinion. Once before I'd been told by a doctor of the "madness" of another approach, yet his approach had carried with it the serious iatrogenic sequelae of continued high-dose steroids. I was very wary of doctors who, in the face of significant controversy, were convinced that their approach was *the only* right one. When the initial orthopedic surgeon who had recommended a live bone graft got furious with me at my audacity for deciding to get a second opinion, my estimation of his medical competence, as well as his personal character, dropped considerably.

Consequently, within a month and a half of leaving one hospital, I returned to another, full of trepidations around yet another bout with surgery. I hoped for the best and feared the worst. Fortunately, the experience went as planned and the medical care was consistently good. A few days after going into the hospital I returned home, still with a very uncertain prognosis and still strongly admonished to get off of my hips if I felt any pain.

This was difficult advice to follow. Using crutches, I could only stand for about three minutes without pain. My only choice was to remain immobile or to use a wheelchair and adapt my house and my life to this. My orthopedic surgeon had told me, "I hate wheelchairs," but, in the next breath, he was adamant about the dangers of walking even with crutches when I experienced *any* discomfort. Initially, after surgery, I could not walk at all. Within several months, I was able to use crutches to get to a car, walk from my car to my office, and get around the office for a few hours. This would, however, exhaust my good "hip time." My hips would ache and I needed to use the wheelchair when I returned home. I got into a pattern of using crutches outside the home for part-time work and using a wheelchair at home and for family excursions.

Accommodating to being handicapped in this way was wrenching. I was used to running up and down stairs about 20 times a day. A 20-second run was now a 3-minute expedition by the time I wheeled my wheelchair to the stairs, transferred to the stairglide, rode myself upstairs, got into my upstairs wheelchair, looked for whatever article I'd left behind, wheeled back to the stairglide, transferred again, and then rode downstairs. Getting myself from our living room to our kitchen was a veritable expedition since it entailed wheeling to the dining room threshold and transferring to my "scooter" chair (a secretary's chair on wheels) so I could get around our small kitchen. Despite having worked with handicapped people, I had no notion of how infinitely time-consuming the simplest chores were, especially in a home only partially adapted for living in a wheelchair. All of the nooks and crannies of the house suddenly were potentially major obstacles.

The adjustment was particularly difficult both physically and emotionally because of the uncertainty of prognosis and the expected period of being so handicapped. We had recently done significant reconstruction in the house and had little desire to move or do major work again if my handicap was going to be time-limited. Not knowing what my course would be was very trying. My frustration turned into angry sadness as the weeks dragged on into months. At times, I was able to pride myself on the amount I accomplished, despite my handicap. As I look back, I can see that this was indeed not a small amount. I had taught myself to crochet. I had returned to work. I had learned rudimentary sign language in order to consult at a school for the deaf. And at home, I was entertaining friends, caring for my 3-year-old, and managing the household. Yet, despite my apparent successful coping, there were many times when I became enraged at the lengthiness of the simplest chores. My pride in my accomplishments quickly eroded when I compared my handicapped self to my healthy colleagues or to my fast-moving, overachieving former self. When I did this, I always came out behind.

Adding to the problem of adjustment for me was the degree of helplessness engendered by being handicapped in the way that I was. I had previously owned a stick-shift car. For a few months, I could not drive at all because of hip pain. Lucky that my right hip was better than my left, I became overjoyed when I could get out to buy a new car. When I first got it, I went out cruising. The feeling of elation was even greater than I could ever have imagined. I buzzed the streets, driving every which way, indulging in the pleasure of deciding where I could go and how I would get there. The thrill of controlling my fate, even in such a minuscule way, was so immense that I felt like I could fly. I had never before had such empathy for teenagers!

Still, in other ways, I remained far from independent. I'd come a long way from the days when I was hooked up to two IV lines and three other tubes, but my mobility was frightfully limited. I could not walk long enough to do any kind of shopping or errands and, as a consequence, whenever I wanted something I had either to order it and hope that I got what I wanted or to ask someone else to get it. There were many things in the house I could not do. My husband, part-time housekeeper, and friends became my legs and arms.

This was not easy for them or for me. The dependence was frustrating and even at times embarrassing. I had to ask for a lot more than others could comfortably provide. If they graciously did something extra for me I felt grateful, indebted, and embarrassed at being so needy. If they grudgingly or angrily acceded to my requests, I felt angry, trapped, and, at times, guilty. As the weeks extended into months, with minimal signs of progress, I became a seething cauldron of raw emotions ready to boil over if the flame were raised ever so slightly. And there were more than enough people around who could do it. When the UPS man refused to climb back up five stairs in order to carry a package into the house for me, I grew infuriated. When an obese man took the only parking place designated for the handicapped, I became angry, and then, when he went on to justify doing so in a laughing, taunting way ("Well, I'm handicapped too; I weigh too much"), I was enraged. These people and others I needed desperately for their help and cooperation. When they turned me down, they became an easy displacement target for all of my feelings about my illness. Little did they know, or could they know, how important a kind word or gesture could be in assisting me with my daily struggle.

The feeling that if only I were smarter I'd be able to get out of my physical predicament, or perhaps have avoided it altogether, surfaced repeatedly. I kept asking friends what they would do if they were in my predicament. I'm not sure now what I was looking for. In response to my question, several friends, my husband, and even, once, my orthopedic surgeon confessed that they probably would have walked despite the pain and the sure collapse of their hips. Often I wanted to do this, but I had been clearly warned of the many limitations of hip replacement. I was too scared and too stubborn. Once having embarked on a course or direction, I was panicked at the idea that I would not deliberately choose any change in that course. I had just enough support not to veer off.

I continued to search for answers. When I was acutely ill in the hospital my stockbroker happened to mention that he'd bought stock a while back in a company that was producing a "bio osteogen" machine for the experimental treatment of a relatively rare bone disease. Within a day he'd gotten back to me; the disease was avascular necrosis!

While in the hospital, I asked my orthopedic surgeon. Yes, such a machine was being used in New York. It provided an alternating electromagnetic signal to accelerate bone growth. My surgeon was skeptical but said he would contact the doctor involved about the possibility of my using it. I kept on the trail even after switching orthopedic surgeons and having hip surgery. The problems in finding out about the machine and obtaining this experimental device were immense. I learned that the clinical trials at Columbia were proving efficacious. My surgeon in Pittsburgh was skeptical, but not opposed to my using the machine. Obtaining it, then, became a new project for me, and for several months I spent much time and energy on the telephone talking to the company, my stockbroker, the team in New York, trying to get on their protocol for using the machine. Finally, I was able to get the machine and add the daily application of alternating current to my treatment regime.

Progress could hardly be called swift, however. Prior to surgery I could not take one normal step with my left foot. One year later I could take about 12 normal steps, but this left me in pain for the rest of the day. I was growing restless, discouraged, and reverted back to my old coping patterns. I decided I needed to have some new experts. At the very least, I figured, they might buttress my sagging confidence in the present course of action. And if they felt hip replacement or some other surgery was my ultimate answer I would consider it. Here again, I was not prepared for the answers I received. The first orthopedic surgeon I consulted in Pittsburgh was of top status in a Pittsburgh teaching hospital. He conducted a cursory exam and refused to look at either of the two bone scans, noting that he did not believe they were of any value. "In reviewing your case," he said, "I can see nothing wrong with your hips. You have no avascular necrosis. Your pain can be explained by mild back strain. Go out and walk!" He was definite. He was certain. He had no self-doubt and conveyed no need to investigate further. He did not comprehend or grasp the facts of my life. He showed no empathy for the fact that he was dealing with someone who had been told by four doctors that she had avascular necrosis, someone who had gone through a life-threatening operation to cut the losses from AVN, and someone who had spent a year hobbling on crutches, confining her life to a wheelchair. I wanted to scream with rage and joy. I wanted to cry, to explode. I meekly walked out, yearning to believe him, but very doubtful.

It took me a day under the influence of my husband's calm rationality to sort out my own opinion. I continued to be cautious and lined up three more opinions, two at Harvard. The most eminent of all the physicians shared with me as a parting comment, "My dear, I can't get too excited about your hips." His opinion, too, was that I'd had back strain. He, too, was adamant and convinced he was right. He seemed to have no feeling for what it must be like to have lived my life and then traveled several hundred miles to Harvard only to get a completely different opinion expressed with levity. I returned home with some stocktaking to do.

As I reviewed things, the score was five to two in favor of the initial diagnosis and four to two for proceeding as I had been. Although the two dissenters had been in the most prestigious positions, their assessment neither concurred with the majority nor fit in with my symptoms or the symptoms of back strain. My limitation in abduction because of joint pain, my hip pain upon walking, always left greater than right, the absence of back or hip pain even when lifting while sitting, did not fit in with the diagnosis of back strain. Bone scans had shown diminished activity in the femoral heads which was improving gradually. Lumbar and sacral X-rays were negative. Using my medical knowledge, I concluded that the diagnosis of back strain as a primary cause of hip dysfunction was absurd, and I elected to continue my slow, conservative course.

Fortunately, my judgment was correct and my patience paid off. Over the next few months, my progress was dramatic, slowing again but not yet leveling off (it has not leveled off to this day). Even now, each new step has felt like a miracle. The first time I stopped my car, walked into a drugstore, spent some time browsing, and walked out carrying a cane in one hand and a package in the other, I felt radiant. I took infinite pride in each new thing I could once again do. I felt like a 6-year-old who had just learned to ride a two-wheel bike. "Look, Ma, no hands!" I wanted to scream to friends and strangers alike when I finally untethered my hands from artificial supports. Two and a half years after the diagnosis of avascular necrosis was made, I got to the tennis courts. That was the only time in my life I cried with happiness.

My husband, my son, and I were exultant. We had won our own Olympic medal. With them and their support, I, and we, had triumphed. Without them, I would have assuredly succumbed. Throughout the entire struggle their encouragement, acceptance, and support had been crucial. As my illness had dragged on, both my physical and emotional thresholds for pain were gradually whittled down. The surface of my emotions had been scraped raw. Each new encounter was a potential abrasion to my very sensitive skin. I desperately needed hope and love to soothe my wounds. Their love had helped contain my hopelessness, my rage, and my self-hatred during the long siege when my body felt like an intractable adversary. They and others who were empathic and steady had kept me from despair. They helped restore my shattered world.

IV

Now, five years after the beginning of the exacerbation of my ulcerative colitis a different perspective emerges as I look back on the tedious coping with ulcerative colitis, the horror of the hospital experience, and the adjustment to a major handicap. Up until a few months ago, the memory of the irresponsible nurse who commanded me to quit moaning pierced me to the core, evoking rage and sadness and terror I did not know was in me. Never would I have imagined the impact of a single word, a single sentence on a person who is vulnerable, helpless, and in pain. I am likewise still moved to tears when I remember the devotion and dedication of three private-duty nurses who trudged through snow, worked overtime, and gave up holidays to see me through. I will never forget them and will remain forever grateful.

My heightened sensitivity accompanied me long after my hips improved. Now, two years after my first tennis game, a personal smile, a kind gesture of help, an expression of empathy still can move me to the brink of tears. I wish that some of my doctors and nurses could have opened themselves up to the empathy in themselves that I have received from such widely diverse people as neighbors, grocers, flight attendants, and dog trainers. Having consulted (before my illness) at a rehabilitation center, I am aware of how draining and threatening empathy with helpless, injured people can be to one's own emotional integrity. Yet to block ourselves off from others' feelings of sadness and vulnerability can be countertherapeutic. At times, it seemed that some of my doctors and nurses reacted to my illness and impotence by retreating to a narcissistic, self-centered stance out of a need for self-aggrandizement. This, then, seemed to lead to their categorical dismissal of other doctors' impressions as well as of my own. Further, their own need for power or control interfered with their understanding of what it was like to be in such a state of enforced passivity, unable to control basic bodily needs. Had my surgeon been so aware, he could never have told me that I was too anxious as my nasogastric tube was draining blood, with me lying in bed, sleep-deprived by continuous, 24-hour care and tethered by five different tubes. And I do not think the two orthopedic surgeons would have been so callous when they told me to "just walk" had they allowed themselves to feel and know what it was like to have been in hip pain and have been warned for a year that if you try to walk while you're in pain you will fracture your hip. Did they know, or even care to know, what it was like to spend the majority of your waking hours in a wheelchair? I doubt it. As a physician, I believe it is especially hard to hold onto a compassionate position because of the painful awareness that all of one's invested power and energy is helpless against the tides of fate. I do believe, though, that as a patient I felt more alone, more helpless, more terrified, and more enraged at my situation than I needed to. I am convinced that the emotional devastation of my illness was much greater than it had to be because many of my doctors and nurses had lost their compassion. It may indeed be true that the ravages of my physical illness might have been diminished had I felt greater compassion from my caregivers. Had I not been so sensitized and sensitive and had my brusque consultant been less abrasive, perhaps I would have chosen to have an ileostomy sooner. Who knows whether I would still have suffered the sequelae of excessive steroids. I still speculate.

As for me, a keener awareness of my own vulnerability and of the vulnerabilities of others has had some very positive and very negative effects. On the dark side of the balance, I'm terrified lest I will lose my regained health and become, once more, tethered, dependent, and vulnerable. This has left me hypersensitive to many small maladies. I am frightened that I might miss a symptom like my hip pain that may, in the end, be of major consequence. That experience has proved to be a difficult psychological trauma to move beyond.

I feel I must be constantly vigilant in order to cut my losses should something bad occur. I know I cannot be omniscient and that I should not have blamed myself when I could not extricate myself from the dilemma of my illness. It is clearly apparent to me how self-destructive that was. Yet I know that it was my sensitivity to my body that allowed for the early diagnosis of avascular necrosis at a stage when it was reversible. And I also know that it was my vigilance and my endless quest to improve my knowledge and find new answers that achieved my contact with the surgeon experimenting with the bio osteogen machine. Had I not been convinced that there were answers out there, I might have overlooked an important therapeutic modality.

The effort to strike a balance between self-informed, careful monitoring of other medical problems and hypersensitivity to minor symptoms is complicated by my awareness of the fallibility of doctors' judgments. I am aware of the dangers of doctor-shopping. I can see clearly the folly in having collected as many opinions about my hip disease as I did. However, I am keenly aware of the risk in trusting the wrong recommendation. I feel very lucky to be able to walk freely and normally again. I ask myself, "What if I'd not received the right diagnosis initially, or chosen the right treatment?" I am also convinced that on at least two occasions while I was critically ill, my awareness of the potential for medical misjudgment and mistakes and my own vigilance actually saved me from life-threatening consequences. My experience with these unfortunate mistakes in diagnosis and treatment have left me even more suspicious and questioning than I was trained to be in medical school.

My own ongoing self-care therefore poses continued problems. I must continually struggle to integrate constructively my vigilance, my suspiciousness, my anxiety about new symptoms, and my own aggressive mastery of medical information. My efforts to work out a healthy balance have led me to seek out for continued care an internist and consultants when necessary who are both respected and respectful. It is crucially important to me that my doctors are open to each other's thoughts and my impressions as well. My current doctors' sensitivity to my special needs have been invaluable in helping me achieve a more healthy, positive attitude about new medical problems as they have arisen.

On the more positive side, I have taken from my illness a vibrant pleasure in my own relative state of good health. Training and then walking my 100-pound dog is a treasured delight. Not once do I walk her around our hilly block without remembering back to the first time around with crutches, and then the first time around with a cane, and then the first time I could walk past two houses without a cane. Each of these repeated memories brings a new and unique joy. Many activities that to others feel like ordinary drudgery are each very special and memorable. Even playing soccer for five minutes with my 7-year-old is enough to elate me for a day. I treasure my mobility, and I value many small aspects of my life allowed by my present health. Wandering through the woods on a hike with my family, planting flowers in my garden and seeing them bloom, driving to my office, and moving freely at work are gifts I now have. I no longer take them for granted.

Also, my tremendous struggle to regain my mobility in a strange way allowed for a much easier transition to living with my ileostomy and accepting myself as I am. I think the adjustment to being disfigured would have been much harder had I not been coping with another problem that impaired me in so many greater ways. To be sure, it has taken time for me to accept the ileostomy and come to feel attractive, feminine, and sexy again. However, for so long my attention has been focused on my mobility that in many ways I did not have time or emotional energy to brood excessively about being disfigured. Now, four years later, I suddenly can realize that I have made tremendous gains in accepting my ileostomy. I do not like having it. But I can live with it and still feel comfortable and attractive in my dress and activities. This was something I could not do when I first came home from the hospital. Before my surgery it was something I imagined I could *never* do. Did it take my hip disease and being so handicapped to convince me otherwise?

In a strange way, my recognition of how much I did take for granted has broadened my work psychotherapeutically with patients. Knowing how difficult life can be, and knowing some of the small joys that are there to be found if we only look, has given me an optimism about what patients can accomplish therapeutically even in the face of much psychological adversity.

Hand in hand with my own renewed pleasure in life and this new optimism goes a much deeper empathy for the struggles of those less lucky. I realize now that there had been many gaps in my empathy for the chronically ill and handicapped. I was exquisitely sensitive to the newly handicapped person's sense of sadness and anger at his or her loss. But I think it took this experience of personal disability to bring out in me a fuller empathy and respect for the continued struggle of the "well-adjusted" handicapped or sick person. I was blind to the fact that each day presents new obstacles; even a "routine" is never quite "routine." A spilled glass of milk, a box left on the front porch in the snow, a flat tire are much bigger undertakings when one cannot move freely, comfortably, and energetically. Like Tennessee Williams's Blanche, the vulnerable have always depended upon "the kindness of strangers." I, too, needed it and depended on it. Now I know what that kindness can mean.

CHAPTER 23

ULCERATIVE COLITIS

"LOUISE SCOTT"

I am a 29-year-old psychiatric resident with a nine-year history of chronic inflammatory bowel disease. To date, I have had at least 40 rectal exams, 13 sigmoidoscopies, 3 colonoscopies, and 40 barium films.

These data are simple to relate; less easy to appreciate is the personal impact of this disease. As I see it now, my decision to become a physician and my attitude toward patients have emanated from my experience with illness. In turn, becoming a physician has influenced *me* as a patient. It has sensitized me to the great vulnerability that comes in being cared for and, eventually, has shaped my response to my doctors, to my care, and, in some ways, toward my colleagues.

I was introduced to chronic illness about ten years ago, sometime during my junior year in college. At this time, I began to have diarrhea several times a day. In the winter of my senior year I noticed blood. I didn't discuss this with anyone; I just went to the student health service. That was a mistake—I could tell, even then, that the doctors were inept. They had problems with the sigmoidoscope, and during the procedure I could detect urgency in their voices: "Stop the machine, are you crazy, the suction's too high." The nurse was rubbing my neck and fighting to stay calm. After all that, the pathology report seemed oddly anticlimactic. It read simply: inflamed colon. Much more difficult, I'm afraid, was the series of barium films. The first study, a set of 15 X-rays, had to be repeated because the originals were lost.

After reviewing my case, the health service physicians imparted their momentous diagnosis: "Probably nerves; here's a prescription for Librium." Their referral to a gastroenterologist, "if you have any more questions," seemed to suggest they had as little confidence in their ability as I did. I consulted this man and, after an expertly performed sigmoid exam and a review of the films and specimen, he told me I had ulcerative colitis. At that point, my reaction was one of simple relief that the diagnostic odyssey had ended; however, therapeutically, nothing had changed. Neither antispasmodics nor steroid enemas were ef-

"DR. LOUISE SCOTT" will complete her psychiatric residency in 1988.

fective in controlling diarrhea, yet I was strangely indifferent to the continuing symptoms.

Soon after, I graduated and moved to the Midwest to attend graduate school. I continued to have at least five blood-streaked bowel movements a day, preceded by intense cramping. Through student health I was assigned to a new gastroenterologist on the staff of the university hospital. He prescribed loperamide, which was somewhat helpful in controlling the daytime frequency of diarrhea.

I was well into the first semester of school when I felt weak and nauseated and had an increase in bloody diarrhea. Three days later I vomited bright-red blood and was admitted to the hospital. The hematemesis was self-limited and minor in comparison to the flare I was having. Never having been hospitalized, I finally felt like a patient; this identity seemed implicit in coming under the control of others. In retrospect, now I realize that I have allowed my doctors' behavior to define me as a patient—the greater their effort to impose treatment on me, the more I feel like a patient, irrespective of the severity of symptoms or of my willingness to accept treatment.

In the hospital I was a very good patient. I think I was actually intrigued by the novelty of it all, and my attitude toward procedures was one of cooperative resignation. I kept thinking of my mother, who had died of leukemia a few years earlier. The knowledge that my problem was far from terminal seemed to relegate it to the status of the medically trivial. Except for the uncomfortable first day, I felt well enough to encourage friends to visit. I asked my doctor to call my father and explain the situation. I was certain I'd get better soon, or at least return to baseline and resume my course work and social activity.

After discharge on 60 mg of prednisone and 2 gm of Azulfidine, I did well for about two weeks. Then I began to have problems concentrating and memorizing. Soon, I realized that I did not understand what I was reading. Thinking was difficult and I felt restless all the time. Eventually, I became so tearful and disorganized that I had to drop all of my courses. Over the next two weeks, things became worse. I couldn't even read newspaper headlines—the words made no sense. Unable to construct complex sentences, I spoke only in simple statements or single words. I enjoyed nothing and could not imagine anything that would ever make me happy again. I slept 14 hours a day, and when I was awake, I would either cry or eat ravenously. The smallest task demanded great effort, and when I thought about killing myself, it loomed like an insurmountable mission.

Every day I called my doctor, who remained infinitely patient and reassuring. He tapered the steroids, a process that took six weeks. When I was down to 15 mg, I felt better and was able to return to school.

But by then I wanted to do something else with my future, something less esoteric and isolated than the kind of biological research that I had planned. For one month I had been out of my mind, and it was the most harrowing experience of my life. I needed to serve that experience in some way, and I began to think about psychiatry.

As I pursued admission to medical school, I continued graduate work. In this interim period, during which I was having five to ten watery bowel movements a day, I largely ignored the problem and coped with symptoms superficially. By then, it had become a routine matter to memorize the locations of nearest bathrooms and to avoid cellulose in any form. I learned to drink clear liquids for 24 hours before a date in order to minimize embarrassing trips to the ladies room.

In medical school, I was able to give the "steroid episode" a formal designation: organic affective syndrome. Minus the toxic component, however, the experience would have a different diagnosis and a radically different personal meaning. It would be major depression, and the idea that I had somehow caused it or was vulnerable to relapse would be unshakable. Now, years later, I find this imagined response reified in the minds of my patients, and it leads me to regard the notion of personal responsibility in mental illness as perhaps the most painful of all.

Parallel, though less intense, is the concept of stigma associated with certain medical conditions. This idea never occurred to me until I learned that ulcerative colitis, in classical psychosomatic theory, belongs to a group of chronic diseases whose etiology may be rooted in personality. Though modern psychiatry largely rejects this "illness as metaphor" interpretation, I've heard faculty refer to ulcerative colitis in the context of psychogenic illness and have since been especially reluctant to disclose my condition. Yet I sometimes wonder if I confuse privacy with paranoia—as when I requested a day off for "medical reasons" but would not tell co-workers that I was having a colonoscopy.

In medical school I developed a certain sympathy for patients undergoing minor procedures. Having once been on the tapered end of IVs, nasogastric tubes, barium enemas, and endoscopes, I hated them. Only after much agonizing and procrastination did I finally approach the patient and insert an IV or an NG tube.

Of course this changed when I began internship. I started with a surgical rotation that demanded I modify my approach to procedures. The swiftness with which I conformed, in attitude and pace, to the other surgical house staff surprised me.

At the time of internship, I had ulcerative colitis for seven years and had my own ideas about how frequently one needed a colonoscopy and sigmoidoscopy. Rectal exams seemed unnecessary, simple as they were, because I could easily test my own stool for blood. I had long ago decided to refuse steroids since I couldn't tolerate the mental status changes. Azulfidine did not seem to help and the fact that it was prophylactic against flares seemed meaningless.

My new gastroenterologist was on the staff of the same hospital at which I worked. I was referred to him by one of my medical school instructors up north. I liked my new doctor very much and took care of several of his patients. As my symptoms worsened in the first few months of internship, he recommended that I take prednisone. I was having 10 to 15 watery, bloody bowel movements a day and lost ten pounds. I drank 2 to 3 liters of fluid a day but was constantly thirsty. I knew I wasn't doing well, but I wouldn't take the steroids and assumed I'd get better eventually.

About halfway through the internship year, I had three nights of shaking chills. On the third night I checked my temperature and found it was 104. The next day, I had a private room in a nearby hospital. I didn't think I was very sick; if I had, I would have been terrified of house staff. As it was, I was preoccupied with my dread of steroids.

I argued with my doctor about the necessity of hospitalization in spite of his disbelief at my resistance and at the extent to which I let myself "deteriorate." Orthostasis, anemia, low albumin, and 50% bands won me 300 mg of hydrocortisone a day plus hyperalimentation. I talked my way out of a blood transfusion and considered refusing steroids but knew that this would completely alienate me from my doctor. Later that day, when one of the house staff asked me if I had been seen by a surgeon, I felt defeated and recognized how much I really did need the steroids.

In contrast to my model behavior during the first hospitalization, I was not a good patient the second time around. My friends who were residents at the hospital told me how to call the lab and read the ID number off my wristband to get results. I called at least once a day and was able to inform the intern publicly of the daily lab values when it became clear he hadn't yet checked them. I removed my IV over the protest of a nurse after I started taking fluids. I knew too many tubes of blood were being drawn and when my hydrocortisone and hyperal were hours late.

I would not change into a hospital gown and I rarely left my room. I did not tell my family I was in the hospital and refused to let my doctor contact my father. I discouraged visits from all but close friends, and I did not want my fellow house staff to know why I was in the hospital. I pleaded to go home after four days and was discharged, reluctantly, three days later.

In short, I made my doctor very uncomfortable. He had let me know from the start that my resistance to hospitalization and refusal to inform my family was "very strange." He became increasingly frustrated when I pressured for discharge so I could return to work in a few days. Still, I sensed his genuine concern for me, and soon a friendly kind of tension developed between us.

I wondered whether his trust in me had been damaged; it should have been, but he never seemed to treat me any differently. In fact, he and his associates spent a generous amount of time with me on rounds. I had previously made them aware of my history of steroid-induced depression (even to the point of giving them copies of articles on the topic), and it became an acceptable joke for them to ask, "Are you crazy yet?"

I was discharged on 60 mg of prednisone and Azulfidine and waited to get depressed. To be compliant, I stayed out of work for another week, though I was impatient to get back. Gradually, I realized that I had misinterpreted anxiety as impatience. The strangeness I had known seven years before became sickeningly familiar. I had trouble focusing on a task and thinking clearly. My body housed a subtle interior panic, as if all my organs were restless and writhing in their cavities. I tried to read some cardiology in preparation for the upcoming CCU rotation, but nothing made sense, and I was reduced to agitated whimpering. I immediately began to taper the steroids on my own, knowing that my doctor would be furious. Within a few days I was calm enough to read and write and began the CCU.

The rotation was disastrous. I could hardly remember who my patients were. My orders were variously incomplete, unsigned, or incomprehensible. When on call, I couldn't follow the other interns' signouts. On other nights, I went home hours after the others. I never understood what was happening in a crisis and once actually left the unit after the code team arrived. Constantly on the verge of tears, I couldn't give coherent presentations. I wouldn't make any treatment decisions on my own, though I did maintain a wheezing patient on a beta-blocker.

I was desperate and demoralized but felt unable to explain my situation to other house staff or attendings because I didn't want them to know I was sick in the first place. My doctor and his associate provided emotional support and, as before, I became my old self after the steroids were tapered.

After the intensity of internship, the pace and schedule in psychiatric residency seemed leisurely. My symptoms improved dramatically, literally within two weeks of beginning residency. After nine years, this was the first time it occurred to me that emotional and physical stress could exacerbate ulcerative colitis.

When I remember the CCU experience, which took place almost a year ago, I envision myself in an orbit of sustained frenzy. After just having been an inpatient myself, emotional distance from the CCU patients was difficult to maintain. I recall being struck by the intensity of their hospital experience as compared to mine. The gravity of their illness, depth of their dependence upon staff, and insult to their autonomy seemed devastating. I tried to be empathic but would overshoot to the point of putting myself totally in their places. Then I panicked; it was as if I were incapable of subtle projective imagination. I remember thinking that this could not happen to someone who had never been a patient.

Now that I am in psychiatric residency, the residue of certain experience is still with me. It is my fantasy that I have special insight into the despair of major depression. Indeed, several depressed inpatients have told me I was one of the few who understood them. I am only partly gratified by such patient comments because they are also poignant reminders that I, too, could have been a patient on a psych ward had my depression not remitted with steroid taper.

All this serves to sharpen the consciousness that I bring to my work as a resident on an inpatient psych floor. But the end result is often frustration—as when I see patients' dignity compromised by the excessive scrutiny of their behavior. Patient credibility is low on the unit and reports of behavior are frequently distorted by nurses who present their own interpretation rather than recount the behavior itself. This practice can be meaningful since psychiatric nurses have a considerable role in patient management.

At staff insistence, higher-functioning patients participate in low-level tasks, such as baking cookies. If they demur, this resistance is generally regarded as unwillingness to participate in treatment. Patients are also made vulnerable in community meetings. In these sessions, with both staff and patients present, certain details of an individual patient's history—marital discord, for example—are mentioned. Though it is not intended, the patient frequently feels exposed and embarrassed after such a disclosure.

I deplore these aspects of "treatment" and suppose it is my tendency to identify with depressed patients that predisposes me to such a reaction. I know I would deeply resent such strategy directed at me.

Extrapolation from my experience with chronic disease brings other issues into focus, such as compliance. For nine years I have been inconsistent in using medication and untruthful about the medication I did take. I alternately ignored or minimized my symptoms. I do not know why I did this, but I do know about the sense of confusion and guilt that arises from the suspicion that I may be sabotaging my own health.

The notion of control is important in illness, but it is especially powerful in chronic disease because the vulnerability persists a lifetime. As someone with a decade of inflammatory bowel disease, I know I am at risk for development of malignancy and that, at the first endoscopic sign of dysplasia, my doctor will begin to contemplate surgery. I view this event as a single point along a spectrum of possibilities and, though it is unpleasant to consider, a part of the larger and welcome realization that I am likely to know what can happen to me. Knowledge is control; the comfort of reasonable prediction outweighs the sadness of what may transpire.

Still, I never considered the acquisition of control, through knowledge or anything else, to be my motivation for becoming a physician. At the core of my decision to enter medical school was a desire to help people suffering from mental illness. And so I was surprised when my doctor said he assumed I chose psychiatry so that I could better understand my emotional reaction to ulcerative colitis.

It is true that psychiatric residents spend an inordinate amount of time thinking—mostly about themselves. Indeed, I have thought about the ways in which my disease has influenced me personally and professionally. Some effects are obvious, and I've written about them here, but others are yet to be felt since insight tends to have a latency all its own.

CHAPTER 24

ULCERATIVE COLITIS

"MAURICE RASKIN"

Most of those ills we poor mortals know, from doctors and imagination flow.

—Churchill

It is an equal failing to trust everybody, and to trust nobody.

—Author unknown

The following is a true tale of the effects of a chronic and acute illness on a young physician and his family. The medical aspects of the story have recently concluded (I hope), but the emotional effects are probably still developing. It is difficult to maintain perspective on a series of events that have so affected one's life. My wife or my physicians might write quite a different account.

I am a 26-year-old medical fellow at a major medical center in the Northeast. I was in good health until late in my second year of medical school, when I developed a moderately severe case of ulcerative colitis—bloody diarrhea without discernable cause. At that time, a sigmoidoscopy exam revealed disease to at least the upper reach of the instrument. This initial attack responded to treatment with salicylosulfapyridine alone, without hospitalization or the use of steroids. I continued to take medication prophylactically after the acute episode, under the care of a physician while in medical school, and did not hear from my lower bowel for the next few years.

At some point during this healthy period, though, I acquired a secretive stance toward my illness. I recall feeling that no one cared. In addition, I was especially sensitive to the generalizations that seemed prevalent among fellow physicians about patients with ulcerative colitis—whining young women with emotional problems. I recall in

"DR. MAURICE RASKIN" is a fellow at a northeastern medical center.

particular my personal physician during medical school taking me with him to see a patient in the emergency room: a young woman with inflammatory bowel disease.

The patient was lying on a stretcher, crying uncontrollably and complaining of abdominal pain. Her exam was benign, so my physician tried to calm her by revealing in a voice loud enough to be heard through the sobs, "See this young doctor here? He has colitis, too!"

I felt my face redden. I wanted to look behind me to see whether anyone had heard him. Could I be compared to a patient who shared only a disease process with me? I felt, "Certainly not," and proceeded to make that clear. My method consisted mainly of denial of illness.

The denial took many forms. One was my lack of curiosity about the extent of my disease. I had many reasons for not getting a barium enema, but it all boiled down to my not wanting to know. Strangely, it was easier to ignore my illness and continue to function as though everything were normal than to be brought face to face with the uncomfortable reality. This is a process we see often in our patients as well.

Lack of curiosity about my illness, however, did not apply to the disease as an abstraction or as something other people had. I quickly became adept in the diagnosis and treatment of inflammatory bowel disease. I took an elective in gastroenterology, learned to do sigmoidoscopies, and never shied away from treating patients with inflammatory bowel disease later as a medical resident in New York.

I suffered a second attack of ulcerative colitis, despite a prophylactic regimen of sulfasalazine as a junior resident. I had coincidentally just finished a rotation on the gastroenterology service.

I felt confident that I could handle my own treatment, provided I could avoid hospitalization and treat myself. I started a regimen of high-dose oral steroids and steroid enemas and continued to work. The treatment was a success in that the attack subsided and I was able to taper off steroids, but only after six months of life-disrupting bloody diarrhea.

Life went on as usual after that prolonged attack had ended. One tends quickly to forget pain and discomfort once it has ceased. To remember it is to renew it. I did live with a certain fear of another attack, though continuing to take sulfasalazine religiously. There is no surer way to achieve 100% compliance with medication regimens than to have a patient galvanized with fear.

My next academic and cultural milestone was a fellowship in gastroenterology at Famous-University Hospital (F-UH). My girlfriend transferred her residency to F-UH, and we became engaged. We both suffered drastic cuts in stipends, but being at Famous was considered compensation enough.

Health was not a problem until March of my first fellowship year, when an attack, much worse than my previous two, began. High-dose oral steroids seemed to be of no benefit and anorexia became a problem. In six weeks I lost over 20 pounds, going from a lean baseline to a walking skeleton.

Still I resisted seeking medical help. Rationalizations now included: "What more can they do, short of surgery?" and "I have to keep going until after the wedding or else I'll be admitted and we'll have to cancel the wedding." My fiancée reluctantly went along with this, with the proviso that I see a Famous gastroenterologist right after our weekend honeymoon.

Meanwhile I continued to work under what can only be viewed now as comical circumstances. During the worst of my attack, I had to plan my day carefully around irregular bathroom breaks. I stuffed bathroom tissue in my pockets (imagine if there were none), had a roll of paper towels under the front seat of my car (less obvious than a roll of toilet paper), and cursed the lack of restrooms in the hospital parking garage. I often could barely make it from home to the hospital lobby.

I took to coming in late every day to conserve my limited energies. I made believe I was somewhere in the hospital if paged while still at home. I was able to get away with this because, as a consultant, I had no primary patient responsibility. Another problem was being paged in a restroom. Why weren't there telephones within an arm's length of the bowl as in all the new Hilton hotels?

As time wore on I became progressively weaker. I began waiting for elevators, even to go down one flight, leaning against walls to rest whenever I could do so without being seen. I also sat on patients' beds whenever feasible during visits. I often experienced light-headedness, but I concluded that it was not due to anemia because the hematocrits I checked on myself were always normal. I did consider that they might be falsely elevated because of dehydration, but I rejected that interpretation because I thought I was drinking plenty.

I must have looked as though I was headed for the wrong side of moribund, because the chairman of my department pulled me aside late one afternoon and asked me if I were having upper gastrointestinal bleeding from an ulcer or something? "Close, but no cigar," I thought, tempted to tell him the truth then and there. But the wedding was less than a week away. He told me to take the rest of the week off and rest up for the wedding. I gratefully assented.

The wedding took place as scheduled. Despite my fear that I would be hauled off in an ambulance just before the ceremony, only a few people, all physician friends whom I had not seen in a while, commented that I looked as if I needed some time off from work. Although it is considered impolite to tell someone that he does not look well, that is an inhibition physicians tend to lose.

The Monday after my wedding, true to my vows, I turned my care over to a Famous gastroenterologist. He promptly admitted me to the hospital. For privacy, I chose to enter a community hospital rather than F-UH. Much to no one's surprise but my own, after hydration I clocked in at a hematocrit of 30 and an albumin of 2.0. I was treated with intravenous steroids and peripheral parenteral hyperalimentation for a few weeks and left the hospital ten pounds heavier, with my hematocrit close to normal and having only two bowel movements per day.

The improvement proved to be short-lived, however. Within a week, I developed fever and anorexia and was readmitted, this time to F-UH. We wanted all the resources of a tertiary care referral center available should I require surgery emergently. There were disadvantages as well, though.

One aspect of university hospitalization is the greater lack of personal privacy, which inevitably obtains owing mostly to the presence of numerous students and house staff. Although there are benefits in having an extra half dozen bright young people involved in one's care, the amount of traffic through the patient's room and across an already tender abdomen is vastly increased. As a physician still in training myself, I found it difficult to limit student and house staff visits, even when I was tired and sick. If the truth be known, though, rarely will the patient be better served by legions of house staff than by a single highly competent attending physician. The unfortunate tendency with too many cooks is to overtest and overtreat.

My F-UH hospitalization lasted three weeks and was marked by a poor response. I was still not psychologically prepared to accept colectomy. I reasoned that I had gotten over long flares before and this one would run its course as well if I could hold off the surgeons for another few days. Had I been more receptive, surely most gastroenterologists would have strongly recommended surgery at that time. I recall that when my primary physician was away for a few days, the faculty member covering him tried to shock me into reality by telling me that the odds were slim that I would improve without surgery, given the duration of my nonresponse to intravenous steroids. My response was resentment. "It's not his body," I thought. I was then even more determined to get better, and that is indeed what happened.

I left the hospital considerably weakened, on moderately high-dose oral steroids, and returned to work after a few weeks' recuperation at home. I never really felt well, though, despite being able to work. I became anorexic and began to have more frequent, bloody bowel movements. Within a couple of weeks, I had lost ten pounds and was having bowel movements every hour through the night. At that point I had had enough and asked to be admitted for surgery.

I considered two surgical options. One, standard colectomy and ileostomy; and two, Park's procedure. The latter involved two operations, was not always successful in reducing the number of bowel movements, and necessitated going to another institution where the surgeons were experienced in it. I decided to hedge my bets by having a colectomy without abdominoperineal resection, but with stripping of the mucosa of the rectal remnant. Thus, the option of having the Park's procedure at a later date remained.

I awaited my cure with a sense of relief. There is an aura of perpetual optimism in the field of surgery that does not exist in medicine. The sword would surely be mightier than the pill. I discussed various aspects of my care with the surgical residents taking care of me (one of whom was a friend). Thinking back, I cannot recall any fear of the operation or its consequences—to operate seemed clearly the right decision. Yet I suspect that fear was indeed present, but kept in check by my insistence on being involved in all aspects of my care. I would not give up control until it could not be avoided.

I refused preoperative sedation—"I'm not nervous"—and had personally chosen both the anesthesiologist and the resident doing my case. I remember the last thing I said before the induction of anesthesia: "We'd better change that IV, it's getting phlebitic." The first thing I asked upon awakening in the recovery room was "How long was it?"

The answer surprised me. The operation had taken five hours, considerably longer than expected. I later learned that the faculty surgeon had done every stitch himself ("skin to skin"), the chief resident and second assistant only retracting and keeping the field clear. In addition, every bleeder was tied rather than cauterized to minimize bleeding and avoid a transfusion.

The first postoperative night sticks in my mind. I was groggy from anesthesia and, later, narcotics, thirsty and sore-throated from intubation and a nasogastric tube, and restless but barely able to move because of pain and weakness. I had asked for a private-duty nurse for the first postoperative night.

My parents, softer touches than my wife or the doctors, wound up staying with me until 4:00 a.m. From childhood I could remember that whenever anyone in my family was particularly ill, he had a private-duty nurse for a while. I was in a sense claiming my birthright, relying on tradition to help me through a period of uncertainty. I was irrationally attached to the idea and could not understand the attempt to deprive me of it. I viewed this as a sign that no one cared.

The first postoperative days were marked by apparently normal recovery, with steady removal of accumulated foreign bodies—urinary and nasogastric. I was even being told of a tentative early discharge date, but, about a week after surgery, I "spiked a fever" of 101 degrees. Initial physical examination, lab tests, and chest X-rays were unremarkable. A small peristomal abscess was incised and allowed to drain.

When the fevers and abdominal pain continued, broad-spectrum antibiotics were begun. A red herring appeared, in the form of a single blood culture, drawn through a central line, which grew Staphylococcus aureus. This delayed the correct diagnosis, I believe. I was now regularly spiking through broad-spectrum antibiotics, acetaminophen, and steroids as my leukocyte count approached 30,000, mostly early forms. My abdomen remained relatively nontender, but I was in nearly constant pain, exacerbated by any movement.

What was most remarkable through this period of undiagnosed fevers and general deterioration was widespread denial by my physicians of the gravity of the situation. It should have been quite obvious that something was seriously wrong, but it took seven days for the correct noninvasive diagnostic test to be performed. My surgical resident-friend even went so far as to declare that I was not having an unusual postoperative course. My wife had to insist on an infectious disease consultation, which also failed to mention the correct diagnosis in its assessment.

With the first temperature elevation, given my persistent ileus and abdominal pain, my wife had asked me what I thought the most likely source of my fever was. I replied, "intraabdominal abscess," and she agreed. I was not pleased with her blunt assessment but began to press for a CT scan or an ultrasound to "rule out" an abscess. My attending gastroenterologist tried to persuade me to back off from involvement in my care, to instead "Read something." My surgeon was more inclined to wait—whatever was causing my fever would eventually become manifest.

I had already built up a silent resentment of my surgeon before this. He had, I felt, breached my trust by never discussing with me personally the nature of the operation he had performed. Each day I waited for him to explain why the procedure we had agreed upon was departed from in one key aspect: He had not stripped the rectal mucosa, thereby committing me to a future operation to accomplish this. I realize that the best approach would have been to ask him about it directly. My mind-set at the time, however, was to trust no one until he or she had proved both capable and caring. The surgeon was from the "old school," though, and told patients only what they needed to know or insisted on knowing. Regardless of the merit, or lack thereof, in my case against him, it was convenient to have a scapegoat for my woes.

As the physician-reader has surmised by now, the CT scan revealed a massive intraabdominal abscess. Water-soluble contrast failed to show direct leakage from bowel to abscess cavity, so the next day a catheter was placed percutaneously with ultrasound guidance, and liters of pus were drained. I had defervesced the day before the abscess was drained, no doubt in anticipation. Improvement from that point on was slow but steady. The catheter stayed in place for at least three weeks as I underwent weekly "abscessograms" to reposition the catheter and assess shrinkage of the abscess cavity. I had been hospitalized for nearly a month, so I completed the last weeks of drainage at home on oral antibiotics and trailing a portable vacuum pump.

A difficult patient to begin with, I became even more so as my hospitalization lengthened and the complications accumulated. One day I noticed that a nurse was injecting into my central line nonsterilely and began to watch more carefully (I had already had central line sepsis, thank you). It happened twice more, despite a lecture by the head nurse reminding everyone to "prep" her lines.

Another pet peeve of mine was prevention of the clogged intravenous syndrome. Some nurses use an automatic pump to administer intravenous medications, which provides safeguards against clogging, while others let the medication run in by gravity and try to come back when the medication has finished running in. If the nurse is late with the latter method, the intravenous may be ruined and a new one has to be started. Cursed by this knowledge and ever-vigilant, for lack of anything better to do, I would switch the intravenous myself if the medication ran out and the nurse had not returned. I became self-appointed Auditor of Nursing Services, a job that required only a flashlight (for middle-of-the-night assessment of line patency) and a sufficiently compulsive nature. I found it very difficult to trust anyone with my care.

I did finally get better, but unfortunately, the story did not end with removal of the catheter draining my abscess. Repeat CT scan showed a reaccumulation of the abscess, though much smaller than the original one. This time the cavity was not conveniently located for percutaneous drainage but abutted the rectal remnant and appeared accessible transrectally.

Resigned to my fate, I reentered the hospital. The next day I was taken to the operating room. My surgeon labored in vain for two hours trying to blunt dissect into the abscess cavity through the rectum. While I was still under anesthesia, he called my wife to obtain consent for an immediate transabdominal drainage operation. (We had not discussed this possibility, so he could not simply go ahead.) Fortunately, my wife demurred, knowing that I would be furious if surgery were performed without my concurrence.

Instead, the procedure was terminated. In the recovery room, I was told my options. The surgeon recommended abdominal drainage with healing by secondary intention to ensure that the reaccumulation would not occur again. The alternative was CT-guided drainage, which we had been told would be via a difficult transgluteal approach. I told him that I was favoring the surgical option. That was a Saturday.

The next morning, the chief of CT radiology came to see me and enthusiastically showed me my films, declaring that by computer reconstruction of the various cuts, he had found a better "window" for a percutaneous drainage. He also brought an article about the favorable success rate of percutaneous versus surgical drainage. Although the first percutaneous drainage had failed, I was not at all enthusiastic about the prospect of another prolonged hospitalization for surgical drainage, especially with healing by secondary intention, and decided to give interventional radiology another try. The radiologist said that he had talked to my surgeon and would inform him that he planned to attempt a percutaneous drainage Monday morning.

My surgeon did not make rounds that Sunday, so I did not see him prior to the CT drainage. That Sunday evening, the house staff on call were unable to start my intravenous line, despite multiple attempts. Knowing that my veins were poor as a result of long hospitalizations, and anticipating an ongoing need for intravenous antibiotics, I felt a central line was in order and called my surgeon for his opinion. He said, "You have my permission to do whatever you want. You've been making the decisions all along." I recognized a hint of anger behind his perceptually even tones but interpreted it as meaning that he did not want a central line. So the intravenous stayed out.

Later that evening I got a call from my surgeon, this time overtly angry. One thing led to another and three months of suppressed hostilities were laid out on both sides. He told me he could not deal with my making decisions then changing my mind. "None of this would have happened if I had been allowed to do the operation I wanted to do in the first place."

Finally, the rejection: "I will see you through this, but, if CT does not work, I cannot just drop what I'm doing and operate on you. You will have to decide, then, who you want to be your surgeon."

This exchange had occurred at the worst possible time. I felt very much alone and fearful that the CT drainage would not succeed.

The next morning, my wife mediated a reconciliation between us, and I went on to the CT scan. Miraculously, the abscess had disappeared over the weekend. I can only theorize that the blunt dissection

Saturday had opened an unrecognized channel that allowed for drainage or resorption of the abscess. In any case, luck had finally found me and I was discharged the next day, this time to continue oral antibiotics for several weeks. I have remained well since that time.

What can be learned from my adventures in the land of the ill? We will all visit this land sometime in our lives, unless we are spared by sudden death or nuclear holocaust. One question is: What is good care, and who gets it?

Despite the ideal that all patients should be treated alike, we know that this does not happen. As physicians, we may spend more time with, and go out of our way to facilitate the care of, patients we have a personal liking or respect for. There is also a tendency for nurses as well as doctors to lavish more attention on young patients with critical or terminal illness than on old patients with the same problem. Patients with rare or dramatic illness also command more and better care.

Standards of care vary widely. As a resident, I have seen many examples of suboptimal care. From that standpoint, it is easy to ignore the lapses, rationalizing that doctors and nurses are human, and that most of the incidents result in no significant harm to the patient. As a patient, it is harder to find excuses for sloppy care. As a patient, I got the distinct impression that we, as physicians, are aware of only a minority of the sloppy care that is delivered. Our patients, of course, are aware of even fewer of these instances.

It is an old saw that physician-patients get poor care. Certainly, unless they choose to disguise their identities like movie idols, physicians fall into the category of patients who tend to get extra attention. This itself is beneficial to the physician-patient. What I think can be detrimental are two phenomena, both resulting from care providers' identification with their patient.

The first is what I call the "bending the rules phenomenon." There was an unspoken tendency in my case to spare me those procedures and tests that were considered uncomfortable or nonessential. For example, there was no insistence for a long time on making a pathological diagnosis of my disease. I did not receive the standard bowel prep at all prior to my surgery. My nasogastric tube was removed a day earlier than it would have been because I complained about throat irritation. I was encouraged to use narcotics freely for any discomfort. Clinical judgment was compromised for issues of little importance.

Second is a denial when things go wrong, as I described in my postoperative course. Why this occurs I can only speculate. One might argue that everyone really knew that I had probably developed an abscess, but denied it so as not to alarm me, just as we would never tell a patient that he probably has cancer until the diagnosis is ironclad. This went a step beyond that, though. The denial was to themselves as well. My care providers did not want anything to go wrong, so they had difficulty seeing things as they were. Taking care of another physician can be like taking care of a close relative. You have something more at stake in the outcome than with the ordinary patient.

What is at stake probably varies with the caretaker. Some may simply identify with their physician-patient (there, but for. . .); others may worry subconsciously that their professional reputation is at risk. It is rightly considered an honor to be asked to care for another physician, because it means to everyone that you are highly thought of by your peers. One must live up to such honors, though. Lots of other physicians at your institution may be following the case with a special interest. A poor outcome, even if unavoidable, reflects badly on the care provider.

How, then, does one guard against the problems inherent in treating other physicians? I think the solution is to recognize the potential pitfalls and to ask oneself at each step, "Is this precisely what I would do for ordinary patients?"

A related issue is: Should a physician care for patients with an illness that the physician has suffered? Again, the answer will depend on the individual and how he has dealt with his illness. One may make the mistake of going one step beyond laudable empathy toward one's patients and become sympathetic, an emotion that can color one's judgment. A personal example of this was brought to my attention by an attending gastroenterologist with whom I had worked while I was healthy. He learned of my recent surgery and said, "Now I understand why you never wanted to operate." It was true. When patients were admitted with ulcerative colitis, I would be the proponent of conservative medical management for longer than anyone else on the team. This was undoubtedly a reflection of my own fears of undergoing surgery at that time. On the other hand, once personal difficulties have been resolved or worked through, the physician who has suffered a chronic illness may be better equipped to deal compassionately and effectively with that illness and with others. One must guard, though, against using one's illness as a means of cutting off patients' complaints. For example, I was once treated to the following enlightened view of what it means to be ill: "I was hospitalized myself once; it was not pleasant having ____. But, I got through it." That effectively ended the conversation.

This raises an important point about the physician's view of the nature of the sick role. I believe that doctors, by and large, associate illness with weakness. We belie our feelings by our preference for certain modes of patient behavior. The dependent, complaining patient is considered weak, stupid, and generally less worthy than the independent patient. The Puritan ethic clearly prevails among U.S. physicians. Patients earn the respect of their caretakers when they are stoical—the "silent sufferers." I recall being complimented by my attending and others when I withstood the obvious pain of incision and drainage of a small peristomal infection without flinching.

Finally, how should one try to behave as a patient, and more, important, does this tell us something about how we should, perhaps, treat our own patients?

Serious illness is something we all fear, consciously or not, because it represents uncertainty and a loss of control. Those who manage their illness with minimal loss of control are admired. Loss of control is particularly dreaded by physicians, who are expected to be in control not only of their own lives but of those of others as well. I don't think one can prescribe proper patient behavior. Your caretaker should be a good enough physician to deal appropriately with a wide variety of patterns. Although it was very trying for my physicians to have a patient who insisted on participating in all decision making, it would have been psychologically out of character, and wrong, for me to relinquish control. I would have been a nervous wreck wondering whether the right things were being done. Other patients, however, might be more comfortable relinquishing more control.

In general, I now believe that patients should be encouraged to retain as much control over their care as they want, and are capable of handling. There is no place in the practice of medicine for paternalism. (In pediatrics, maybe.) We do no public service by fostering dependency in competent adults.

Has being ill changed me as a person? I went through an experience as a young adult that most people do not encounter until they have reached an advanced age. In a sense, then, I have been aged by my illness. I have become more appreciative of the world around me and less concerned with what people think about me. I am more self-reliant.

I feel closer to the relatives and friends who have shared my plight. And I hope that I have become just a bit wiser. After all, it would be quite a shame to have been at the gates of hell and not learned from the journey.

CHAPTER 25

ULCERATIVE COLITIS

MALLORY STEPHENS

I was not an average child. I suppose I really was, but I didn't feel like one. When I was 4 or 5 years old, I realized that my father had a special position in life. He was a politician! And a very active one, to boot. He was a farmer, a businessman, and an assemblyman. His district included an entire small county.

When he was first elected, he knew the first names of his 3000 constituents. At the end of his 27 years as a New York state assemblyman, he represented almost 30,000 people and he still knew most of them. But I remember the slurs, accusations, and nasty remarks that I overheard about my father. He was also the committee chairman of his political party for the county and eventually became chairman of the influential Ways and Means Committee. He befriended elected officials and worked closely with the Speaker of the Assembly and the governor. He was an influential man.

All this affected me in a way that I am still not sure I understand, except that in my mind, he could do almost anything, and perhaps I felt unable to live up to such a level of achievement. With his political influence, he "arranged" an internship for me at a municipal hospital which I felt wouldn't have been possible to obtain on my own merit.

Within a week after graduating from medical school, I married one of the most beautiful and wonderful women a man could ever want. We honeymooned at a small private hotel in Bermuda. Shortly after returning from this paradise, we plunged into work—my wife as a secretary and I as a green intern. The patient load was large and I was extremely busy.

As everyone knows, an intern's hours are long enough, but because of my guilt regarding my father's influence in obtaining the internship, I felt the need to perform above and beyond the call of duty. Therefore, I did everything possible to enhance the welfare of all my

DR. MALLORY STEPHENS is a 57-year-old rheumatologist who has a solo practice in Mt. Kisco, New York. He is affiliated with the Hospital for Special Surgery.

patients. The hospital I worked in gave almost complete responsibility for the care of each patient to the assigned intern. At that hospital over 30 years ago, the residents were treated and regarded as consultants. I can remember the times when I desperately wanted help for an acutely ill patient and had difficulty locating the resident on call.

In the medical school I had attended, I think the largest responsibility given to me was starting an intravenous infusion in a patient. Perhaps the stress of all this new responsibility, the long working hours, lack of sleep, and the guilt I felt regarding my appointment to this municipal hospital helped bring on my illness. Or perhaps it was related to my being a country boy who was plunged into a busy, demanding, inner-city hospital where microorganisms were waiting to invade.

In 1954, all interns at the hospital where I worked wore high-collared white shirts, white pants, and, unless we were doing some particularly active work, white coats. One day, I had eaten a hurried lunch of a hamburger and large strawberry milkshake. While riding up the elevator to the ward where my patients were bedded, I felt a violent cramp across my lower abdomen and the urge to move my bowels. If I had been able to move toward a toilet, I would have done so instantaneously, but this was impossible, as the old elevator with at least half dozen other people in it moved slowly upwards. Within seconds, I felt another giant cramp unlike anything I had ever felt before grip my lower abdomen and, to my surprise and chagrin, I felt a bowel movement being expelled. Immediately, my face flushed with surprise and anger. Never before had I lost control of my bowels!

As the elevator finally came to a stop, I rushed to the nearest bathroom to find the back of my trouser leg bright red. My embarrassment escalated while cleaning them, because the red color would not disappear and there was no way to change them for a clean pair. All my other trousers were at our apartment, over an hour away, and I was already 10 or 15 minutes late. I cleaned my clothing as much as possible, put them on again in their wet condition and walked like a whipped pup to the ward, fully expecting that on seeing the red stain on my pants, everyone would suddenly stop, stand back, open their eyes widely, raise their eyebrows, and shout, "Ugh!"

I was relieved when I got past the first few nurses, interns, and patients without any of them expressing surprise or scorn. As the afternoon progressed, my ever-perceptive resident asked me if I was all right, and I assured him and myself that this was just a case of acute gastroenteritis. One of my fellow interns offered to cover while I went and changed, but I gratefully informed him that that was impossible.

The next day I brought an extra uniform to the hospital and made sure to have a ready change if need be. As the weeks wore on, the bloody diarrhea continued but the lower abdominal cramps were not as severe as in the elevator. The amazing thing is that I generally felt well and never missed a day of work. Perhaps that helped me convince myself that I need not see a physician. Since the bloody diarrhea had continued for weeks, I realized that this was not acute gastroenteritis. It could not even be attributed to my internal hemorrhoids, which I had had for years. Could it be ulcerative colitis or was it a curable disease—something like amebiasis, maybe? After six months, with considerable ambivalence, I made an appointment to see the hospital physician at the employee clinic. Why I went to him I don't know. He was not a gastroenterologist.

During the initial interview, which lasted no more than five minutes, I described my symptoms and the physician examined my throat and abdomen. He told me to come back for a sigmoidoscopy and gave me a slip for a barium enema, which was performed before the sigmoidoscopy. The barium enema was within normal limits, which should have relieved me, but instead it raised my curiosity.

The two-week wait for the sigmoidoscopy drove me into a mental frenzy. If the barium enema was normal, what could possibly cause this problem? Could it be cancer? If it was malignant, I was prepared to raise hell with the employee clinic physician for putting the sigmoidoscopy off for two whole weeks.

I was expecting the worst. To my surprise, he performed the procedure expertly and gently but rapidly explained that I had ulcerative colitis that was localized in the rectum. He prescribed Azulfidine, which I took for a month or so without any noticeable effect and then stopped.

During the year of hard work and long hours (often I worked through the entire night for 35 or 36 hours straight, stopping only for brief periods to rest), I learned to live with my condition and adjust to it. My wife, who looked forward to the little time we had together, grieved at my long absences and the lack of communication, which she had been so used to in our small town. Not infrequently when I would come home late in the evening, I would fall asleep at the dinner table while eating. What a joyful spouse I must have been! Any other woman would have walked out and said, "Good riddance!"

In spite of my illness, my work was above average. I was one of only a handful of over 100 interns whom the chief of medicine commended with a letter for a high rate of autopsies.

In general, this internship was extremely demanding—far more so than most others. The hospital had over 3000 beds and they were full most of the time. One busy day, I personally admitted 16 patients. We had attending rounds six days a week, chief resident rounds every evening, chief of service rounds weekly, grand rounds weekly, and—if you had any time and interest left after all these, which were more or less mandatory—there were the subspecialty rounds.

In addition, we were required to do all the basic laboratory work on our own patients. Every time we gave a patient a blood transfusion, except in an extremely rare situation where it was considered more important to keep the patient alive at that instant, we checked the type and cross-match to make sure the blood bank had done it properly. In addition, we quite frequently had to wheel our patients to the X-ray department. We almost always took the electrocardiograms. In addition to room and board plus our uniforms, we actually received a check from the city of New York in the amount of $50 per month.

I mention the above because even for an intern in the best of health, life was difficult. And my health was—to say the least—not the best. Diarrhea afflicted me daily—usually 4 to 12 bloody bowel movements a day. The more stressed and fatigued I felt, the more severe the diarrhea. The malaise I felt was profound. I would feel tired for weeks, even months, at a time. Many people noticed that I did not look well. I looked pale, sallow, and thin. My weight dropped about ten pounds.

Ignoring my feelings, I continued to work as hard as, or harder than, my confreres. Frequently, it was a race to the nearest bathroom to avoid soiling my clothes. I wasn't always successful in keeping them clean, but if necessary, I could go to nearby quarters for a change to fresh clothes. Throughout the first year, I kept hoping that this condition would somehow remit and allow me to feel better, but it never did. Interestingly—and perhaps this was discouraging too—beyond a certain point, rest did not seem to affect the disease much.

I read the textbooks regarding not only ulcerative colitis and regional enteritis but anything else causing diarrhea and bloody stools. Then I surreptitiously sent my stool under a patient's name for culture. To my disappointment, instead of returning as *Salmonella, Shigella,* or something curable, it returned as *Escherichia coli*. The examination for parasites was also unrevealing. Several years later, I relearned that amebiasis has a cycle and stools have to be checked every three or four days at least three times, or the cysts can be missed. As soon as possible, I examined my stools every day for two weeks but never found anything that even looked close to a parasite. Although I am a rheumatologist, my familiarity with the gastroenterological literature far exceeds the average physician's, probably because of the constant hope that something helpful will be discovered.

Somehow with all my problems, I was able to obtain a medical residency in another municipal hospital in a different part of the same city. I obtained this completely on my own, without any help or even the knowledge of my father. Perhaps this should have relieved me and unburdened some of the guilt I was so laden with, but my symptoms continued.

The hospital was associated with an outstanding medical school, the Albert Einstein College of Medicine. There was a certain excitement and pride in being associated with an institution that had so much hope and potential. The teaching exceeded my expectations and was of consistently high quality. As the year progressed, my intellectual stimulation and enjoyment reached heights I had never previously known. For the first time in my life, I realized that the academic and theoretical realm was inextricably linked with the real and practical world.

Perhaps because of this environment, I immersed myself almost totally in the care of my patients, learning everything possible to help them.

My wife had continued to work in Manhattan to support us. One evening after work, she expressed her feelings about our life and its effect on her and on us as a couple. We both felt that life for us could be better. Shortly thereafter, I spoke to a friend who was a resident in psychiatry. He saw her and helped her through a difficult period. Following this, she decided she wanted to enter into psychoanalysis. After considerable discussion and consideration of our finances, arrangements were made with an attending physician and she began.

The year passed rapidly and it was necessary to enter the army. The Selective Service had been trying to induct me into the armed forces since shortly after graduation from medical school. I had successfully avoided their clutches, but now the time had come to pay the dues. We spent the next two years in Maryland at Fort Detrick, which was then the biological warfare center for the U.S. Army. Life was different. It was so much easier than anything I had known since college. We only worked 40 hours a week plus every fourth night. Even on the nights we were on call, the physician slept most or all of the night. It was unusual to admit even one or two patients to the hospital during such a period. In general, life was so easy that I could hardly adjust.

I read the current medical literature extensively. As part of an assignment at work, I reviewed the world literature on typhoid fever and then wrote an extensive summary. During our stay there, my wife developed pain and morning stiffness in the proximal interphalangeal joints of her fingers. After several months of these symptoms, she saw my immediate commanding officer, who was an internist. After a physical exam and blood tests, he informed her that she had rheumatoid arthritis. Later, he informed me of his findings and diagnosis. In his attempts to lessen the impact of this information, he indicated that it might be best if I did not think about what the future would be like regarding my wife's health. This unnecessarily concerned me for a long time, whereas now, 30 years later, I know she has done relatively well.

After completing the mandatory time, I went back to the same hospital and medical school as a second-year resident in medicine. I was one of only three residents chosen by the chairman of the department of medicine to continue the program and complete the residency. I was a rather formidable house officer, easily able to discuss most topics with the third-year residents, attendings, and professors. After spending most or all of the night caring for acutely ill patients, we would stand and discuss all the diagnostic measures done and to be done, and then the choices of therapy. Occasionally, to my surprise and delight, I ordered or did something for a patient that a senior resident or attending did not understand or was not familiar with. It was a pleasure to explain to them my reasoning underlying such measures and to banter the pros and cons of a certain test or treatment.

A man was admitted one night and, with my background, I quickly made the diagnosis of typhoid fever before the cultures or antibody titers returned. The stool and blood cultures actually grew out *Salmonella choleraesuis*, but the treatment instigated so promptly probably saved the patient's life. As a resident, I was honored to be asked to discuss *Salmonella* infections at grand rounds shortly thereafter, since the discussant at such occasions had always been an attending physician or professor.

The year of hard work and intellectual stimulation was suddenly over. I felt somewhat disappointed at the time because my wish to become chief resident was not fulfilled. Instead, much to my gratitude in later years, I became a fellow in rheumatology, the first to hold that position at the new medical school. The section chief, who was my mentor, was a wonderful person. Not only was he exceptionally pleasant, but he was a brilliant investigator and teacher. We spent most of our time in the laboratory trying to understand all we could about the synovial membrane. To the best of my knowledge, I was the first physician in New York City to perform a closed joint biopsy.

During this year, my wife, who was undergoing psychoanalysis, encouraged me to do likewise. I resisted her efforts for several months but finally realized that our relationship might be better if I, too, were to enter it.

With my residency and fellowship completed, I began work at the Rockefeller Institute and began the emotional process first instigated by Sigmund Freud. In the beginning, I was awed by the beautiful buildings and laboratories, the easy availability of animals, the relative freedom of designing and running my own experiments. Among the most pleasant features were the lunches served at Founder's Hall. At that time, every scientist could eat in the main dining room and be served excellent food by waitresses. In such a way, each person was exposed to the multiple and exciting ideas of leading investigators from many different scientific disciplines. Several were Nobel prize winners.

My work was basically involved in two studies. My mentor was Rene Dubos. Dr. Dubos had a lifelong interest in tuberculosis, so I fed hundreds of mice diets high in unsaturated fatty acids and then infected them with the tubercle bacillus. I found that the more highly unsaturated fatty acid diets increased the animals' susceptibility to TB.

The other aspect of my work was even more interesting. Mice would be checked with stool cultures and then given various antibiotics. Their stools would be examined during and after the periods of antibiotic administration. During the three years spent doing research in this laboratory, I thought a great deal about the gastrointestinal tract. I came to feel that man has only begun to scratch the surface of what might become known regarding the gut. Reflect, if you will, that the gut is man's direct connection with the rest of the world. Depending on what he eats and/or drinks, he lives or dies. Enzymes help digest food, but why do we and other animals have billions of bacteria in our gut? Surely they help digest our food so it can be absorbed and converted into energy, but is that their only function? Why do the bacteria that usually inhabit the GI tract remain localized inside the lumen? And why are some bacteria such as *Salmonella typhosa* capable of invading the intestinal wall and migrating into and up the lymphatic vessels into the nodes and even the bloodstream?

After three years of this fascinating place, I decided to enter private practice. Although I enjoyed the research work at the Rockefeller Institute, I came to realize with the help of my psychoanalyst that caring for and helping patients is what I really wanted to do.

I decided to subspecialize and just practice rheumatology. To my surprise and delight, my practice doubled within a few months and tripled and quadrupled not long after.

Late one afternoon, after a year of being considerably busier, I spiked a fever to 104 and developed a large inguinal node on the left side. After phoning a friend who had also been a medical resident in the Bronx and was a practicing internist in Mt. Kisco, I followed his advice and went to the emergency room, where another friend who is a surgeon met and examined me. He diagnosed a perirectal abscess. Within a few hours, I had been started on antibiotics and IV fluids, and was whisked to the operating room, where a large incision and drainage was performed.

Upon awakening in the hospital room, I can remember the excruciating, searing, knifelike pain inside my rectum and perineum. I must have screamed, because shortly thereafter a nurse gave me an injection of morphine sulfate with relief in about five minutes. This promptly put me to sleep, but within two hours I was awake again, screaming in pain, only to be relieved by morphine again. As this cycle was repeated, I feared and had already convinced myself that I was a hopeless narcotic addict. It was with great relief that I heard my physician say that I was having pain from the inflammation in and around my rectum and that the injections were necessary for relief. Within a few days, the abscess ruptured through my perineum on the right side, causing a fistula that became permanent. To my consternation, after the abscess drained, the pain persisted. I remained in the hospital as a patient for several weeks, which seemed like an eternity. Even at the end of the hospital stay, I would have periods of excruciating pain relieved only by an injection of meperidine. The only way I could explain such intense pain was that perhaps the perineal muscles went into spasm.

When I went home, I was concerned that I might need an injection and would be unable to get it quickly enough. Fortunately, when I would feel the pain mounting, I quickly immersed my trunk in a tub of warm water with relief. For several more weeks, I remained in bed at home, wearing gauze bandages over my anus and perineum. Altogether, I lost six weeks' worth of work owing to this complication of my disease.

Sometimes it seems that disaster strikes doubly. Within a few days after returning home, while I was still confined to bed, our son fell down a fireman's pole at the village playground and fractured his femur. In the emergency room of our local hospital, a friend who had trained with me in the Bronx and was in practice in orthopedics placed him in a body cast extending from under his arms to his toes on the side of the fracture and to his knee on the other side. He remained in the hospital overnight but the next day was home in his own bed, lying supine like his father.

My wife performed like a true Florence Nightingale, running back and forth ministering to both of us. She would pick up our son with his heavy cast, bring him into our bedroom, and place him on her bed so that we could be together. I would read and tell stories to him and we would watch television together.

Finally, it was time to remove his cast. To my deep chagrin, when our son was brought home without his cast, instead of being more active, he lay in bed barely moving. As this profound passiveness continued all afternoon, all evening, and even the next morning, my concern mounted to the point where I telephoned the orthopedist. He reassured me that a child incorporates a cast into his body image, and when it is removed, the child reacts almost as if he or she has had an amputation. This made me feel much better. Shortly thereafter, our son began moving his legs and later his body. Within a few days, he was back on his feet.

I felt extremely grateful that my son had made such a miraculous recovery and that I was able to return to work. Of course, my bloody diarrhea continued and the usual course of the day was characterized by two to eight bowel movements that were coated with blood and pus. In addition, I now had a perianal fistula, which drained small amounts of mucus. I went to see a leading Manhattan gastroenterologist in his Park Avenue office. After examination and sigmoidoscopy, which he had to perform with a pediatric scope, he informed me that I had a rectal stricture as well as a perianal fissure. The barium enema showed evidence of disease other than in the rectum. He felt that the diagnosis was Crohn's disease rather than ulcerative colitis. Another course of Azulfidine was tried for several months, again without any noticeable effect.

As the visits to the gastroenterologist became less frequent, the work of private practice and the pleasure of my wife and family absorbed me.

My stools were now narrow due to the stricture, but at times, this was to my advantage in that even before the abscess, the control of my anal sphincter had been lost. Now if a violent lower abdominal cramp gripped me, I would lose control and soil my trousers only if the stool was loose or liquid. Oh, how many times I had to rush from wherever I was to clean myself and change into clean undershorts and trousers! How many hours were spent in this most menial and distasteful task? I would hate to calculate them.

Life continued in this pattern more or less for 25 years after the onset of the original symptoms. At age 50, I developed a nasal abscess. I went to an ENT specialist and took erythromycin regularly. However, after 10 or 11 days of taking this antibiotic, I developed abdominal cramps, bloating, and excessive flatus. These symptoms cleared quite rapidly when I took yogurt. I ate yogurt, usually a different flavor each time, with every meal and before going to bed.

Years before, a lactose tolerance test had demonstrated a moderate lactose deficiency, and although I knew milk and milk products were to be avoided, somehow I felt yogurt was all right to eat. Within two weeks, my gut exploded and I became violently ill. Ever since leaving the hospital I had not felt well, but late one afternoon, two months later while working at the office, I had repeated abdominal cramps and almost continual diarrhea. I was sweating and had a low-grade fever. I went promptly to see my friend and internist, who fortunately happened to be a gastroenterologist.

He gently suggested a sigmoidoscopy and then admitted me. The next day, a barium enema showed extension of the disease and involvement of the entire descending and most or all of the transverse colon as well. IV fluids and hydrocortisone were administered and my old friend, the surgeon, came to visit frequently. Both the physician and the surgeon recommended surgery, but remembering vividly the six weeks of pain following the surgery for the ischiorectal abscess, I politely but firmly refused. I was not about to undergo surgery without at least a trial of medical therapy.

After a week of hydrocortisone 300 mg IV daily, plus other supportive measures, improvement was minimal. The weakness was profound, I could barely walk, and my weight dropped from 125 pounds to 110 pounds. Surely, I had a long way to go, but my optimism, as always, was at a high level. After one week, I left the hospital, probably as ill as when I entered, but my symptoms were masked by 60 mg of prednisone daily. Shortly after arriving home, I awoke one morning with pain and swelling in the left knee, to a degree that made it impossible to bend. Indomethacin, even 150 mg daily, seemed of little help, but fortunately, the symptoms subsided spontaneously within a few weeks. While on these two medications, I took antacids on a regular basis. Having treated many patients with connective tissue diseases, I was well aware of the many side effects of corticosteroids. As time went on, potassium, calcium, and Vitamin D were added and anything else that might help prevent complications from these drugs. In the hospital, oral supplementary feedings had been started and I continued them at home. Anorexia seemed to lessen but the weakness increased, as did the bloody diarrhea. Prednisone was increased to 80 mg daily and I felt some improvement.

Perhaps the most unusual feature was the muscle weakness and wasting. At about the age of 18, I weighed approximately 138 pounds. Even though my appetite had been good and I had eaten 4000 to 5000 calories a day, my weight had gradually dropped to 125 pounds. When walking up only one flight of stairs, I would slow down and feel tired upon reaching the top. My muscles had shrunk, most noticeably in the thighs and quadriceps. My quadriceps were atrophied, and I could not rise from a squatting position. The only way I could negotiate the one flight of stairs was to stop and rest at least twice on the way up. This was present within the first few weeks after starting corticosteroids. After months of taking prednisone, I probably also had some steroid myopathy, but as the months went by and my general condition improved, so did the strength of my muscles.

Shortly after leaving the hospital, I took the films of my barium enema to the gastroenterologist in New York. I expressed my feelings that this exacerbation could be controlled by conservative measures and that surgery could be deferred. He concurred and thus began the following saga. It would be 14 months before I was well enough to return to work. Fortunately, there was enough insurance to pay the bills and my office nurse. Television became tiresome and I read long novels such as *The Winds of War, The Thorn Birds,* and *War and Remembrance.*

Although my physicians were constantly trying to reduce the corticosteroids, after almost four months, the dose of prednisone was still 60 mg daily. For the next five months, we varied the prednisone dosage, but nine months after the exacerbation, I was still unable to work and still on a potentially hazardous dose of prednisone, 30 mg every two days. At this point, my gastroenterologist and I agreed with my local physicians that surgery was indicated. Time had helped me accept the thought of living with a colostomy or an ileostomy.

My fear began to increase, first because of the possible complication of steroids and second because of the possible, nay probable, complications of surgery. I went to see the surgeon again. For my wasted, almost cachectic state, he ordered a high-calorie diet supplemented by liquid feedings. The gastroenterologist in New York felt that I was in such a compromised condition that he recommended surgery be done in several stages. The general surgeon disagreed. He felt that a proctocolectomy with complete removal of the rectum could be performed. At this time, I felt that surgery of some type had to be done, and the sooner the better. When the surgeon informed me that the first opening in the operating room schedule was in six weeks, I called him and begged him to do it as soon as possible. At my request, the surgeon telephoned the New York specialist and discussed my general condition and what type of surgery should be done. Not until later did I learn that they still disagreed about what kind of surgery should be performed. Meanwhile, I kept eating as much as possible and drinking the oral supplements until they began to lose all flavor.

When I was admitted three days prior to surgery, my weight had increased approximately five pounds. The gastroenterologist felt that because of my weakened general condition and the large dose of steroids that I was on, it would be too risky to remove my rectum. The surgeon felt that after the colectomy, a proctectomy should be performed. As I had considerable respect for both men, it was very difficult to decide. In the beginning, I agreed totally with the gastroenterologist, but as time went on, my feelings changed. Even though it may be more painful, I reasoned, who wants two or more operations if it could all be done in one procedure? Two days before surgery, I telephoned the gastroenterologist from the hospital and, after discussing the pros and cons, informed him that if it was possible, I would be willing to undergo a proctectomy as well as a colectomy.

Following this, the surgeon then said that he would use his judgment at the time of surgery, and if the tissue was not too friable, he would do both procedures. On June 25, 1980, my entire colon was removed, a permanent ileostomy was fashioned, and my rectum was removed.

Within a few days, I was up walking with the catheter and drainage bag in one hand, the tube hanging out of my nose, and pushing the IV pole with the other hand. Soon I began to eat and everything was going smoothly. Surely there would be a complication soon.

I remained in the ICU for about seven days. With the help of the nurses, I learned how to empty and change the bags and base plate.

In approximately three weeks, I went home, all sutures and wires having been removed. The steroids were changed to oral prednisone, which within one month tapered and within two months discontinued. The pain for the entire hospitalization and postrecovery period was less than the pain following the incision and drainage for the rectal abscess.

The internist informed me that the pathology was that of ulcerative colitis and that the surgery may have been curative. Having believed for so many years that this was Crohn's disease, I withheld any final judgment on both of these statements. The abdominal wound healed rapidly but the perineal area remained red and raw, draining bloody fluid for weeks.

The surgeon had been very direct and forthright prior to the operation. He had explained most of the complications that can follow an abdominal perineal resection, but the one that concerned me most was impotence. My wife and I had discussed this prior to surgery but we both felt that the need for surgery was so great that we had to take the chance. During my entire hospital stay, no erection occurred. About six weeks after I arrived home, one day while I was lying in the reclining chair, my penis became slightly enlarged for about 30 seconds and then shrank back to its usual size.

What would our life be like if I were impotent? Would my wife leave me? Would I go to a urologist for help and possibly get an artificial penis? My wife was marvelous throughout the entire illness. She never expressed her anger and the frustration that she must have felt in a personal way that might have offended or worried me.

Within a few days, a second and then a third erection occurred. At this point, I realized that maybe, just maybe, my potency was returning. Wait and see, wait and see. But I did inform my wife that I had had an erection. Within a few weeks, erection followed by ejaculation had occurred and at last my potency had been restored. What a relief! My wife and I smiled broadly at each other. Happiness was here again.

As my recovery continued, I returned as soon as possible to the big city to visit the gastroenterologist. After he had examined my perineal wound, still draining at that point, I informed him that the pathology report was ulcerative colitis rather than Crohn's disease (regional enteritis). He expressed surprise and asked me to obtain the glass slides with the microscopic specimens for him. Several weeks later, he said he had reviewed the slides with his pathologist at one of the large teaching hospitals, and it was their feeling that the diagnosis was regional enteritis. I expressed no surprise since he had felt that was the diagnosis for many years. Who was I to believe—the internist and the pathologist at the local hospital or the gastroenterologist and his pathologist at the large medical center? When I expressed my quandary, the gastroenterologist gave me the names of three pathologists who were outstanding experts in the field of inflammatory bowel disease and suggested that a slide review by one of them might be helpful in resolving this dispute. After several weeks, the pathologist at our local hospital mailed the slides with an accompanying letter to the pathologist at the Lenox Hill Hospital in New York City. After what seemed like an interminable wait, his report returned with the diagnosis of "active chronic ulcerative colitis with pseudopolyps." I smiled broadly as elation filled my chest!

By the time this good news came, the surgeon had said I was well enough to return to work and, although still feeling weak, I did so. As the months passed, my strength would increase and then plateau, increase again and plateau, and to my surprise and delight, increase even more. It felt in some ways like being an adolescent again as my muscles became larger and the ability to walk normally, to squat and do a deep knee bend, and even to walk up a flight of stairs without stopping returned. Oh, how nice it felt to be able to function again in a normal way!

Some people find it difficult to adjust to a colostomy, ureterostomy, or ileostomy. They feel alone, isolated, and different, with a rubber or plastic device that hangs outside their abdomen, into which their waste is excreted. To help those people, there are specialized nurses, called enterostomy therapists, psychologists, psychiatrists, and even an organization called the United Ostomy Association. Perhaps the ten months of illness during which I was unemployed gave me time to understand what it would be like to have an ileostomy. Perhaps the unquestioning love received from my wife and children and other family members, or perhaps the generally good feeling about myself, made it easy to adjust to the ileostomy.

In the beginning, the bag would fill and require emptying once or twice each night. Even puncturing the top of the bag with a pin to make one or several holes to release the gas did not prevent the problem. At a local meeting sponsored by the United Ostomy Association, during which lectures were given and exhibits were put on, mostly by the manufacturers of the various devices, a salesman gave me an ileostomy bag that measured 29 inches long and 7½ inches wide at the top and 3½ inches at the bottom. After wearing this for several nights, which were filled with rest without interruption, I realized that the regular container was adequate, and I have been wearing it every night since, and sleeping well. One learns that such disposable plastic bags can be torn or damaged by carrying heavy objects on the right side, and to prevent this you carry them on your left. A regular man's bathing suit with trunks can be worn without showing an ileostomy. Swimming is no problem for the ostomate, but if one dives from a distance of three feet or greater above the water, the plastic bag is often dislodged and torn away from the base plate. However, if one dives at a distance of less than three feet, the bag will usually remain adherent to its connection.

In general, I feel an ileostomy is a small price to pay for the well-being accompanying it. During the long ten-month period preceding surgery, a saying occurred to me: "For every disadvantage, there is an advantage." These words perhaps offer some comfort when one feels under stress. But even now, after five years of being well, when I think about a ureteral or renal calculus as one of the complications occurring in some patients with an ileostomy, I also realize that cancer of the rectum, which is relatively common; diverticulitis, which has occured in so many members of my family and, in some instances, so severely; and cancer of the colon need be no concern to me any longer. Furthermore, I shall never need to be proctoscoped, sigmoidoscoped, or colonoscoped!

My present physical condition is excellent. My gratitude concerning the recovery of my health is profound. One of my college classmates died from ulcerative colitis two years after graduation. Another friend in medical school developed ulcerative colitis while interning. He died the following year from complications of his disease, shortly after starting a residency in psychiatry.

One of my major concerns when ill was the effect on my wife and children. How they coped with it as well as they did I shall never know, but my love and pride regarding them are even deeper than before. When they needed help, I was unable to give it. Perhaps my recovery has helped reassure them that I wanted to be near them and love them. Also, it must have been difficult for some of my patients. To have a physician you depend on become suddenly ill and close his practice temporarily can be upsetting. My office assistant tried to help our patients in as many ways as she could. We referred patients to the physicians we felt would be best for them. After being out of the office for a total of 14 months, I was surprised that in a highly competitive area, almost 50% of my patients returned when my office was reopened.

There seems to be a strong association between the psyche and the soma. They are intertwined in an interestingly complex way that perhaps no one fully understands. The association between disturbed emotional feelings and ulcerative colitis has been known for many years. Several decades ago, there was a feeling among some physicians that the disease was caused by an abnormal psyche. Surely stress and emotional conflict can exacerbate the disease, but this is true of many other diseases. There is little doubt in my mind at this time that ulcerative colitis starts as a physical disease. Like any other chronic disease, it causes anxiety, frustration, and anger, and the psyche and the soma become inexorably intertwined. The patient, as a human being, may or may not express some or all of the feelings to loved ones or to the physician. If the physician understands the disease and, more importantly, a little about human nature, he is better able to accept the frustrations and difficulty of treating such a patient. It is my strong wish that an effective medical treatment will soon be found for this disease.

CHAPTER 26

CROHN'S DISEASE

"R. F. SPOONER"

When I was 12 years old, approaching my Bar Mitzvah, I was sitting on the floor with a group of children in my Boy Scout pack. Suddenly I felt a strong urge to go to the bathroom. I barely made it. When I got home that night, I kept this little problem to myself and did not think much of it until the problem became more frequent. In addition, I began to have belly pain that kept me up at night. I would roll in bed from side to side to minimize the discomfort and usually would stay up the whole night, distracted by the constant cramps. During the day I was always fatigued. It was not long before my appetite diminished and I was eating less and less at meals, unable at times to take more than a few mouthfuls. Eating caused belly pain and nausea and even vomiting.

Until the onset of my illness I was the fattest one in the family. This changed quickly, though, when I shed more than the extra pounds. My linear growth should have been taking off, but it seemed frozen in place. I was thinner, and people around me thought I was taller as well. "He's going through puberty," neighbors would comment. After the first summer it was obvious that I was not growing as I should have.

After two months of weight loss, diarrhea, abdominal pain, and midprandial vomiting, as well as what must have been a great deal of silent unhappiness, my parents finally decided to take me to see the doctor.

Our pediatrician, a college friend of my father, was well known in the community primarily because of his father. A generation earlier he had brought the field of pediatrics home to our town from what was then the "Mecca"—New York City. By now, though, our pediatrician had acted upon his own disenchantment with his profession and had entered politics. He maintained his practice on weekends and the rest of the time sat in the legislature.

"DR. R. F. SPOONER" is a 30-year-old physician practicing in New England.

I distinctly remember visiting him with my parents on a Sunday morning. He measured my height, weighed me, and scribbled the numbers in a small, black, wire-bound notebook that he kept in his right hip pocket. My pediatrician had always been reserved; his friendliness and playfulness were always strained. Even as a younger child, I remember having the sense that here was someone who didn't like what he was doing. But at this visit, my doctor seemed preoccupied, more quiet than usual, and bored. He looked at me quickly and, since he was in a rush, patted me on the head and said, "Oh, he's just growing up. No cause for concern." The irony in this statement was too great to overlook.

My parents were not satisfied with my pediatrician's answer and were quite pleased that he was out of town when I developed a fever. The physician covering him examined me and immediately admitted me to the hospital for tests. That same afternoon he took me into his office and told me what he thought was wrong with me. I remember sitting across from a three-dimensional plastic cutaway model of the gut. He pointed to the distal small bowel and explained that all the inflammation was there. He said the condition would wax and wane but that I would probably have it the rest of my life. He called it regional enteritis and told me that it was the "President's disease," an allusion to the intestinal ailment that afflicted Dwight D. Eisenhower. I liked the association of my disease with such a famous person. It gave the disease some meaning and made the embarrassing symptoms I had to endure less upsetting. I realized later what a clever comment it was to make to a patient.

Although I don't remember my exact reaction to this new diagnosis, I recall viewing the whole matter as a challenge of sorts. I was somewhat fearful because now that my symptoms had a name, my illness had become real and permanent. It confirmed the isolation I had felt until that time. I realized that now I was truly on my own. I was growing up very quickly now, if only emotionally.

My understanding of the disease was that my body was digesting itself. I didn t have a good idea of what inflammation was and, among other projects, I set out to learn as much about this process as possible.

My sense of challenge and excitement, rooted in naivete, was quickly squelched when I met my hospital roommate. Steven was about five feet ten and gaunt. He was, as my grandmother would say, like a glass of water. He had wispy dull hair and cheeks that were terribly sunken. His eyes were glassy and recessed and his skin was ashen. He was only 16, but he looked 90. He shuffled around unsteadily, leaning on his wheelchair. One hand would always be pressed inside his gown, Napoleonlike, holding his colostomy bag in place. We became friends the way prisoners condemned for life in the same bleak cell become friends. It was clear to me that Steven was frightfully ill, but I would not let it occur to me that I could end up like him. Our diseases were somewhat different: He had ulcerative colitis and I had regional enteritis. Nonetheless, the day Steven died, I stared in the mirror for 20 minutes, wondering how much longer it would be before this image would fade as well.

After I was admitted to the ward, tests were done, house staff examined me, and rounds were made on me. Everyone commented on how precocious I seemed. I recall the house staff standing at the foot of the bed as I explained to them that, yes, I did have "nocturnal" diarrhea. Their amazement at my intellectual precocity was due only to their failure to recognize an important aspect of Crohn's disease in children: stunted growth. I was 13 years old but looked 10 or 11.

A gastroenterologist who was to become my physician for the next several yars came to see me. He did a proctoscopic exam and, I think, told me that I was too stressed. It was not until later that I understood exactly what he meant by that.

I improved in the hospital and after three weeks went home on prednisone and Azulfidine, a sulfa drug. I ate about 12 meals a day, and I think all the food was going straight to my face. It was round as a beach ball. The Azulfidine tablets were enormous; I gagged on them every time and rarely had success in swallowing them. I decided that the medication made me nauseated and that must have meant that I didn't want to get better.

I had become what I thought was terrifically independent. I treasured my privacy more than before. Only later did I realize that my desire for independence was simply transmuted isolation.

Although I was happy that I was eating again, my bowel habits did not improve significantly. In addition, I was having nightly sweats and fevers. Occasionally the pallor of my iron deficiency anemia would be masked by an endogenous flush of fever.

It seemed to me that exacerbations of my illness corresponded with the seasons. I remember reading about such an association with stomach ulcers and wondered whether the same might apply to Crohn's disease. My bouts of disease seemed to recur each April, and for the longest time I searched for significance to this observation but have been unable to find it. Two months after my first hospitalization, I was readmitted because of persistent symptoms.

During the second admission I enjoyed the hospital environment—or, at least, the lack of the home environment. My gastroenterologist and pediatrician must have perceived that I was greatly upset because they arranged for me to speak to someone. For about a year I saw a psychiatrist. He was a strapping man with a passion for shooting white-water rapids in the Yukon. He was also very skilled. While I thought we were having great dispassionate intellectual discussions, he was subtly pointing out to me my enormous anger and impatience. Of course, it was only much later that I made these insights, but on some important level the psychiatric intervention was crucial to me in coping with my illness. While I insisted on focusing on the palpable aspects of my illness, he would focus more on emotions revolving about the disease itself. I would demand a precise definition of "inflammation," and he would say that he went to medical school too long ago to remember what it was.

My main contact with physicians throughout the early years was with my gastroenterologist. I looked forward to my appointments with him. His appointments were interesting primarily because he did not focus on my disease. Rather, he focused on himself and his own problems, professional and personal. I thought this was somewhat odd but took his confidences as a compliment. Whenever I would appear in his office, he would ask me how I was, and after I lied and told him that I was doing fine, he would shrug his shoulders and start to recount anecdotes from his New York days or list examples of incompetence or stupidity on the part of his colleagues. He would examine me, weigh me, do proctoscopy, and announce whether or not there was a "little blood" in my stool.

Sometimes he would put me on prednisone and sometimes he wouldn't. I don't think he really believed in Azulfidine, but he used it anyway. It was only later in my career that I experienced this paradox myself: We often do things to patients for some vague anticipated benefit even when we are convinced that the modality itself is probably not effective.

Despite what had become almost chronic pain, frequent diarrhea, and an inability to eat socially because of fear of exacerbation of pain, I became furiously ambitious. In addition to holding every major extracurricular leadership post in school, winning writing competitions, and getting into the only Ivy League schools worth mentioning, I managed to pursue a relatively healthy social life. All this time, though, my doctors were telling me to slow down. They said that my condition was one that required rest and relaxation and that I should minimize stress. Only my gastroenterologist had a different view about the dispensation of such advice. Much to my amazement I now find myself using the same example. Whenever I would ask my gastroenterologist if he thought my illness would improve if I weren't so active, he would look at me with an expression of resignation, shrug his shoulders and say:

> I had a patient once who was very unhappy in his marriage. He had a condition which I was convinced was made worse by stress. Every visit

> he would ask me if he should get a divorce. Well, there was no way that I could tell him to get a divorce. What would have happened if he went ahead and ruined his marriage and then didn't get any better? A person has to do whatever makes him feel better, and he has to make his own decisions.

My doctor wasn't convinced that for me being inactive wouldn't be more stressful than a more ambitious life-style.

After I saw this doctor for over a year without much improvement in my condition, he finally told me something that had a profound effect on the way I viewed my prospects for the future. He confided in me on one visit that when he was in medical school, he, too, had an illness identical to mine. For once I was relieved. This meant, by analogy, that I, too, would be able to live at least till age 50 and pursue a normal career. It was the therapeutic value of this comment that made me realize that the degree to which a physician treats a patient as a friend and confidant should not be guided by archaic notions of the hierarchical structure of medicine but by the way the physician, as a person, feels about his patient.

One day I told my doctor that I thought, given the size of my brothers and parents, that I should be a bit taller. I was, after all, 17 and probably nearing the end of my growth phase. I also asked him why he was ordering barium enemas every year if my disease had always been limited to the small bowel. His answer to the first problem was to send me to an endocrinologist—"The smartest man I ever met. He could sit at rounds and follow three or five conversations at once." This smart physician examined me. He told me my bones had grown as much as they would, that my testicles were the right size, and that I would be very short the rest of my life. The next week my doctor sent me a Xerox copy of his letter, which reiterated what I had already heard but contained the phrase "His keen intellectual ability is likely to compensate him well for any social deficit he might suffer." "Social deficit"—what social deficit? I was 17 and probably had more experience than most of my friends. Was this guy in touch? Or was he warning me of some special disadvantage that was likely to accrue to me because of my stature that I had not yet discovered? Was he setting up a situation for a self-fulfilling prophecy?

Although I had never thought about my stature in a negative way prior to this visit, I certainly gained from this renowned endocrinologist a brand new stigma to integrate into my character.

At one time, when my doctor felt that I wasn't doing as well as I might, he arranged for me to see his mentor in New York. I arrived there with my parents. The appointment was for 1:00 p.m., and we entered the waiting room about that time. Several hours later, and after we made several visits to the receptionist, the consultant finally appeared and apologized profusely.

After an hour of talking to this specialist of specialists, it was clear he was going to tell us nothing new. My parents paid him $100 in cash, as requested, and we went on our way. One week later my doctor sent me a copy of his report. In it was a blatant error. He recommended that we try an every-other-day prednisone regimen. The problem was that I was already on that regimen. It was obvious that this doctor had not even assimilated the information of the case, let alone proofread his letter before signing it. Two unforgettable lessons had been learned: The relationship between reputation and quality is not always a positive one, and sloppiness and failure to follow through on plans are inexcusable for a physician.

I went away to college and did relatively well without any modification in my frenetic level of activity. By this point I had read extensively on my disease and knew that eventually I would have surgery. My daily routine included pain and diarrhea, but I had adapted. Occasionally, drenching night sweats would develop, but I kept these a secret. I think I might have even convinced myself each time that it was the "flu."

My doctor's commitment to his laissez-faire approach was finally strained when I asked him if I should go to medical school. He thought for a moment and then blurted out, "I just don't understand why you keep on pushing yourself. I never thought that it was good for you in the long run." I learned later that week that he had just rushed home early from a vacation because of an attack of ileitis. Although I didn't realize it at the time, his highly personalized advice was probably good for me. Although I didn't heed it, I valued this outburst of honesty. It was rooted in experience and had more meaning to me than most of the platitudes that we as doctors serve our patients.

After college, I did not let my illness interfere with my career goals, and went on to medical school. My performance there, I believe, was limited by chronic pain, multiple recurrent obstructions, and diarrhea. Finally, the decision was made with my new gastroenterologist to have an elective resection of the diseased bowel. Just as the arrangements were being made for me to have the operation in another city to protect my privacy (I was still exceedingly jealous of my right to privacy and increasingly aware of the numbers of petty, gossipy people who percolate through hospitals), I had an acute obstruction while rotating through surgery clinic. I turned livid with pain and fled secretly to the on-call room. There I had shaking chills, uncontrollable bilious vomiting, and pain more severe than I had ever experienced. My gut was about to burst. My body had finally rebelled against my ambition. I knew the jig was up. For the first time in my life I knew real fear: I saw myself tethered indoors to vinyl tubing and an intravenous nutrition pump the rest of my life. On the other hand, I was enormously relieved that that rotted mass of gut would finally be torn from my belly, where it was causing only harm. My only problem now was to get to my gastroenterologist's office without being seen by colleagues. I called my doctor on the in-house phone, and he told me to get to his office right away. After sneaking around hallways and down stairwells, I made it to his office, where he was calmly waiting for me. He looked at me and instantly called the surgeon. I walked down alone to the surgeon's office, feeling sick and anxious. I had never met him before, and the one thought that went through my mind was whether or not he was a conservative surgeon. In his office he placed a nasogastric tube. I was later to detest in my own patients the same commotion I made over the tube.

On my way to the private wing, I lay on the guerney, hiding quietly under the sheets for fear that classmates would recognize me. Once I was in my room, a resident took my history and examined me. I was started on intravenous therapy and developed an awkward relationship with the blue pump box that delivered my liquid nutrition. Its regular beeping became a very comforting sound.

After three days of this parenteral nutrition, I was taken to the operating room. The last thing I remember was telling the anaesthetist that I thought I smelled garlic. When I awoke in the recovery room, I did not feel the least bit self-conscious. Gone was my intense need for privacy. In a very interesting turn of events, I was happy that my problem was no longer my private secret.

All along, my desire to keep my illness to myself was rooted in my need to be judged solely on my merits. I was always fearful that if anyone should discover my ailment, he or she would make allowances for my performance and I would never receive full credit for my efforts. I suppose having passed a successful four years in college and now medical school, I had earned the right to relax my stringent standards. By now, people who knew me would judge my accomplishments on their merits. And if they didn't, I could now feel comfortable saying, "Tough luck for them." All along, I knew that my accomplishments were all the more respectable because of the hidden handicap with which I had to contend.

The following morning my surgeon came around with his troupe. He told me he took out more bowel than he had ever done before in someone my age. I asked him if I would be a bathroom cripple from short gut. He nodded. I cried briefly, somehow thinking that the world had just been stolen from beneath my nose. Once my spasm of self-pity had waned, I learned the most important lesson of this ongoing ordeal: Nothing heals like time. What seems unconquerable today will, five years from now, often be completely forgotten. Not only is our ability to remember unpleasantness limited, the tendency of our bodies to remodel the source of the unpleasantness is extreme.

I believed that time would heal because I had no choice. My own expectations in this area were supported by articles that my roommate fished out of the library on gut adaptation. After three weeks in the hospital, during which I regressed completely and felt relaxed for the first time in my life, impatience finally got the better of me.

I was discharged from the hospital 15 pounds heavier than I had ever been and feeling like a human being. I had no pain for the first time that I could remember, and I don't think that I will ever forget that sensation.

The months and years after were years of adaptation. I did have the short gut syndrome and, although my surgeon refused to allow me codeine to decrease diarrhea, my gastroenterologist felt that physiologic addiction was a small price to pay for a socially viable existence.

The medications, together with several therapies for fat malabsorption that I developed myself, worked well enough for me to go on to a residency in internal medicine. This was the first of many compromises I would be making. My surgeon told me to get out of medicine altogether. He said my disease would certainly recur and then I would really be in trouble. I abandoned my strong desire to become a surgeon and quickly found reasons why internal medicine would be better for me anyway.

The training program I had selected turned out to be grueling. This choice was probably not especially wise, but I did well in it anyway. I never missed a day of work and was able to conceal my illness from everyone except an astute program director. It especially galled me when people would take days off for colds or sore throats. But I decided early that I was not going to let other peoples' work values alter mine.

A chronic illness touches every facet of a person's life. When one is afflicted with an illness so early in life, its role in personality development must be great. But there are probably many other effects, some of which I list, as they relate directly to the topic of this paper.

1. Did being ill early on affect my decision to become a physician? Is it true that we emulate that which we know best—and if this is the case, did I lose out because I didn't consider other career choices?
2. Did my negative experiences with doctors affect my respect for physicians and my own self-image once I became a physician?
3. Did my illness affect my understanding of "quality of life" and, hence, the way in which I relate to patients?

Although I came from a professional family—a family without physicians—and although my family was extremely healthy, without much contact with doctors or hospitals, there was a great respect for physicians, so great that often I felt too intimidated to talk to my doctors. Eventually, by virtue of my testy disposition, I would explore the limits of my relationship with them and discover that mostly they were interested in talking to anyone who was bright and was not a nag. Still, I recall feeling very hesitant about asking questions, feeling that it would put the doctors off and I would gain their disapproval.

I'm sure my experience was not unique. I believe most patients are nervous when they come to see a physician because they are afraid of the unknown. Doctors generally mean bad news, and there is nothing a physician can do to change this. His or her personality can make things easier, but in the end, a person does not see a physician unless something is wrong. That nervousness leads to another common problem: the failure to understand simple instructions given in the doctor's office. The good doctor adapts his practice to compensate for these unalterable behaviors. My own experiences in doctors' offices have made me very sensitive to the patient who is there in body but not in mind or spirit.

It is likely that my time spent in and out of doctors' offices and hospitals during the years when my career was being planned probably influenced me to go into medicine. This is not so surprising. The real question is whether I was motivated by conventional altruism, greed, or intellectual curiosity. I long ago comfortably dismissed the first possibility because I had always felt so consumed with my own survival that I did not feel I had energy to spare for altruism. The truly selfless physician could end up expending all his emotional energy on patients' problems and be left with nothing for himself or his family. We are all familiar with examples of this.

The goal of greed would have been better attained with an MBA than with an MD, and I confidently dismiss this motivation. I must say, though, that the fear of disability has always weighed heavily in my goals, and medicine was a satisfactory choice for me because I knew that if I ended up tied to an intravenous nutrition pump, I could always be a psychiatrist. At any rate, the third possibility—that of intellectual curiosity—had always seemed to me the most direct stimulus to choosing this profession. I was consumed with the naive notion of knowing many facts. Knowledge was power, and power, in a broad sense, was a way of controlling one's environment. Because my internal environment was so obviously beyond my control, modification and direction of my external environment was highly desirable.

The notion that knowledge of the illness would allow me to control it found an interesting form of expression very early. Soon after the diagnosis of Crohn's disease, I visited the university bookstore to find a medical textbook that would explain what I wanted to know. There I found a textbook of gastroenterology and read everything about the disease. The sentence that I was looking for and the one that stood out the most was "Despite the inconveniences of the disease, most patients go on to lead relatively normal lives." Well, I could settle for that.

If my choice of medicine as a career was based on intellectual curiosity buoyed by some rather close relationships with doctors, how did my respect for doctors bear up in view of the episodes I cited earlier?

I think that every child, and every part of every adult that is a child, seeks a hero. That is obvious in our collective cultural experience: in the tales we tell children at bedtime, in the movies we watch, in the people we vote into public office. Doctors have been heroes in society's eyes. We are all familiar with the common refrain (at least it was in an affluent suburb where I did my training) that, "My doctor is the best in the city." And often, the physician to whom the patient was referring was someone to whom most informed people would not have given any awards. Yet the patient's attestation was simply a symptom of the need to believe that he was being swept away by someone who would take care of all his problems. It is regression in illness in a subtle form. Dr. X is the greatest doctor in the world, and he will take better care of me than anyone else. Through this form of regression, the patient mistakenly absolves himself of any responsibility for getting better and, at the same time, places his physician in the impossible position of being solely responsible for healing.

This positioning of the physician on a pedestal is changing rapidly. It is the luck of my generation that we have come along at a time when there is such an upheaval in the profession that the notion of hero in medicine may never again apply. Doctors have become businessmen or partners of businessmen, and, as a result, everything they do may be held suspect. Profit motive lurks behind each barium enema, each test for blood in stool that might signify cancer. The basis of doctors' heroism in the past—selfless devotion—has been crumbling. It was not until college that I became aware that there was another, older view of this—one that predated the showy opulence of the Mercedes-Benz era. After reading *The Doctor's Dilemma* by George Bernard Shaw, it jarred me that this, too, was an acceptable view of physicians for some. Greed was not a problem unique to physicians of the second half of the twentieth century. The play shook me but not my dedication to my goal.

My experience with physicians has been tainted by sloppiness, mild negligence, professional fatigue and disaffection, greed, and lack of wisdom. Despite the negative experiences with some physicians, I must have developed an overall positive impression of the profession, or I would not have chosen it for myself. More important, I must have derived a realistic idea of what is reasonable and what is unjustified expectation.

It was with the recognition that doctors were not perfect and that this was not a crime that I applied to medical school. And it was with a significant degree of cynicism that I viewed doctors and their motives during my own medical education. There was no question that financial satisfaction and security was a motivating factor for many of my peers. I have no problem with that. It is no less offensive to me to be a lawyer or a shoe salesman and to want to be rich. In our society there is only one profession where one need take an oath of poverty—and the ranks of that humble group, I have read, shrink daily. There is nothing wrong with wanting to have the best for oneself and one's family. What is wrong is when a physician performs unnecessary tests in order to make that money or sees more patients than he can handle and still do them all justice.

As a group, physicians are not heroes, nor should society expect of them heroic sacrifices. If, from day to day, they can perform small acts of heroism with individual patients and family, then perhaps they will have fulfilled their professional obligations.

My only expectations from a physician and from myself is that we strive to do our job perfectly most of the time and that, when mistakes are made, we have the courage to correct them promptly.

I learned from my own experiences as a patient and as a trainee that it is not the role of the physician to judge his colleagues. He must only judge himself and have the strength to correct the faults if he finds them. I think it is far better for a physician to be a fellow man to his patient than some unattainable amalgam of god, pater, and hero. Such a role is probably more emotionally draining but in the end is likely to be more rewarding.

My recognition of the fallibility of doctors has made things easier for me personally: My expectations of myself are tempered, and guilt is not a frequent problem.

My contact with doctors and hospitals defined my early life the way the basketball court might define the life of an inner-city youth or the library the life of a paraplegic. Where we spend our time, for whatever reason, guides us into a particular cubby hole or down a particular mail delivery chute. It is not surprising that many disabled people or sick people choose the medical profession. In some there must be motivation by guilt: "As bad off as I am there are those worse off and to do penance for my wicked ways I will devote my life to helping them."

Certainly, feelings of guilt and worthlessness are common in patients with diseases of the gut—the powerful metaphor of spending much of their life preoccupied with the disposal of waste must not be lost.

But what is the effect of all this contact with hospitals on how the physician sees and treats his own patients? There are probably two schools of thought. The first might say that physicians who have a particular illness are least qualified to treat others with the same illness; the lack of objectivity would be damaging. The other school might say that that group of doctors is the most qualified because they know about the problems that these patients have. This is similar to the argument that the best obstetricians and gynecologists are likely to be women because they best understand the needs of women. I think that what often distinguishes a good doctor from a bad doctor is the interpersonal skill and knowledge of healing. But I believe that doctors who have been sick have a more precise perception of what being a patient is all about. There is no substitute for being there. The physician who suffers a particular ailment is much more likely to understand instantly what a patient may be going through and, hence, be in a better position to be helpful. A gastroenterologist may intellectually understand that it must be socially crippling continually to be in search of a bathroom, but he truly understands this problem only when he himself has, for example, an abbreviated infectious diarrheal illness.

Empathy is a capacity that can be cultivated through observation, but it is the reflexive appreciation of the practicalities of disease that distinguishes the ill physician from the well physician. And with chronic illness, it is often the resolution of practical problems that makes the difference between worthwhile life and life not enjoyable enough to live. I assure you that a chairman of a department of physical medicine who is a paraplegic will go to great lengths to make sure that the subtle needs of his constituency are attended to. He will also know which suggestions proposed by people not in his exclusive group might be frivolous.

I cannot emphasize enough the importance of attending to the subtleties of living with disease. It is often mundane work, work that we, as physicians, would prefer to relegate to assistants. But physicians need to identify ways that can improve the life of their patients to help them move to symbiosis with their disease.

I think my own illness has made me a good doctor. There are colleagues who have never been ill who are clearly superior clinicians and who perhaps have an even greater store of empathy than I. But illness is not something for which one wishes. And it is the responsibility of the patient to make the best of his life under the circumstances. The experiences that I have had as a result of my sickness have shaped my value system as a physician. They have also guided my choice of a specialty. When I was caring for several people my age who had the same illness I did, I discovered that although I could identify with them very well, I did not want to. Fears about my own prognosis were enough of a burden. I did not want to wonder how much closer I was approaching the actuarial curves for recurrence of disease every time I admitted a patient who was status postresection for ileitis.

On the other hand, whenever I encounter young patients with potentially chronic diseases, I have made it my business to talk to them and to be as encouraging with them as my own doctor was with me. I still hear doctors tell patients that they should change their job or marriage and they will get better. If asked my opinion, I categorically tell the patient to do whatever will allow him to enjoy life and the people around him. You must beat the disease by not allowing it to confine you any more than the routine of therapy or symptoms already do. If you die earlier as a result of your chosen life-style, at least you will have died with a smile on your face.

Probably the greatest and, to me, the most rewarding confirmation of this approach came when I read the latest edition of a textbook I had read when I was 14 years old. The advice in that early edition was that Crohn's disease patients should choose a profession that will not be physically demanding. In the latest edition that statement is gone and is replaced with a view that more closely approximates mine. When I was told by the author that he changed that paragraph in part because of his knowledge of my experience, I felt that my ambition hadn't been for naught.

CHAPTER 27

CROHN'S DISEASE

DAVID E. HEIN

Picture a 13-year-old boy, physically well developed, an above-average student, a very good athlete, and a leader among his peers. He suddenly discovers inside his anus a draining sore that does not go away. At the same time he suffers loss of vigor and gains no weight. Three attempts at incision and drainage result in recurrence of what proves to be a fistula. The local surgeon, at a loss to explain the failure of the surgical treatment, recommends a second opinion from the Mayo Clinic.

I was that 13-year-old adolescent. For 50 years I have lived with Crohn's disease. As a physician, especially a gastroenterologist, I am able to look back over the phases of my illness and picture behavior characteristics that have persisted—although at times disguised—throughout the 50 years of my chronic illness.

Robust and larger than most of my classmates, I had enjoyed excellent general health throughout childhood. My greatest interest was in sports and I excelled. My athletic and scholastic abilities made me more a leader than a follower. I was an only child of upper-middle-class Jewish parents. My mother was a third-generation American, my father emigrated from Germany in 1893 at age 2. My father was a hardworking traveling salesman who was gone from home much of the time. He did not participate in any activity other than work, nor did we enjoy an ideal father–son relationship. He loved me deeply but displayed his love primarily in material ways. My mother was the dominant, but not domineering, parent who made most of the decisions. She was a vital part of my day-to-day childhood experience. Intelligent, sensitive, warm, energetic, and both physically and emotionally strong—it was

DR. DAVID HEIN is in private practice of internal medicine and gastroenterology in Atlanta, Georgia. He holds appointments on the clinical faculty of Emory University School of Medicine and the Medical College of Georgia. His special clinical interests include inflammatory bowel disease and diseases of the liver. Dr. Hein is a fellow of the American College of Physicians and the American College of Gastroenterology.

she, of course, who carried most of the load of my illness from its onset.

My maternal grandfather was the most dominant figure of my early childhood. Although he died shortly after the onset of my illness, I recognize that most of my response to, and behavior during, my illness stemmed from his influence. He was physically and psychologically domineering. Victorian and idealistic in his approach to life, he expected all of his family (and especially me) to perform at the high level of his expectations and within the narrow limits of his tolerance.

My earliest memories of my illness are related to the presence of that draining sore on the skin just outside my anus and the discomfort that followed bowel movements—a "bearing-down," aching sensation that lasted from a few minutes to an hour or two after defecation and then gradually subsided. Initially the area was drained but later a fistulectomy was performed. I went away for eight weeks of summer camp, and shortly after my arrival, the drainage and postdefecation pain recurred. I dreaded having bowel movements because of the discomfort that followed. In spite of this, I had an active, happy, and highly productive experience. I participated and competed vigorously in all sports and camping events.

After I returned from camp I underwent my first medical evaluation for my failure to gain weight and the recurrent fistula-in-ano. Among the assorted programs that followed were treatment for amebic dysentery, premeal insulin injections, and ingestion of four quarts of cow's milk per day "to stretch the stomach," and increase caloric intake. Needless to say, all of these programs had significant undesirable side effects and were worthless. I was unable to participate in sports for the first time in my life because I lacked the physical strength and heeded the medical advice not to get "overtired."

Around the time of my 15th birthday, I underwent a third surgical procedure for the rectal drainage and discomfort. Since this treatment was more extensive, it was decided that I should enter the Mayo Clinic in Rochester, Minnesota, for evaluation and treatment.

At the clinic I was evaluated by two surgeons who operated on me and made the diagnosis of extensive anal ulceration probably due to tuberculosis. I remained in Rochester for about 16 weeks as an outpatient, undergoing twice-daily rectal irrigations and weekly proctologic examinations. No specific treatment was available. After three or four months, I returned home to continue the rectal lavages with witch hazel three times a day and did not return to school for some months. For the following year and a half I was asymptomatic, insofar as the anorectal disease was concerned, but I failed to gain weight and grew very little. My school attendance was regular, and I took additional courses, which enabled me to graduate with my class.

Because I was deteriorating physically, I returned to the Mayo Clinic for evaluation by a prominent gastroenterologist, Dr. B. By that time I was having frequent abdominal pain with accompanying embarrassing noises, significant anorexia, and weakness. At age 18, my weight was between 90 and 95 pounds—my top weight had been 115 pounds at age 16. I was hospitalized upon my arrival at the clinic. I remember Dr. B.'s coming into my room later that day and telling my parents and me that I probably had an uncommon condition known as regional enteritis and that surgery should take care of my problem. This was early June 1941, some nine years after Dr. B. B. Crohn and his colleagues had described the disease for the first time.

Surgery was performed and the diagnosis was jejunitis with almost total obstruction of the midjejunum extending for approximately 45 centimeters. I have forgotten details of the postoperative course, but I know it was stormy. I was shocked when my mother was asked to donate blood for me but felt better when told that I did not have a malignancy. After the early postoperative period I recovered my strength rapidly. During this time I was allowed to go into the amphitheater of the hospital operating suite and observe the surgeons performing operations similar to mine, as well as thyroidectomies, gastrectomies, and similar procedures.

When I was discharged from the clinic we were told that while there was no specific treatment for regional enteritis, convalescence involved prolonged rest and proper diet. I was told to avoid cow's milk and to eat a low-residue diet. I was also advised to postpone entering college for another year.

I spent the following year out of school with limited physical activity. During the early months, I was able to participate in minor sports events, such as umpiring college intramural softball games.

I entered Northwestern University as a 19-year-old freshman in September 1942. I quickly realized that physical and emotional stress created more diarrhea. My weight dropped some, but I was physically able to carry a full load of academic subjects and also participate in extracurricular activities.

The last two years of college found me in fairly good physical condition. I gained no weight and participated in no athletic activities, not even physical education on campus. A three-day physical examination for my draft board in 1944 found me unacceptable for military service and I was classified 4F. I entered Emory University Medical School in September 1945, joining a class of 66 students, one-third of whom were navy, one-third army, and one-third civilian.

The competition was fierce and never let up during the entire four years of medical school. I felt as well as I had since beginning college. In June 1947, between my sophomore and junior years of medical school, I got married. Approximately two months later I had a sudden onset of severe abdominal pain, which persisted for over 12 hours before I consulted a local surgeon.

Surgery proved that the problem was not appendicitis or appendiceal abscess but ulceration and perforation (with moderate necrosis) of the previously isolated jejunal loop diseased by regional enteritis. The diseased segment of jejunum was removed without additional small bowel resection or further anastomosis. The postoperative course was uncomplicated. I returned to medical school.

As I recall, nocturnal diarrhea began to occur during my clinical clerkship in the third and fourth years of medical school. I blamed this on the long days and frequent nights "on call." I felt more bloated and distended at times, and again I associated it with the diet (hospital food) and the long hours put in each day. My weight did not increase, though I was consistently trying to put on a few pounds. I finished medical school in the top third of my class and went on to internship, medical residency, and fellowship in gastroenterology at Cincinnati General Hospital and the University of Cincinnati College of Medicine.

I experienced the first of several partial bowel obstructions during the latter part of my fellowship year in 1952. After two more episodes of small bowel obstruction, I agreed to surgery. In early September 1952, only three months after reporting to my residency, I underwent resection of approximately three feet of terminal ileum and the right colon with a classical ileocolic anastomosis. Except for an episode of rectal bleeding, my postoperative course was smooth. Pathology reported Crohn's disease involving the ileum and cecum, with no disease at either end of the resected bowel.

I enjoyed good health for the next seven to eight years. For the first time since the onset of my illness in 1936, I had significant remission, I gained weight to 165 pounds, and I was physically strong and painfree. Postprandial diarrhea became a part of my living pattern but seemed a small price to pay for all of the positive factors.

I entered the solo practice of internal medicine–gastroenterology in July 1954. Eighteen years had passed since the onset of my disease, and I hoped and believed that I was one of the 40 to 50% who are "cured" or permanently arrested. This, however, was not the case. In the very early 1960s I suffered significant diarrhea (up to nine to ten stools per day) with afternoon and evening abdominal discomfort and distention. Once again my weight began to fall despite a voracious appetite. There were several episodes combining fever to 103, generalized aching, and profound watery diarrhea that lasted two to four days.

By early 1970 I had developed acute arthritis in both knees requiring steroid injections and physiotherapy. Ankle and leg edema increased markedly by 1971. It was difficult to ascertain my true weight because of the edema. When periodic laboratory tests were performed and GI X-rays taken, their interpretations varied from moderate small bowel abnormalities to severe inflammatory bowel disease of the small intestine with probable blind pouch involving the midjejunum. By 1971 my blood albumin, cholesterol, calcium, and indices had become decidedly abnormal. The edema was generalized and my energy hit an all-time low. I was eating huge quantities of all sorts of foods, and I was nearly exhausted. I would fall asleep whenever I sat for a few minutes.

I was forced to accept the reality that professional help was badly needed. My situation demanded a complete medical evaluation. When I entered a distant and major university hospital, my serum albumin was 1 gram%, and other extreme biochemical abnormalities were present. My average daily intake was estimated to be about 7000 calories! X-rays revealed a large blind pouch in the midjejunum with markedly abnormal small bowel distally. Tests for malabsorption were positive, steatorrhea was present, and there was minimal impairment of pancreatic excretory function. In one week of minimum activity and near total bed rest, I lost 15 pounds of fluid and by the second week my true weight was 110 pounds. Diagnosis was (1) recurrent Crohn's disease involving all of the small bowel distal to the midjejunum, (2) a jejunal pouch secondary to the previous side-to-side anastomosis, (3) malabsorption with severe malnutrition secondary to (1) and (2), (4) severe hypoalbuminemia producing edema, (5) eating habits compounding the problem.

Conservative (nonsurgical) treatment was indicated. I was told that various combinations of treatment—primarily diet and drugs—could be tried and that should the medical program fail, there was probably a surgical approach. Total parenteral nutrition was considered as one alternative. This technique, however, fairly new at the time, was associated with complications and thus was rejected. My diet was to be small quantities of low-residue, lactose-free food eaten in six meals per day. Steroids were begun in fairly large dosage. Tetracycline was chosen as the antibiotic to treat the bacterial overgrowth in the jejunal blind pouch. Imodium was used to control diarrhea. I received B_{12} injections every two weeks. Salt-poor albumin was begun intravenously while I was still in the hospital and repeated on three occasions after my return from the hospital. In addition, I was taking 10 mg Synkayvite subcutaneously every other week and folic acid by mouth daily. Instructions regarding my return to work were nonspecific and left up to me and my personal physician in Atlanta, but rest and diet were emphasized as an important part of this treatment.

The results were astounding! Edema was controlled and serum albumin remained normal. Steroids caused me little trouble except for reducing my sleep markedly. I spent many a night reading rather than tossing and turning in bed trying to fall asleep. With the changed diet, stool frequency diminished and was appreciably less fatty. My weight gain was slow but steady. My most bothersome symptom was profound muscle weakness, which continued in spite of my general improvement and feeling of well-being. I began simple isometric exercises to aerobic exercises, which I continue periodically today. Reduction and discontinuation of steroid dosage after 12 months also helped the muscle weakness. My weight now varies between 150 and 160 pounds. I began psychiatric counseling in 1970 and have utilized it intermittently ever since. Over the past ten years there have been two perirectal abscesses requiring incision and drainage. I live comfortably with a single anal fistula which drains periodically. A rectal stricture at 6 cm has developed and is digitally dilated twice a month. Flagyl in low dose controls the disease adequately. I continue the vitamin K and B_{12} injections twice a month, plus daily Imodium, tetracycline, and a vitamin with iron. My diet remains moderately restricted for fiber and lactose. My energy and vigor have returned to a level not achieved since my illness began in 1936. I play tennis twice a week and enjoy a full-time private practice in two offices and patient care in three hospitals along with my three partners. All of my laboratory studies are normal. Barium studies of my gastrointestinal tract have been done at appropriate five-year intervals and have been unchanged. I do see my physician on a yearly basis for a physical examination. Except for respiratory infections, I am rarely ill.

As I reflect on the past 50 years that I have had Crohn's disease, I see that my 1972 illness and recovery offers me a fine opportunity for analysis and comparison of my feelings and behavior patterns. I suspect that the most important feelings that motivated my behavior were, respectively, determination, denial, and depression. I shall begin my analysis of these "three *D*'s" and their impact on me at the nadir of my illness—the decade before I went to the major university hospital as a patient.

As early as 1960, my physical health was declining. The changes were so gradual that I did not recognize the warnings. I had been in solo practice of internal medicine and gastroenterology since 1954. My practice pattern was typical for my community at that time. My office was adjacent to my primary hospital, but I had privileges in six other general hospitals in metropolitan Atlanta.

Every day was long and, in addition to my developing office practice, included visits to several hospitals in different parts of the city. I was also involved in the medical community, actively participating in the local medical society and state specialty societies. A cofounder in 1957 of the Georgia Society of Internal Medicine, I was an officer and member of the executive council and a charter member and soon to be president of the Georgia Gastroenterological Society.

By the mid-1960s, much was going on in my life. I moved into a larger office, sharing space, expenses, and weekend call with another physician, and my overhead increased. My wife and I and our two teenage daughters had a beautiful home and the life-style to which we were accustomed was costly. As my activities and responsibilities increased, so did my symptoms of diarrhea, steatorrhea, polyphagia, and fatigue. I simply pushed harder and longer. I was not infrequently gone from home 15 to 18 hours per day. I allowed myself to exist on three to four hours of sleep most nights. My eating habits became indiscriminate and self-indulgent.

During this period I was aware of my situation. I had a physical examination, including both a barium enema and a gastrointestinal series with a small bowel follow-through. There was clear-cut evidence of Crohn's disease of the distal small bowel and a blind jejunal pouch from the old anastomosis. My internist recommended that I see a gastroenterologist for further care. I chose to consult with my close associate about my medical problem.

In many ways the choice of my closest medical associate as my gastroenterologist seemed quite natural because I considered him one of the most competent in Atlanta. He had known me for many years and it certainly was convenient to "receive" medical care right in my own office. In retrospect, this decision was not necessarily a wise one, considering my attitude and approach to my symptoms. I do not fault my care or my colleague, yet there were only minimum studies undertaken and I certainly did not suggest others on my own. All decisions were made and advice given after discussion between the two of us. This lack of objectivity presented (what I now consider) major delays in control of my symptoms. Advice was given in a nonauthoritarian manner—from colleague to colleague or friend to friend—and there was little actual follow-up regarding results of the recommendations. I now know that subconsciously I was protecting myself from the reality of my situation. Getting objective medical opinion from any gastroenterologist probably would have necessitated my leaving Atlanta. I wished neither to take the time nor to face the probable outcome of such an evaluation.

My denial is obvious to me now. I was refusing to accept my illness while getting more ill all the time. Denial had influenced my life and behavior from the time I was 13, but at no time before the 1960s had it been so compelling. I became defensive about my weight loss and general appearance. I detested being told how thin I was. Among my friends and acquaintances, my failure to gain weight despite my huge appetite was frequently mentioned and discussed. I became self-conscious about my diarrhea and steatorrea. Not only was I constrained to know where the toilet was located—especially at restaurants—but I had to devise methods of disguising or eliminating the terrible odor that emanated from the stool. I would light matches or cigars, or on occasion would burn paper in attempting to eliminate the smell in the restroom. For a while I even ingested chlorophyll pills. I became anxious whenever comments were made in public restrooms about the awful stink someone was making, and I believe my concern was an early symptom of my increasing depression.

The changes that occurred in my marital relationship at this time played a significant role in both of our lives. Whenever I complained to my wife, Virginia, of being tired (a horse would have tired with the hours I was working) and under too much stress, she would naturally suggest and even urge that I make some changes in my life and work pattern. I would tell her that I likened my commitments to the passenger-filled jet airliner streaking down the runway beyond the point at which takeoff can be stopped or deviated. She rejected my logic and insisted that I was not beyond the point of changing. In spite of the encouragement, I really felt as though I could not significantly change my course or speed. Virginia was, of course, intimately involved in my illness. She had seen me growing increasingly ill yet refusing to do anything constructive about my situation. She found herself waiting hours for me to come home for meals with rare calls from me that I would be late. When I did call I rarely came home anywhere near the time that I set. I know she had mixed and conflicting emotions ranging from sympathy and guilt to anger, anxiety, and fear. For years she was supportive. However, while I was outwardly and publicly denying my illness, I was privately—in actions and words—telling her of my fears of permanent disability or death from advanced disease. My behavior imposed a huge burden upon my wife and our marriage. Virginia became increasingly depressed. In the mid-1960s, with my encouragement, she sought psychiatric help. As a result of this counseling, she realized that she could not carry the load of my illness and peculiar response to it. She told me it was *my* problem and *I* should do something about it. She would no longer feel responsible when I indicated my fears and feelings of despair without attempting to alter my life-style. Our daughters were now in high school. Virginia went back to college and into graduate school. This opened to her a totally new and challenging life of her own. I do not imply that she cared any less for me or was less concerned about my health and feelings, but it was clear that she would no longer allow herself to be victimized by my pathologic response to my illness.

Why did I—a physician who should know better—react as I did to my illness? Initially I didn't want to admit to myself that I was going downhill physically. I feared what might happen to my practice, my finances, and my image. If my patients and colleagues knew of my illness and if I stopped or gave in to my symptoms, my practice could end or be severely damaged. I knew that the prognosis for advanced Crohn's disease was not good, and I actually feared what I might learn about my physical state. On the other hand, I had had little pain and few physical symptoms during the early period of this exacerbation. After all, I had been through significant problems with this disease for many years. Furthermore, the day-to-day and month-to-month signs and symptoms changed so gradually that I did not recognize fully the overall course my body was taking.

This response was self-destructive, but it was not the only adverse behavior that I was practicing. Eating had long before assumed a major role in my life. With my terrible malabsorption problem, high caloric intake—which I equated with large quantities of food—seemed the best way to maintain my nutrition. I spent hours shopping for, preparing, and eating food. This preoccupation with food consumed enormous amounts of time. My eating pattern became my "trademark," a significant part of my life-style.

My personal life was taking a bad turn. My wife's depression had been significantly improved with psychotherapy. By 1970 she was a full-time graduate assistant and seemed less involved in my life. Though no less self-destructive, I became more depressed. I felt more and more trapped by my situation but still avoided making any important decisions about my health. The more I procrastinated, the worse my emotional state became. I was often agitated and ill-tempered at the office, at hospitals, and at home.

I reached the "low-water mark" in my emotional state in late 1970 and finally went to see a psychiatrist. My experience in relationship-type therapy was good. Since the therapist was the same one Virginia had seen a few years before, he was aware of our relationship and my illness. In my psychotherapy I learned that much of my behavior—especially toward Virginia—was passive-aggressive. I further learned that much of this stemmed from my own anger and depression. I began taking a more realistic approach to my abnormal preoccupation with food. I continued eating large amounts, since my appetite remained insatiable, but I spent less time in buying and preparing food. My visits to the psychiatrist decreased during 1971 as reality pierced consciousness.

Physically I suffered from muscle weakness to the point that climbing stairs became an effort. The edema, recurrent bruising, and subconjunctival hemorrhages continued, but somehow I lived with my symptoms. My patients, colleagues, friends, and family seemed to accept me. I never discussed my appearance and behavior with anyone.

Looking back today, I see myself carefully avoiding any dialogue that dealt with my looks or my health. I didn't want to appear impaired or to be treated differently. I didn't want my patients to think of me as being unhealthy and, therefore, less able to take care of their health.

At that point I was unable to give of myself to my patients or to anyone else as I would have wanted. It was all I could do to survive. My own problems probably resulted in my becoming more deeply involved in their situations than was necessary or in my best interest.

I continued my inevitable "crash course" until an event in late 1971 shocked me into action. A colleague and friend who had not seen me for several months called me aside and told me that I looked dangerously ill. He advised me to get medical attention soon. Until that moment no one had actually "laid it on the line" in the way he did. Jim was an academic gastroenterologist and I accepted his advice with confidence. His objectivity, frankness, and unmistakable concern for me and my health struck a chord within me for the first time. I knew that he was correct and that I needed help badly. I was finally conscious of the fact that I might not survive my illness if I didn't do something about it soon.

Thus awakened, I made several decisions that I had failed to face at all. I had to decide when and where to go for my evaluation, how to plan for day-to-day care of my patients and the financial loss. Whether my wife should continue in graduate school full time was also considered. I questioned the probabilities of my recovery. If advised that surgery was indicated, I pondered whether I would survive. Would I become much more disabled? I knew I might even have cancer. I was frightened and realized that I had a real reason to be depressed. Was I willing to undergo the rigorous tests and examinations that were necessary for proper evaluation? Contrast media, venipunctures, enemas, nasogastric tubes, and the like were not new to me, but they were nonetheless objectionable. Then there were the familiar but never personally experienced procedures like needle biopsy, endoscopy, and percutaneous central feeding catheters, to mention just a few. Virginia and I had frequent discussions. None of the problems that we talked about really seemed insoluble. She urged me to visit my psychiatrist for further counseling and support, which I admitted needing very badly.

I did return to the psychiatrist and was finally able to voice my underlying anxiety, fears, and pessimistic outlook for my future. For the first time I allowed myself to deal with the seriousness of my illness and my advanced state of malnutrition. I received immeasurable support and practical suggestions during my sessions with the psychiatrist. This relationship has continued to the present on an intermittent basis and it has made a major contribution to my health and happiness.

In considering the options available for my major medical evaluation, a distant location seemed to provide personal privacy.

When I am being treated, particularly in the hospital, I try to be a cooperative patient. Being at that top-ranked institution was no exception. However, I shall never forget my doctor's parting advice on his first visit to me in the hospital. To paraphrase, he said that this was an excellent facility and that my floor was well run with highly competent nurses. Mistakes and miscalculations occur regardless, and a physician-patient can expect the traditional foul-up. Thus, he warned me to be alert and not hesitate to *question* or *refuse* any given treatment or preparation for or participation in a test if I thought there had been a mistake. Furthermore, if I was concerned I could call him at any time, and he gave me his home phone number. This was most reassuring. There *were* one or two significant mistakes that were corrected when I questioned the nurse in charge.

As a physician I was treated with special care while at the institution, particularly by the professional personnel. I appreciated this consideration. There were a few times when I sensed that technicians were uncomfortable carrying out procedures on "a doctor." They either mentioned their discomfort or made inappropriate remarks such as, "You can probably do this better than I can since you are a doctor." The special care I received from the GI fellow assigned to me was marvelous. Whether a physician-patient receives good hospital care is directly related to his behavior, which is not much different from any patient in the hospital. Twice while there I attended the weekly GI teaching conference. Once I was the patient whose case was presented for the opinion of the gastroenterologists there, but I was not allowed to stay for the discussion of my case. I was later briefed as to what had been recommended. This was reassuring, although I wasn't certain that my doctor had given me the whole range of opinion expressed at the conference in order to spare me some of the unfavorable points.

After two weeks in the hospital, our final meeting with the doctor took place in my room with Virginia present. I was told of the major findings. I was relieved that the medical situation was no worse. I considered the report on my current state of health favorable. I was also relieved that I had not stressed my body or neglected my symptoms to the point of no return. I did not have cancer. At the same time I recognized that I did have some options and that the future did not look as bleak as I had anticipated.

Euphoria followed my return to Atlanta. I am sure that some of it was steroid-induced, but my basic attitudes toward myself, my illness, and my life in general had taken on a positive and optimistic air. I was determined to follow the medical program "to the letter." I continued the psychiatric counseling I had restarted before leaving Atlanta, and I found it even more helpful than before.

Positive influences on my recovery were (1) a physician who served as an authority figure for me, (2) an excellent communication channel through my local physician and concerned partner who could work with me in carrying out my doctor's specific recommendations, and (3) reported follow-up information that kept my program active and current. This was in distinct contrast to the preceding years of casual care. I am certain that this change was possible principally because my attitude and approach to my illness was different. I needed strict and positive guidance from afar plus ongoing and enthusiastic contact locally. By this time I was receptive to it.

I have always believed in God or a superior being or force responsible for order (disorder) in our universe. Having lived with the highs and lows of my illness has not changed my beliefs. I have not been, on the other hand, a frequent or regular participant in the formal aspects of the religion into which I was born. (Incidentally, if free to choose any religion, I believe I would choose Judaism.) I pray whenever I feel the desire or need to do so. I do not feel the need to attend a house of worship to have my prayers heard. I am not certain that my illness has increased my faith, but it has not lessened it either. Surely humans have a huge power to influence their own destiny. My feelings and experiences as both patient and physician have strengthened this conviction. I have utilized the love, skills, and interest of other human beings to help me through the years. I have no doubt now, or ever, that the driving force which has made me better physically and emotionally, and a more whole person, has been my own willingness to utilize and synthesize all of the forces and skills available to me. I cannot rule out a "superior being" as one of these forces. Prayer has, in some way, afforded me the inner strength to help myself.

Determination has been the driving force in my life. In retrospect, it is difficult to separate determination from denial. In the earlier days of my illness, my behavior was the outgrowth of my determination to perform well regardless of physical handicaps. My decision to pursue medicine was made during 1941—the year that I was out of school following surgery. I have no doubt that this decision was heavily influenced by my illness. The handicap that my illness imposed on me could not have been overcome without driving determination.

The working formulas for much of my life appear to have been:

ILLNESS + DETERMINATION = DENIAL

ILLNESS + DENIAL = DEPRESSION

In high school I wished very much not to be different because I was physically ill. It was important for me to get my share of physical hazing with my peers during pledgeship and initiation into high school and college fraternities. Paddling the buttocks was a significant part of this hazing, but if I revealed my problem with that portion of my anatomy a different form of hazing would be applied to me. It was not easy for me to convey this information to those involved; so frequently I simply "took my share" of the paddle and ignored or "forgot" that I had been warned not to allow such to happen to me.

During medical school I experienced many instances of denial: not wanting to discuss my illness with anyone, not wanting special consideration because of illness, and proving my strength to myself by working longer hours on the wards or in the emergency room than most of my peers. In spite of the advice from friends, physicians, and others that I should pursue a less strenuous specialty, I chose the field of internal medicine. While my choice was certainly influenced in part by my illness, it also involved denial to myself. That I should consider my physical condition in planning for my future would be an outright admission of my illness.

The roots of my depression extend back as far as high school when I felt anger at being unable to participate in sports as I had always dreamed I would. Being different limited and changed my relationships with my peers. Teenage narcissisism made me angry that my body failed to develop. Although I accepted my inability to enter college with my peers, I felt resentful that I could not take this major step toward maturity with them. In fact, I was lonely during that long year, and I often felt cheated by not being a participant in college activities. Of course, all was not bad. I met the girl who would later become my wife, and I did enjoy some of the social activities at Georgia Tech and the University of Georgia during that year. Still, it was somewhat as an outsider—I never felt fully accepted by the students.

I shall try to place in perspective what my experience with a longstanding illness has meant to me both as a physician and as an individual. I know that I have grown emotionally. While one normally matures with experience, I am certain that my maturation occurred largely as a product of psychotherapy, prior to which I was up to my ears in denial. Understanding myself and accepting myself is perhaps the bottom line of most of the positive results. Although I seemed to deteriorate physically and emotionally at the same time and recover similarly, there is no way to determine how much each influenced the other.

I am certain that psychotherapy has been beneficial in my relationship with Virginia. Worn down and depressed by my constant denial of my illness and by my passive–aggressive behavior toward her, Virginia developed an independent posture toward me and my illness which gave me more substantial support, while protecting her at the same time. My depression and passive-aggressive behavior has diminished significantly. Virginia's reaction to my behavior had a positive influence on me. I have learned to relate to her in a more mature and direct fashion. I rarely forget to call when I'm running late, and I am realistic in estimating the time I will get home. We enjoy each other's company, interests, and activities. I have always supported her work and now find that sharing in her academic life affords me much pleasure and has been a broadening experience. I never have objected to her nice income—we have fun sharing it!

I am sure that being a patient influenced my decision to become a doctor—a gastroenterologist in my case. Naturally, I see many patients with inflammatory bowel disease, particularly Crohn's disease. I am able to relate to most of these patients and empathize with their concerns about weight loss, diarrhea, pain, etc. I especially care about these patients as individuals and probably spend more time with them than with many others, listening to their physical and emotional problems and suggesting practical and pharmacologic remedies. My interest in state-of-the-art management of inflammatory bowel disease is more personal than that for other diseases.

As a rule I do not discuss my medical history with my patients, but there are times when I find it useful to inform a patient that I have Crohn's disease and have had it for most of my life. I must admit that I have felt frustrated by those rare patients who attempt to use the disease in claiming total disability when such is clearly not the case. Although I see total denial as an abnormal approach for any individual in dealing with the disease, I do feel that more determination and less self-indulgence are often necessary.

My experiences as a patient have made me more aware of physician behavior. I try to be totally honest with my patients in dealing with complications and unexpected problems, although today, medicolegal factors do not make this easy.

I enjoy my life and enjoy living. Although I continue to work full time and put in the usual 10- to 12-hour days, I am learning to pace myself. I know that physical and emotional fitness add up to keeping well. When I overdo, push myself too hard for too long, and don't conserve my energy, I feel lousy! I no longer ignore my exhaustion or deny its existence. I am more productive because I am physically stronger, so I accomplish more in less time. Medical checkups and laboratory studies are important and regular features of my relatively new "health care program." The bottom line of all this is acceptance of the fact that I am totally responsible for myself.

I recognize that I am not cured in any sense of the word. At the same time, I feel very happy with myself and my life-style. I enjoy people and my relationships both in and outside my practice. Being able to be more open and having a good self-image are important ingredients in the recipe of life's enjoyment. My family is a major source of happiness and support to me. Both of my daughters are in medical-related fields and are productive and happy. That I am the grandfather of a spunky, adorable little fellow of 18 months has given me immeasurable happiness and strengthened my commitment to the future.

Who better than I can attest to the truth of the oft-quoted biblical passage "Physician heal thyself"? My dictum now, taken from Dr. Oliver Wendell Holmes: "[Formula for longevity:] Have a chronic disease and take care of it." Although late to embrace either of these wise pieces of advice, I think that there has been sufficient time for me to enjoy my total environment, grow with my experiences and give back something of worth to this world. I truly believe that having lived these past 50 years in the shadow of personal health problems, becoming aware of my reactions to them, and working through difficult solutions have been of much greater advantage than disadvantage to me as a physician and as a human being.

CHAPTER 28

DUODENAL ULCER

HARRISON F. WOOD

In October 1938, at the age of 19, I was admitted to the Presbyterian Hospital in New York City. For two days I had noted weakness, dizziness, and shortness of breath accompanied by dark, tarry stools. I was seen by a friend's physician, who diagnosed gastrointestinal bleeding, phoned the admitting office of Presbyterian, and instructed me to proceed there immediately by taxi. I did so and was promptly admitted to a medical ward, where I was thoroughly worked up by the resident, who informed me that I had lost a significant amount of blood via my GI tract. This resident was both competent and reassuring. I was kept at total bed rest, given morphine and intravenous fluids. I had no abdominal pain or tenderness. I confess that I felt unique. None of my friends had had similar experiences or long hospitalizations, except for one who sustained a broken femur with subsequent osteomyelitis in a motorcycle accident.

At the time of my bleed I was at loose ends. My father would not send me to college unless I could give him a good reason for his doing so. He remembered his time at Amherst as one of frivolity and riotous living, though he did have loyalty to the class of 1910. In 1936 I was graduated from a progressive private school in Greenwich, Connecticut. A few of my classmates had gone on immediately to college. Two of them had gone successfully into the theater. One had gone for a postgraduate year to Le Rosay School in Switzerland. I had vague thoughts of becoming a writer. I had little interest in science. A niece of Robert Koch had been my science teacher but failed to impart an interest in bacteriology despite her "relationship" to the tubercle bacillus. I feel that I received an excellent liberal education in high school, but it did not provide me with any incentive to enter any useful or learned profession. My father was an architect, but I had no wish to follow in his footsteps. I spent the academic year 1937–1938 in Europe

DR. HARRISON WOOD is a 66-year-old retired internist. He has a special interest in rheumatic fever and acute phase proteins.

partly with a classmate who had run away from Dartmouth and partly with my mother, who was a good linguist. When I returned from Europe, I lived with my family in New York. I went regularly to almost every museum in the city and to the Metropolitan Museum of Art, which was only a few blocks from home. I was continuing my education on my own, but I was at loose ends and did not know what I wanted to do with my life.

In historical perspective, several aspects of my hospitalization are worth mentioning. An upper GI series was not done until two weeks after admission. Such procedures were then postponed until well after the acute phase. I was transfused with blood taken from my sister just before it was administered to me. I developed urticaria after the transfusion. Gastroscopy employing the inflexible metal gastroscope of that era was carried out. I remember lying with my neck dorsiflexed over the edge of the examining table while the rigid tube was passed down my esophagus into my stomach. I vividly recall reading a large billboard stating, "I'd walk a mile for a Camel," from that examining table. Another procedure done was a cholangiogram. Repeated stool specimens were examined for occult blood. Hematocrits were done every few days. Finally, at the end of two weeks, I was out of bed on a graduated schedule.

Two patients on that ward remain vivid in my memory. One man in his early 20s had Hodgkin's disease. He had bitterly resigned himself to an early death and talked of his thwarted hopes and ambitions and of all the joys of life he would miss. The other was a man in his early 60s who had contracted encephalitis in Vienna in 1917 and who constantly fell asleep in the middle of conversations. Nothing could be done to help him.

I was given the diagnosis of duodenitis, but one of the attending physicians, Dr. George Draper, was convinced that I had bled from a duodenal ulcer. Draper was a distinguished and charismatic man. His grandfather Draper had been professor of chemistry at Bellevue Hospital Medical School in the nineteenth century, and his grandfather Dana was the editor of *The New York Sun* who wrote the famous "Yes, Virginia, there is a Santa Claus." His sister was the noted monologist, Muriel Draper. George Draper was interested in constitutional medicine and wrote several interesting papers in the field. He had written a monograph on poliomyelitis with Dr. Simon Flexner when he had been at the Rockefeller Institute. I had long talks with Dr. Draper about my life and illness and about the medical profession. He told me to avoid any stressful occupation, citing the high incidence of gastric and duodenal ulcers in New York taxi drivers and policemen. I had never dreamed of being either.

Dr. George Draper was a towering figure to me. Through my illness, hospitalization, and contact with excellent physicians, I became increasingly interested in medicine. Doctors seemed like powerful figures to me. They did things to people. At the age of 5½, I had had an extremely traumatic surgical experience. As I later learned, I had begun to identify with the aggressor.

I remained in the hospital one month, which in the context of today's medicine was an inordinate length of time. However, the prolonged hospitalization provided me with ample time to contemplate my life, its lack of direction, and possible long-term goals. I decided that I wanted to become a physician, not so much to treat patients as to learn about the mechanisms of their illnesses. I decided I wanted to go into medical research. That illness appeared to me to be a unifying, maturing experience.

My father became convinced of the validity of my motivation and consented to pay for my college and medical school education. I started college at NYU in September 1939, just days after World War II began in Europe. I found college highly stimulating and rewarding, in some ways almost a continuation of the intellectual ferment of the unusual high school I attended. I majored in chemistry and minored in German in college. A chemistry major was designed to get me into medical school. I was actually more interested in English and German than I was in chemistry, though the logic of organic chemistry was beautiful. As the tempo of the war increased, college and medical school curricula accelerated. I went through summer semesters at college and was admitted to NYU College of Medicine after three years of college.

From internship I went into the Public Health Service for two years. I spent the following seven years at the Rockefeller Institute and its hospital.

My GI tract had been mostly quiescent for 21 years until 1959. I had avoided highly spiced foods and heavy alcohol intake, but I was a fairly heavy cigarette smoker. In August of that year, I felt some epigastric discomfort experienced as a gnawing sensation. I did not consult my physician. I drank a large amount of milk but took no antacids. I recall a Labor Day cocktail party after which I had severe epigastric distress for two days. I still did not see my internist. During the last week of September I experienced the onset of rather severe upper abdominal pain. I remember working in my laboratory at NYU on the third day of severe pain when I told a young Dutch physician friend about it. He told me what I already knew. "You *must* see a doctor. It sounds to me as though something major is going on." Early that evening when I got home my wife telephoned my physician, who was also a friend. He was a former chief resident at the Hospital of the

Rockefeller Institute who had opened a practice in internal medicine in Manhattan. He came to see me about 7:00 that evening and examined me thoroughly. He told me that I had a surgical abdomen and should be admitted to a hospital immediately. He thought acute cholecystitis was a good possibility. Within two hours I was admitted to the New York Hospital. Thirty-six hours later I had an exploratory laparotomy done by a surgeon whose competence I trusted. As I came out of anesthesia in the recovery room I said to a nurse, "Was this operation really necessary?" She replied, "Yes," and I dozed off again. I had had perforation of a tiny posterior duodenal ulcer. The surgeon had done a plication and given me the bonus of an appendectomy. Bowel sounds returned, and four days after the surgery I had the most explosive bowel movement I have ever had. I remained in the hospital ten days before continuing convalescence at home. My internist gave me detailed instructions on diet and graduated activity. He saw me several times during my convalescence. We had a 5-month-old baby son at home, which did not make my convalescent period easy for my wife. I was supposed to drink about as much milk as he did. By the time I was well I never wanted to see milk or custard again. I remember writing research grant requests and working on clinical research papers while I recovered.

In 1960 I moved from Manhattan to New Haven, Connecticut, to teach immunology in the Department of Pediatrics at Yale. I continued my research on C-reactive protein until 1967. During that year my interest in laboratory research waned, and I was faced with the realization that I had done all the research I wanted to do. I wound it up after 20 years of dedication to it. I felt no void as a result of abandoning the laboratory. By then I had learned that my true gifts lay in the fields of human relations and art.

In 1969 I moved from Yale School of Medicine to the Veterans Administration Hospital. In the spring of 1977 I began to experience growing discomfort in my epigastrium. I went on a bland diet and treated myself with antacids. Despite this, the epigastric distress continued. Although I had an excellent internist, I again denied my symptoms. I still do not understand my evidently strong need to deny symptoms that would have alerted any good internist, let alone myself, to a probably underlying disease.

I came home from work one mid-April afternoon and had a black, tarry bowel movement. I phoned my internist, who was still in his office. He told me to go immediately for admission via the emergency room to the university hospital. The resident had not completed her work-up when my physician arrived. I had an NG tube in place. My hematocrit was low and intravenous fluids had been started. Largely because I had had a small cerebrovascular accident the previous summer and had labile hypertension, I was admitted to the intensive care unit for close monitoring. I remained there for two days and received two units of packed red cells. My blood pressure was taken every half hour for 12 hours and hourly thereafter. My hematocrit was closely followed. On the third hospital day I was transferred to a medical floor. An upper GI series showed a duodenal ulcer and old scarring of the pylorus. My internist told me, "It looked as though an army had walked over it." I remained in the hospital ten days and afterwards had a convalescent period of two or three weeks before returning to work. My medical care had been superb. I did not like being a patient and ardently hoped that my duodenum would be quiescent for the remainder of my life. However, this was not to be. The worst was yet to come.

On October 22, 1980, I went into New York to hear the New York Philharmonic perform the Verdi *Requiem*. It was a magnificent performance with Placido Domingo as the tenor soloist. I must have been bleeding during the requiem, for when it was over I took a taxi to 68th Street and First Avenue near the garage where I left my car. I went into a Greek restaurant on the corner, went to the men's room, and vomited blood. I felt faint and broke into a cold sweat. I sat down at a booth in the restaurant. Two men looked at me, came over, and asked, "Are you all right?" I told them what had happened. Plainclothes New York City policemen, they drove me to the emergency room of a nearby hospital. I was admitted with hematemesis.

I was assigned to a staff gastroenterologist, who did endoscopy. He visualized an active duodenal ulcer, which was also seen on an upper GI series. This physician urged surgery. I was seen several times by a surgeon during that hospitalization. There was an eagerness about him that stimulated mistrust in me. I wanted to get back to New Haven to get opinions from physicians who had treated me before. I was permitted to return to New Haven ten days and two units of packed red cells later. The care at the hospital in New York was good, but I wanted to see my trusted regular internist, especially in view of possible impending surgery. When I saw him he referred me for repeat endoscopy by a gastroenterologist who two years previously had done colonoscopy on me. He, too, saw an active duodenal ulcer. The consensus was that I should have surgery. Three bleeds and you're out. I chose for my surgeon a physician of excellent reputation who two years earlier had removed a benign villous adenoma the size of a walnut from my lower colon. He was noted in the New Haven medical community for his good judgment and skill.

Surgery was scheduled for November 17, 1980. It was hoped that this would be a pyloroplasty. However, the pylorus was too scarred for such a procedure and instead a gastrojejunostomy and truncal vagotomy were done. I was returned from the recovery room to the floor with a full bladder and, groggy as I was, I recall the extreme discomfort and long wait for a house officer to catheterize me. The immediate postsurgical days were very painful and stressful. I was instructed to cough at least hourly during the first few postoperative days. That was agony. With each cough I felt as if I were being stabbed in the belly. One day about a week after the surgery I developed severe hiccoughs only partially controllable by Compazine. They lasted two days. Ten days after surgery I was discharged home, where I completed my convalescence.

During that period I thought back over my medical history. Overall, I had not been a very good patient. Within a few months after each acute episode I resumed living as though nothing had happened to me. I did not slow down, did not particularly watch my diet. I continued to be a heavy cigarette smoker. I worked hard. My interest in the profession of medicine lessened. I felt that my duodenum had betrayed me, had made me more vulnerable than others. I asked, "Why me?" I felt that my life had been sabotaged by my gastrointestinal tract and that it ultimately rendered me a less effective physician and person. These were very difficult feelings to come to terms with.

I feel that being a physician did not affect the quality of medical care, which, overall, was excellent. However, it may have speeded up appointments and procedures and influenced care in subtle ways that I am not aware of, as, for instance, quality of nursing care. The only major gaffe that I recall was the failure of the recovery room staff at one hospital to check me for bladder distention before sending me back to my room. If I had it to do over again I would choose the same physicians. They were all competent and caring. Some of them became friends.

It is now 47 years since I had my first gastrointestinal hemorrhage. I am 66 years old and have been retired from the practice of medicine for two years. True or not, I feel that I have entered old age. I have frequent gastric reflux, sometimes accompanied by severe pain in the region of the splenic flexure. Two upper GI series in the past three years have demonstrated no marginal ulcer. The badly scarred duodenum is still patent and barium passes into an apparently normal jejunum. Reflux of barium from the stomach into the esophagus is evident, though there is not a hiatus hernia.

Living with my GI tract over the years has not been easy. It has bestowed on me four sudden and totally unexpected hospitalizations. I believe that my illnesses made me a more compassionate physician than I would otherwise have been. They taught me to really listen to patients and to try to comprehend them as total beings in the context of their families, work, and strivings. It changed them from isolated cases to people with medical problems in a social context. I am not describing holistic medicine but rather medicine as a humanistic as well as scientific discipline.

Religious faith was of no benefit to me during my illnesses. I have none but envy those who do. I have a good friend, a retired physician in California who is a very active, practicing Episcopalian. He is now running a busy soup kitchen in a large city under church auspices. His concern for the hungry and homeless stems from a truly religious concern for his fellow man. I envy his belief and commitment.

In retrospect I believe that my decision to become a physician was at least in part neurotic. Nevertheless, I accomplished a good amount and had my share of real satisfactions. The greatest satisfaction was teaching medical students. Their enthusiasm was stimulating and infectious. Their questions, both substantive and general, were always challenging.

I have a bibliography of 45 papers in the medical literature. Though none of them is a milestone in twentieth-century biological investigation, some of them are very good and they are often cited in the current literature.

If I had it to do over, I would probably not choose to become a physician. As a group, I find them quite limited in their interests. Too many of them have become arrogant, perhaps unconsciously, in the confines of their specializations. I think that most practicing nonacademic physicians have too much interest in high incomes, sometimes to the detriment of patient care. I know an internist who used to be in solo practice with ample time for each patient. He has joined with two competent younger physicians in as automated an office as possible in a modern "medical center" with all ancillary services, a radiology center, a complete clinical laboratory, etc., in the building. He sees at least three times as many patients as he saw when he was on his own, usually briefly, and misses some diagnoses that would not have escaped him when he devoted more time to each patient. He hears, but he no longer listens. His income has probably tripled as his patient load has tripled. He is still a good physician but not as good as he used to be.

My illnesses have turned me inward and have also sharpened my observing eye. If I were again 19, I would probably become a curator of prints in a museum or a print dealer. Over the past 15 years I have acquired considerable knowledge of prints and have bought and sold a fair number of them, from Dürer to Jasper Johns. Unfortunately, I never had enough capital to build a major collection. I am left with a Benedict Arnold gastrointestinal tract, a completed medical career, and a small collection of major prints. I also have two fine sons in their late 20s. Neither of them is a physician.

PART V

CANCER

CHAPTER 29

ANAPLASTIC CARCINOMA OF NECK

"ALBERT LUTHER"

The pronouncement was made so abruptly, Al didn't appreciate its significance. "Your blood pressure is still all right," his friend had said. "The insurance company shouldn't have turned you down. But I don't think you should go back to them until you get that lump in your neck removed or at least biopsied."

Lump in his neck? Al had felt so well all year, he thought that his increased collar size had meant he was settling comfortably into middle age and finally gaining some weight. It only took a few hours to resume his compulsive behavior. Without appointment and without even a telephone warning, he bolted into the examining room of a surgical colleague. Stripping off his shirt, Al approached his friend like a tattered ensign in an autumn storm. "I want it off. I want to be on tomorrow's OR schedule." If bad news lay ahead, he would meet it promptly and head on. How else could one handle a crisis? The next day was his wife's 40th birthday. That could wait.

His next Rubicon was on the first postoperative day. Al's surgical colleague was standing at the foot of the bed, oozing platitudes about speedy recovery, pain medications, and other irrelevant drivel. "What's the path report?" queried Al through his dressings.

The attending tried to put him off. Surgeons never have the stomach for bad news. "We'll discuss that tomorrow, when you're feeling better."

"The hell we will," replied Al. "You'll tell me right now, you bastard, or I'll climb over the end of this bed—chest tubes and all. I'll beat the holy hell out of you until I have the answer. I want to make my plans—good or bad."

"DR. ALBERT LUTHER" is a professor of medicine emeritus at the Harvard Medical School and former chairman of the Department of Medicine at the New England Deaconess Hospital in Boston, Massachusetts. He still maintains his research interests in coagulation and allied problems in hematology and oncology.

Al had spent the bulk of his years in hematology-oncology. He had learned by trial and error that patients with malignant disease fell into three broad groups. He knew which one he fitted—the small group that constituted the "I-want-to-know" type. He was like that. Nothing was worse than uncertainty. It was essential to make plans, even for death. He could arrange for an orderly disposition of property. No need to be sloppy. And perhaps the surgeon or pathologist was wrong anyway. He might outlive their prognosis. The second group was a bit larger—maybe a quarter of all patients. They faced the future by not hearing what you said. These were the ones where it was important to talk with the family. After all, someone had to know. But the largest group was the one where the patients played games with the doctor. These patients suspected the diagnosis but weren't quite ready to face its reality. Al had found that the kindest way to handle this group was to let the patient set his own pace for hard facts. Whenever Al performed a bone marrow aspiration or other procedure on a new patient, he would say, "Tomorrow I will be back with the results of these tests. Ask me anything you want to know about your diagnosis at that time, and I will discuss it with you." Almost invariably, the latter group would go to great lengths to delay the results of the studies. They would ask how the Red Sox or Bruins were doing. They would ask about the weather. They would keep the conversation on any topic but the important one. Al had decided it was cruel to bring their house of cards crashing about them. They secretly knew what the problem was anyway. They just wanted some time to become intellectually prepared for the inevitable. Eventually, they would get around to an attitude of acceptance. When they did, they too would become cooperative and grateful. When they finally asked the specific question—Is this cancer, leukemia, lymphoma, or whatever—they were now able to say, "and what will *we* do about it, Doctor?" They already had transferred part of their burden to the helpful hands of the physician. He or she was part of a team. He or she was fulfilling the true role of a physician: to heal when possible, to help always, to harm never.

Al's surgeon was distinctly uncomfortable. How could he tell Al, a physician who knew most of the answers, that it was an anaplastic carcinoma; that it already had metastasized out of the neck, down into the mediastinal nodes; that they didn't get it all out? "It was a growth, a malignancy," he mumbled.

"Hodgkin's?" inquired Al.

"No."

"Cancer?"

"Maybe."

"Stop the crap. Where did it come from, thyroid?"

"We're not sure."

"You're lying through your teeth," Al replied. "Damn it, I want facts."

It was days before he got the full picture. After a brief convalescence, he would have to undergo various tests and procedures. Bone scans, neck scans, node scans, barium swallows, everything short of a homogenization. If all systems were "go," he was then to be readmitted for a sternal crack and total mediastinal node dissection.

Three months later, the procedure was performed: three hours of radical neck surgery followed by three hours of open chest dissection. The postoperative period was more stormy this time: early spontaneous pneumothorax—salvaged by an alert ICU team; late thrombophlebitis and pulmonary embolism—salvaged by a less-alert medical team. Again, he survived, this time blinked back into reality by a miniature Christmas tree with tiny lights that flashed every few seconds on the bedside table.

Finally, he recovered enough strength to go home for rehabilitation. For the first time, he began to understand the Book of Job, which he vaguely recalled from childhood. Job had endured everything—the loss of his family, the loss of his income, the loss of his ego. He even had outlasted boils and the ash heap. It wasn't until his friends appeared and began to commiserate with him that Job's patience had snapped. It was just so with Al.

Well-meaning medical colleagues began to appear at his home. "I think you've got at least a year before it recurs," stated one. Small consolation at 45, Al thought. "You must have immediate radiotherapy," said another. How do they know I want to live so badly? he thought. I haven't complained or even asked for a reprieve. "I'd lay all my chances on radioactive iodine," said another. "It may have started in the thyroid no matter how anaplastic it looks." Al could remember having received repeated courses of X-ray therapy to the skin of his neck and face as an acne-prone pubescent teenager. Maybe that had caused it. No one knew anything about filters in those days. They didn't even know X-rays were harmful. Why try something for treatment that might have caused this mess in the first place?

"No," he replied. "I'm not going to do any of those dumb things. I'm wiped out financially. I'm beaten into the ground physically. I'm a basket case psychologically. I'm going to take my chances and let nature run its course. Meantime, I'm withdrawing the last few hundred dollars from the bank, and I'm going to drive to Florida with my wife and children and sponge off my parents until I either die or get well."

They had just about reached Georgia when the next crisis occurred. Al was lying on the back seat of the car enduring headache, fever, and chills. He felt so awful he wished he could die. That night in the Beachcomber Motel ($8 per room, no extra for children), he had gotten up in the night to vomit and void. His urine was bright orange. Serum hepatitis had begun.

It was six months before he got out of the hospital. This time his weight was under 100. Hyperal was not available in those days. There was little left but a hank of hair.

This new illness was different in all aspects from the recent cancer operations, he thought. Surgery was tangible—something he could get his hands on. He could discuss the diagnosis, think about it, and plan accordingly. Even though the news had been bad, he had been able to modify his life-style, develop a reaction pattern, and then live with it day by day. He had neatly filed his new program into a cluster of synapses in a remote gyrus, not unlike a floppy disk awaiting a summons. But hepatitis! What a miserable affliction this was! He couldn't think clearly. He couldn't concentrate on any subject more than momentarily. Most appallingly, he didn't give a damn. No wonder the Greeks had given the "humour" of black bile the malevolent moniker of melancholia. For week after week, Al lay in a hospital bed with his life barely supported by saline and glucose. His muscle mass—puny to begin with—melted down to the point where his bones were about the only structure remaining. And they were encased in orange-colored, parchmentlike skin. Then, almost imperceptibly, the process began to reverse. His icterus lightened ever so slightly. He drifted out of his coma. Within another week, he began to sit up and take light nourishment orally. Slowly, he recovered from the wipeout of hepatitis B viremia and its attendant cell lysis. As recovery proceeded and he took an interest in his surroundings again, Al's first request was for the transfusion records of the dozen donors whose blood he had received during the thorocotomy several months earlier. But that proved a wasted pursuit. He learned he had developed either DIC or primary fibrinogenolysis immediately postop. For this, he had been given two boluses of 4 grams of fibrinogen a few hours apart. The fibrinogen was derived from three commercial LOTs. Each LOT was fractionated from a pool of plasma from about 1000 donors. No wonder fibrinogen was later removed from the commercial market, he thought. One might as well take an infusion directly from a cesspool.

The time interval was about one year from his diagnosis of cancer and the first neck surgery, through the second operation with the radical neck and mediastinal node dissection, and finally his bout with hepatitis. But eventually, Al returned to work. Once again, his well-meaning friends and colleagues came to offer unsolicited advice. Maybe he could be "cured of the residual cancer which indubitably was still present," they said. Some of them reiterated the virtues of radiotherapy. "You simply must do it," they averred. "It has a reasonably high success rate with this histology. You're not being fair to your family if you don't." Others pushed equally forcefully for chemotherapy. "The more combinations we put together, the higher the success rate," they said. "It's more than 1+1+1+1 equaling 4. It equals about 8 or maybe 12."

Al was unimpressed. And he still felt unreasonably tired. His friends meant well. But they were so anxious to cure his tumor, they were willing to kill him to do it. Maybe it was a residue of posthepatic depression, he thought; too many Dane particles were still circulating. Everywhere he turned, there was evidence to support the advice of his pessimistic friends. The very first grand rounds he had gone to after recovery had been a review of treatment results in people with the same illness. On one of the slides, the speaker had constructed a grid outlining the histologic types of malignancy of this organ, plotted against the number and location of metastases. According to the calculations of this colleague, Al was already dead.

Al remembered distinctly the morning he firmly made up his mind to have no further treatment and take his chances, whatever they might be. He had never been a good sleeper. This night was no exception. He had wandered into the bedrooms of each of his children. Three were at home, two girls and one boy. Another girl was away at school. He watched them sleeping peacefully and wondered whether his wife would be able to raise them by herself. He guessed that she could. After all, she had pretty much done so already. He had been so wrapped up in his career and his work, he had neglected his family shamefully. Then for the past full year, he had been no help at all.

Along about 4:00 a.m., he had gone into his son's room and sat on the red leather window seat. It was summer. The sun came up early. It rose like a giant fried egg on the northeastern horizon. Al was shocked by its beauty, by its majesty, by its unfailingness. It had always risen in that spot at this time of year. And it always would. Here he was worrying about his own microcosm in a background of grand and immutable forces that were so much bigger, more important, and more vast as to make a caricature of his concerns.

And never before had he appreciated the nascent beauty of a new day. Maybe there wouldn't be too many dawns left for him. He must search them out. See everything that he could see. Smell them. Feel them. Try to touch the mist and listen to the birds begin their first morning noise. Always before, he had been angry if he was awakened at this hour. Why couldn't he just lie down and snore like others? Maybe because they worked harder physically than he. But Al wouldn't admit that to himself. His newly awakened interest in nature has lasted since that time. It proved a greater soporific than any pill or formula for deep breathing that he had tried. Once his strength returned, he got an additional boost from taking long walks. He loved the smell of freshly mowed grass and to feel it compress under his shoes, especially if he happened to be swinging a 5-iron on a fairway.

The postrecovery hiatus was not without its humorous side, too. He kept driving his old car back and forth to the hospital and the office. First the tailpipe fell off, then the battery went. The transmission groaned and the brakes squeaked. Why saddle his wife with a new car if he was only going to live a short while? She had one of her own and obviously couldn't drive two. And money would be scarce. It wasn't until the inspection station refused to renew his certificate that he came to his senses. "Doctor," they had said, "if you only live until Monday, you've got to turn in this junk heap for another car."

He often wondered whether his long struggle with uncertainty and expectancy of early death and slow emergence from this presumption had affected his religious life or convictions. Or, more likely, had the opposite been true? Reflecting back on the ten years that had passed since an apparently erroneous pronouncement of fatal cancer, he couldn't recall any great moment of spiritual revelation. There had been no flashes of light, no bells, no tinnitus, no great moment when he suddenly felt courageous instead of afraid. About his only thoughts of death had been the fleeting egotism of thinking what a loss it would be to the world if he died so young. He had led a reasonably good, moral life. But this reflected his conservative demeanor and was done more from habit than from preplanning. Moreover, he had been raised "in-the-church." His clergyman father had set high standards toward which Al instinctively had strived. But his father wisely had avoided any overt pressure for Al to profess his religion publicly or even to attend Sunday services. Al went through a decade as a teenager, then collegian, then medical student during which he rarely darkened a church door. Later he found himself as an intern and house officer going to occasional church services on the rare Sunday he was off call. But it was not until the war that he got into the habit of regular worship. He happened to share a tent with the hospital chaplain of an evacuation unit. The chaplain held services each Sunday wherever they were—the dust of Africa, the mud of Sicily and Italy, the numbing cold of the French and German winters. Generally no one came. Al felt sorry for the chaplain and at first attended out of loyalty to his tentmate rather than an awareness of the needs of his soul. Unintentionally, Al had acquired a new habit. But he was honest enough to know that this did not represent true religious conviction.

Many years later, when his illness occurred, there was no noticeable change in his behavior. He didn't suddenly become more religious, nor did he give up the church out of disappointment over the fate that had been dealt him. He could recall nothing in the Scriptures that promised a life that was easy, comfortable, safe, or even tranquil in exchange for simple faith in a higher being. Even if there had been such a promise, it is unlikely Al would have changed his life-style, and he probably would have skipped church services completely. People of Gaelic extraction didn't change easily.

As the years began to lengthen and he failed to develop any physical evidence of recurrent malignancy, Al felt pangs of embarrassment. Why should he be so lucky? Whom should he thank? His mother insisted he was alive because his friends and loved ones had prayed for him. He wanted desperately to believe that, if for no other reason than gratitude. But as a rigid biochemist and physician, he always had been unable to accept intercessory prayer as a physical phenomenon. Surely there was no all-powerful God that would reach down into an ordered universe and say, "Let's save this one—but not that one. Let's let this one die, and oh, yes, the 360 on that plane which will soon crash." God would be too busy to keep track of all three billion people on this planet. And He wouldn't have time left over for the fish and the trees or the trash with which man littered his environment. But despite these protestations, Al sensed that maybe his religious life was different now. For one thing, he cloistered himself for a few minutes of prayer each morning, even on the days of early grand rounds. He tried to tell himself it wasn't a sense of duty or even of thanks for his apparently good health. He simply liked to do it. It seemed to exteriorize a lot of his frustrations, and even if prayer didn't alter physical events—maybe his thought processes did enter the minds of those for whom he prayed and thus became helpful in some esoteric way. After all, hadn't Rine done that with playing cards? Extrasensory perception he had called it.

Al saw himself acting like his own father more every year. He would never forget one of the last times he had talked with him when the old patriarch was nearly 90 years of age. "I have nothing to fear," his father had said. "I've had my doubts off and on as to whether there really is a life after death. I didn't voice my uncertainties, but I had 'em. Yes, indeed I did. But whichever way it turns out, I can't lose. If there is nothing after death, then there's nothing. That's that. I won't know the difference. On the other hand, if there is immortality, I'll probably do well. I've lived a good life and a moral one ever since I was old enough to make my own choice."

Al's father died happily.

CHAPTER 30

BRAIN TUMOUR

JOHN A. McCOOL

It was the beginning of December 1982, halfway through my final year of medical school when it started. I had just shifted accommodation to commence an obstetrics course. After my first night's sleep at the new hospital, I awoke normally but, on sitting up, quickly developed a peculiar, throbbing headache: six or seven beats, in time with the pulse, each beat progressively more severe, then suddenly disappearing. As I got out of bed, the same thing happened again, and over the next couple of hours it became clear that it was *head movement*, especially standing up from sitting or vice versa, or a sudden glance to the side, that brought on this crescendo of pain. A couple of hours later the headache went away, and I thought no more of it. Till the next morning that was, when the pattern of the previous day's headache repeated itself exactly. And the next morning, and the next, and the next...

I wasn't worried at this stage about the headache; I was too busy wondering what was causing it. A friend there had also developed a morning headache, so we thought at first that maybe the rooms were too stuffy. That night we slept with the radiators off and the windows open. But the next morning the headaches were still there—the only difference was that we were now freezing as well! Soon after this my colleague's headache disappeared, but mine persisted, unchanged. I tried changing every variable factor in my room—pyjamas or no pyjamas, foam pillows or feather, position in bed, heating, ventilation—but none of them made any difference; the headache remained.

After a while I got used to its being there in the morning and largely ignored it. I carried on, ostensibly as normal, over the next three months, but all during this time, the headaches were becoming more severe, often lasting till late afternoon or evening.

There was one occasion, about a month after the headaches had begun, when I seriously considered its implications. I knew that the

DR. JOHN MCCOOL is a 27-year-old houseman in the Royal Victoria Hospital, Belfast. He intends to specialize in psychiatry.

temporal pattern of my headaches was characteristic of raised intracranial pressure; I knew that the most likely cause of raised intracranial pressure was a brain tumour; I also knew that I could offer no circumstantial explanation for the headache. Logically, then, it seemed that I might actually have a brain tumour. However logical this conclusion may have been, I immediately dismissed it as being impossibly unlikely and dropped my search for the cause of the headache forthwith. I had, now and again, discussed my headaches with a good friend, also a medical student, but in any of these chats, as soon as it seemed that the headaches might be serious, he carefully steered away from the subject.

Then things changed abruptly. I awoke one morning, around the middle of March, to blindingly severe headache—constant, boring, completely confidence-sapping. From that morning, I also developed a more or less permanent nausea with bouts of "effortless" vomiting and a mild unsteadiness on my feet. This was, of course, alarming, since I knew there to be no obvious reason for it, and very unpleasant. When, a couple of days later, I put these symptoms together, there was really only one conclusion: that I had raised intracranial pressure—and that meant brain tumour! Naturally, this was not a comforting thought and my mind recoiled from it automatically.

I hadn't been to see a doctor about the headaches. Why not? I don't really know; perhaps I thought they would go away of their own accord, perhaps there was an unconscious inability to admit that something was actually wrong, or perhaps I just didn't want to bother the doctor with a mere headache (not wishing to appear a hypochondriac), or probably a combination of all these reasons and more—but now it was a different story. I was still reluctant, however, and eventually it was my girlfriend who insisted that I see about it.

Being a student, I went to the general practitioner at the Student Health Service. He immediately realised the seriousness of the headache and sent me with a covering letter to a consultant neurologist of the Royal Victoria Hospital (the main teaching hospital in Belfast). I met the consultant the following day, and after listening to my story and examining me, he asked what I thought was wrong. I replied, "Raised intracranial pressure." He then explained that he had given me a thorough examination and that he could find no abnormality, and also that he had particularly studied my fundal veins and found them to be pulsating normally. This meant, he said, that I could not have raised intracranial pressure. However, he continued, he considered that I was a calm person, and he believed me that these headaches were not functional. To this end, therefore, he arranged some blood tests and a skull X-ray and told me to return in three days' time, when we could discuss the results of the X-ray and blood tests and see whether three days' "reassurance" had made any difference.

Unfortunately, his well-meaning words did not cheer me. Okay, he reassured me that I had no raised intracranial pressure (and, therefore, no brain tumour), but I was instinctively dubious about his means of ruling this out; i.e., that my retinal veins were pulsating normally. And, if I did not have raised intracranial pressure, what, then, was causing the headaches? Consider my position: I had no physical signs whatever to corroborate my history, and I was complaining of headaches only two months prior to my final exams. It was understandable that any doctor in the circumstances, asked to make a diagnosis, would probably have said, "tension headache." The snag was, I knew that they were not tension headaches; I had never got particularly nervous before exams and had previously done many important ones without getting headaches, and, anyway, I wasn't that type of personality. *I* knew all this, but everyone else remained to be convinced. On one hand, logically and objectively, I could understand those who were saying that these were tension headaches, but on the other, because I *knew* that they were not and because it was happening to *me*, I couldn't.

I went back to the consultant after three days and described to him how I had been no better since I last saw him. He told me that had I been other than a medical student, he would have admitted me to hospital at our first meeting, but that he was now doing so and that he would arrange a computerised tomography (CT) scan immediately. At that time there was only one CT scanner in Northern Ireland, and since the waiting time for an outpatient scan was one month, it was necessary for me to be admitted to hospital so I could qualify for a scan within five days. I received no treatment nor underwent any investigations during that period.

The admitting doctor examined me conscientiously and confidently declared that I had no physical signs and that I could not, therefore, have a brain tumour. I was under stress, he said, and had been suffering from tension headaches, though, he "generously" added, this could be *muscular* tension. Later, other doctors who examined the central nervous system (CNS) found nothing and, blithely ignoring my history (of vomiting and unsteadiness), dutifully reassured me that all was well: that I was suffering only from "tension" headaches. My friends from the same year, who visited en masse the night before my CT scan, agreed. They clearly thought that I had lost my nerve, that I was "chickening out" of finals.

By the morning of the scan, faced as I was with this tide of opinion allied with my natural reluctance to accept that I had a tumour, I had convinced myself that it was going to be normal. The trouble was that since I could not convince myself that I had a tumour, and since deep down, I *knew* that the headaches were not functional, what on earth was causing them and how the hell was I going to get rid of them? If the scan was normal, the only alternative was that the headaches *were* functional—yet I knew, quite categorically, that they were not. Was I going insane?

(Writing now, it seems easy to say that I had, in fact, a tumour, but that obviously my defence mechanisms were denying it and would not let me admit it to myself. But at the time, of course, this was not apparent, and consequently, the above dilemma was very real and worrying.)

Following the scan, I returned to my bed and waited impatiently for my release. I had arranged for my car to be left outside the hospital and was eagerly anticipating a rapid acceleration away. I felt no apprehension at all about the results of the scan; I didn't conceive of being told anything other than that it was normal and that I was free to go. My consultant appeared around two o'clock. When he asked me to accompany him to a private room and even when he told me to have a seat, it still didn't click with me—I was still waiting to hear him say that everything was normal and that I could go. What he said was, "As I'm sure you expected, a lesion has shown up on the scan. There is a tumour in the cerebellum."

Thinking about it now, I would like to see the expression on my face at that moment to understand better what I was feeling. I suppose there was disappointment, disbelief, desperation, fear, and many other emotions, but I don't remember too well what went through my mind. The consultant assured me the tumour was virtually certain to be benign and that he was hopeful about the prognosis, then left rather quickly. It's difficult to describe what I felt as I stood there. Perhaps it was nothing—it seemed as if half of my mind was detached from it all and was telling the other half how I should react in such a situation. I suppose that it was similar to the "numbness" that bereaved persons feel on hearing the news of the death, and that my rational mind was trying to tell the "numbed" rest of me what I was expected to do. I remember being surprised that I wasn't sobbing with grief.

The consultant returned later that afternoon to see how I was and remarked that I appeared to be a lot calmer. This was true—I had, in the meantime, been transferred to another ward, and once the intolerable red tape was over with and I could get settled into bed without being pestered, my mind seemed to withdraw to another place, and there, oblivious to all that was going on around me, I somehow came to terms with the situation. I seemed to have accepted the fact that I had a brain tumour and that there was nothing I could do about it; the only possible way out of the situation was to put my complete trust in those who were looking after me.

The next day my consultant informed me that he had asked one of his neurosurgical colleagues to see me later that afternoon. I immediately liked the man; to me, he gave off an air of immense confidence in his ability. I felt happy that he was the one to whom I must entrust my life.

My friends also turned up that afternoon, looking pretty sheepish, but also appalled that such a thing had happened. I suppose it made them aware of their own mortality. Nevertheless, they were determined to cheer me up and proceeded with the usual good-natured banter until one of them, a renowned wit, said he had a present for me, and produced a short little book. It was short, he explained, because he didn't think I would have the time to read a long one!

The day of the operation came eventually, to my relief. Though I knew I might die during the operation, I was not at all anxious that morning—more glad to be getting it over with. The surgeon had done his best to scare the hell out of me with tales of maybe ending up with a paralysis or a permanent speech defect or a cough or an abnormal gait, but deep down, I always thought that I would survive the operation intact.

My memories of the immediate postoperative period are very hazy and incomplete. Apparently, when my girlfriend arrived in early evening, soon after the operation, she took one look at me and promptly fainted! Later she told me that I was so white, she thought I had died and no one had told her—she thought that no one could look so dead and yet be alive. I was astonished to hear this, since in my conscious moments during that early postoperative period, I felt no less vital than ever previously. Similarly, I never felt a moment of great relief that I was still alive; I suppose because I had never expected to be dead. Looking back now, it seems as if it took a long time for me to get over the operation, though at the time I remember thinking that things were going much better than I had expected them to preoperatively. I had very little headache and, even though the tumour was cerebellar, very little ataxia.

From the beginning of my experience of being a patient, I was aware of being treated differently from other patients by my doctors because I was a medical student. No procedures were practised on me by junior staff; I was given a private room, if one was available; but most importantly, I was always satisfied that my consultants were being totally open and honest with me, that I was being kept fully informed at all times. I would have found it intolerable had I suspected otherwise. Having now been a patient, I fully understand and endorse other patients' grievances about the withholding of information from them by the doctors. It is the patient's body, the patient's illness, and the patient's right to be made aware of the full picture.

Naturally, following the operation, I was keen to discover the diagnosis, and each time the surgeon came to see me, I asked him about it.

On each occasion, he replied that he didn't know yet, that he was awaiting the pathology report. Of course, he *did* know, since a frozen section done during the operation had shown the tumour to be an astrocytoma, but I guess he was waiting till he decided that I was ready to hear some bad news. A day or so later, as he was removing the huge bandage at the back of my head, he delivered it. He told me that the tumour had been malignant and that I would shortly have to undergo a course of radiotherapy. I was very disappointed. I felt that I had exhausted my resources in recovering from the surgery and that I just would not be able to take a further four weeks of debilitating treatment. Furthermore, I was becoming increasingly intolerant of the relentless noise surrounding me on the ward. Televisions blared constantly, cleaning women with their whining, clanking machines self-righteously barged about all day long, typewriters clattered incessantly; I felt sure that another four weeks of it would drive me round the bend.

But the therapeutic process was ineluctable, and after five days' rest at home, I found myself back in hospital, this time in the radiotherapy unit. As I arrived, the staff were at pains to assure me that I would enjoy my stay, in the "relaxed atmosphere," as they called it, of the unit. However relaxed they may have thought it was, it didn't prevent me being woken at 6:30 sharp every morning. I simply could not fathom the reason for this; it was at least a full hour before my breakfast was brought. Meanwhile, it was made impossible for me to sleep since the awakening nurse had, most deliberately, switched on the light, pulled back the curtains, fully opened the window, and finally, having made sure I was well and truly awake, stomped out, leaving the door wide open. I was surprised she didn't empty a bucket of cold water over me for good measure! I found this deliberate taking away of my very much needed sleep extremely discouraging and unnecessary—and yet it was only one example of the wholly illogical and ridiculous rituals inflicted on hospital patients by the nursing profession.

Luckily, I was obliged to remain an inpatient for only the first week of the four scheduled for my treatment. I seized the opportunity to come as an outpatient as soon as the week had ended, and even though this meant a 60-mile round trip every day, it was, nevertheless, a great deal less demoralising than having to suffer such stupid nursing practices.

The therapy itself was painless, but shortly after it began, I developed a familiar headache and vomiting. The radiation was causing oedema around the cerebellum and blocking the cerebrospinal fluid, giving rise again to raised intracranial pressure. I, therefore, had to go back onto dexamethasone and stay on it for the duration of my treatment. However, the effects of the radiation persisted long after the actual treatment period, and it was a full five months before I could get off the steroids completely. I was furious with this problem since, firstly, no one believed that I could be having any difficulty in stopping the drug and, secondly, I almost ended up with a stomach ulcer. I had been prescribed cimetidine in an attempt to alleviate the constant stomach upset I was having, but when I began to develop nipple tenderness, well—enough was enough!

It is funny that now I don't mind in the least talking or writing about my illness, because I remember being upset about the lack of confidentiality as a patient. The importance of the concept of confidentiality had been repeatedly drummed into us throughout our medical education, but it seemed to me as I lay there in the hospital to be nothing more than a charade; it existed only as a concept, not as an actuality. The experience was good for me, though; I myself am now very much more wary about letting slip any information about any patient I may be involved with.

Two years have now passed since I was told that I had cancer; a prominent milestone on the highway of recovery, one is led to believe—yet the subject refused to die. Two years later, a great many of my daily activities are dominated by the fact that I have had cancer. Nevertheless, the matter does not terrify me; I can, and do, talk about it with equanimity. It fascinates me now to observe patients and relatives break out in a cold sweat when the prospect of the word *cancer* looms, to look pleadingly at the doctor to speak the word, to accept the responsibility, to spare them the horror of the dread word having to cross their lips. It's as if a curse would befall those incautious enough to breathe "cancer" in other than awed, whispered voices.

But one-twelfth of the world's population are born in the sign of Cancer—they see the word, even look purposely for it, every day in the newspaper. Obviously, it is not the word itself that terrifies but the disease.

Although myocardial infarction is a much bigger killer, people have no difficulty in saying the words *heart attack*. They just do not provoke the dreadful fear associated with *cancer*. I find this surprising since a heart attack is often more sudden, more unexpected, more dramatic, and surely, for the bereaved, more devastating in its abruptness than any cancer. In addition, many cancers are now completely curable; an episode of myocardial infarction is likely to imply widespread vascular disease and a lifelong vulnerability to sudden death. An enduring horror, it seems, still surrounds the topic of cancer.

So, what have I learned from the experience of cancer?

I've learnt what it is like to be a hospital patient, learnt how vitally important caring nursing staff are to patient morale. For my first 48 hours postop, I was completely helpless and totally dependent on the nursing staff to keep me in one piece. I shall be eternally grateful to those nurses in the neurosurgical ward whose tremendous kindness, sympathy, and professional competence carried me through those first few frightful days.

However excellent were the full-time nursing staff, the part-time night staff who came in for one or two nights a week were another matter entirely. There were undoubtedly exceptions, but in my experience, these women were largely unfeeling and concerned with little more than getting the night over with as painlessly and as comfortably for them as possible. From one of these women, I witnessed extreme callousness and actual physical abuse of a frail old gentleman next to me whose only crime was to call for a bottle in which to pass his water.

It seems to me that the attitude of the nurses looking after one is really of *vital* importance in determining the speed and extent of recovery from serious surgery, certainly whilst still in hospital, and perhaps even later, when at home convalescing.

I learnt what was for me, a future doctor, an important lesson regarding physical examination of a patient. Being subjected to it was an odd experience—you surrender your body to the doctor for him to poke, prod, press, thump, scratch, as he wishes, and you have no control over any of it; you simply lie there as "relaxed" as possible and yield up your innocence to the doctor's questing hands. It is a very trusting thing do do. I learnt to respect the extent of this trust in any patient whom I may be required to examine in my future career.

I learnt that to experience cancer is not necessarily to undergo a radical or sudden change of personality. Of course, I am no longer the same person; my attitudes to life *have* changed, but this has been a slowly evolving process over the last two years. The appropriate cliché, possibly, is that I should rejoice with each new dawn, rejoice that I have been lucky enough to have been granted another day of life. I *am* very glad to be still alive, but this thought is not uppermost in my mind. I still struggle out of bed each morning with the same fretful reluctance.

It is often said that those who have had a close brush with death are no longer concerned with the petty worries of everyday life, gliding above them serenely. This has not been my experience, perhaps unfortunately; neither have I learnt to accept the unpleasantries of life as being better than nothing, better than being dead.

I have imbued the entire episode of my illness with a personal religious significance. I had spent eight days in the neurological ward waiting for the operation and, to my amazement, I never once felt bitter about what had happened to me, never once thought, "Why me?" or "What have I done to deserve this?" If previously someone had told me that I was going to suffer from a brain tumour, I would have imagined that I would have reacted bitterly, but when this actually did happen, there was no trace of bitterness, no thought at all of "Why me?" Also, during those eight days I remained in very good spirits and not once became depressed or anxious.

I only realised the above sometime after the operation and there seemed to be only one explanation—that God had sent me His grace to carry me through this immensely stressful period.

Many people in my situation, I imagine, would have reacted angrily to God and would consider that He had betrayed them in letting such a misfortune come their way. I didn't, at the time, really believe in God—the question of His existence was impertinent—and was completely areligious (by this I mean that I wasn't for or against religion; it just had no relevance to my life). But naturally, during this preoperative period, with the prospect of death threatening, I thought about God. And as I reflected on these matters and on God's purpose, all my inner grudges, resentments, hard edges, and nastiness seemed to melt away and I was left with an inner peace and a warmth embracing me. I felt some kind of union with God and knew that if I died, I would not fear to meet Him.

I decided that God had seen how arrogant I had become and had sent me the tumour in retribution and concern, to remind me that He was my creator and that I was subservient to Him and must not set myself up as my own God. He dealt me a bad hand in allowing the tumour, but He did not let me die and He furnished many supports along the way to facilitate my recovery. I don't know if God let me live for a particular reason, for some particular purpose, but I do believe that He never meant me to die, that He saw that I had become my own God and sent me a severe jolt to remind me of His deity and to set me back on the right path.

Secularly, it has taken until very recently for me to appreciate that I must insist (to myself) upon my physical health as my number one priority, that all other goals must become subordinate to this aim. It has taken me till now to appreciate that without your health, you have nothing.

But what of the surgeon, the man who held my life in his hands, who saved my life? What does it take to accept such responsibility, to live with the knowledge that a less than perfect job may spell the difference between life and death for his patients? What does it take to accept as his workplace the human brain, the "tabernacle" of our bodies? Is it simply a question of doing the job he was trained for to the best of his abilities, or can he be aware of the awesomeness of invading the essential core of humanity, our "inner sanctum"? And if he is, what sort of courage does this require?

I find it hard to understand that such a man, whose talent and skill are so prodigious, who spends his working hours saving the lives of others, is still a man like all the rest of us, beset with all the hassles and mundanities of everyday life. His dedication and ability don't seem to exist in the same world as keeping his car filled with gas or paying his electricity bill. Surely, I feel, such a man should be spared such trivialities, such indignities.

And how could I possibly thank him, possibly repay what he has done for me? The only way is to become as well and as healthy as I can, and give him the satisfaction of knowing that he has salvaged a life, that whatever I do or become in the future is due to him, and that his work will never be forgotten.

CHAPTER 31

MALIGNANT MELANOMA

HARVEY MANDELL

Almost 25 years ago, when I was in my late 30s, I was busily engaged by a growing private practice of internal medicine. I admitted my patients to a sleepy community hospital in southern New England whose medical staff was made up of about 25 to 30 private practitioners. Because there were relatively few of us, we worked closely together and usually knew about each other's patients and quickly knew when anyone else's patients had life-threatening or particularly trying illnesses. At the time, one of our general practitioners was caring for a prominent local citizen who was having a painful and lingering course of metastatic malignant melanoma. The disease had been diagnosed when a solitary axillary lymph node was excised for biopsy, and it was clear to everyone that the young man would soon be dead. Pain control for cancer was not well worked out then, and the patient was rarely if ever pain-free during his many admissions to our local hospital and to the teaching hospital of Yale Medical School. Because of this patient's dreadful course our medical staff frequently discussed the distressful vagaries of melanoma and the stresses of caring for such patients.

At this time my practice was such that my wife and I felt we could take our first vacation outside the continental United States and made arrangements to visit a Caribbean island. For several weeks I had watched with little curiosity a small nubbin growing on the back of my neck. It was attached by what I took to be a tiny stalk, although it probably wasn't, and skillful arrangement of mirrors showed it was nonpigmented. I toyed with the idea of twisting it around its real or perceived stalk until it fell off but never did it. Since a nonpigmented lesion on a stalk could only be benign, I saw no reason to have a physician look at it despite its increase in size.

DR. HARVEY MANDELL spent 22 years in the private practice of internal medicine until 1976, when he became medical director of The William W. Backus Hospital in Norwich, Connecticut, a post he still holds. He has a clinical faculty appointment at Yale and enjoys writing about the American medical scene as he sees it.

One day, to my surprise, I found my collar wet with blood. Self-palpation showed that it was the lesion that had bled. Since I did not want our island holiday to be marred by bloody collars, I asked a surgeon to remove the offending lesion. He performed the minor surgery in our emergency room and sent the tissue with an ellipse of surrounding normal skin to the pathology laboratory.

A few days later the surgeon removed the sutures. I thought no more about it until I realized ten days had passed since excision and I had not seen the pathologist's report. When I saw my surgeon making rounds one morning I jokingly asked him about the pathology of my "skin cancer." He didn't join in the joke and mumbled something almost unintelligible, but I thought he was complaining that all the path reports were coming out late. I stopped by the pathology lab and asked our pathologist about my "skin cancer" and found that he too failed to join the joke and mumbled something about a backlog of reports to get out.

The next afternoon when I was in the hospital I answered a page and found it was my surgeon calling me. He began his conversation with "Dr. Mandell, this is Dr. A." Although we had shared the care of many patients and saw each other almost daily, it was his way to address his colleagues and identify himself formally. "Yes, Fred," I answered assuming he wanted to discuss a patient. It turned out that I was the patient to be discussed. The conversation was brief.

"It's about the lesion I removed from your neck."

Pause.

"Well, what about it?"

Longer pause.

"Not too good."

"Well, what is it—a basal cell?"

"No, worse—go up to pathology and review the slides with the pathologist."

"Can't you tell me what it is?"

"I don't want to discuss it over the phone."

End of conversation—one speaker relieved to have somehow delivered part of the message, the other bewildered and a little shaken.

I immediately went to the laboratory and found the chief of pathology. He must have seen me coming because he continued peering into his microscope without raising his head to greet me as he usually did. Ordinarily he encouraged practicing physicians to come into his office and chat about pathology, the Boston Bruins, and almost any other topic.

"Jim, can I go over my slides with you?"

"What slides? Do you mean the liver biopsy you did last week?"

"No, I mean *my* slides, the lesion removed from *me*."

"I don't remember the results. I sent the report to Dr. A."

"Jim, I'm not leaving until I see the slides and you describe the pathology to me."

"Christ!"

Finally, after a fumbling search designed to get rid of me, the mysterious slides were on the microscope stage and I had a chance to see them. My skills in pathology were never particularly striking, but peering down the barrel of the microscope at the slides I could see that something was obviously wrong. The pathologist said very quietly, "Most of the normal tissue here is replaced by melanoma cells. The necrotic area on the surface must be where you bled from." Of course I immediately thought of the young man in town who was dying of the same disease at that very moment.

Always private, I discussed the diagnosis with no one until a week later, when I tracked down my surgeon and asked him what I should do. I had decided to do whatever my doctors told me to do and not enter into the decision making. He said I should take the slides and see a surgeon at Yale in consultation. He added that if further surgery was needed I should have it done at the university hospital. I wondered if he really felt he needed consultation or if he was relieving himself of the difficulties that occur when taking care of colleagues. He asked which surgeons at Yale I knew best and we decided the consultant should be a certain professor of surgery whom I liked and admired.

The appointment was quickly made, vacation plans were canceled, and for the first time I told my wife. I have never known why I didn't tell her immediately—we have always been closer than any couple I know. I guess I couldn't bear having her see me mortal and flawed—like other human beings. She knew only too well that I was both and gave perfect support. She seemed to know instinctively when to be silent and when to talk. Her timing was never wrong.

At Yale, the surgeon sent the slides off to pathology, poked all over me for palpable nodes and masses, and looked to see if there was a lesion elsewhere to which this could be a metastasis. He said he could see nothing beyond the local disease, went over my chest X-ray with the chief of radiology, and asked me to wait until the pathologist called with his diagnosis. When the pathologist called to say he agreed with the diagnosis of malignant melanoma, my surgeon said he wanted me to take my X-ray and the slides to a certain cancer clinic in New York, and he would arrange a consultation with the head of the clinic. I asked wryly when my doctors were going to stop dumping me on each other and stated firmly that the head of the clinic would be the last consultant to see me, and then they should decide who was going to be my "real" doctor. So much for staying out of the decision-making process. We both laughed and my surgeon said he would be my "real" doctor with help from my very good local surgeon.

My appointment at the clinic was for 9:00 a.m. We arrived at 8:45 a.m. and found the waiting room filled with an assortment of cancer types. One person had a tracheostomy, another was practicing esophageal speech, one had a leg amputated, and another an arm. One woman had an extensive dressing over one ear, and a middle-aged man was talking quietly about his colostomy to the woman sitting next to him.

I noticed that they all had plenty of reading material with them, and many had brought snacks or lunch. These were the veterans who had learned that although everyone was given a 9:00 a.m. appointment, we would be invited in according to some mysterious order that no patient had ever figured out. There seemed to be equal chances that you would see a doctor at either 9:00 a.m. or sometime toward evening.

After a bit, I was asked to provide a urine specimen and to turn my slides over to someone who would presumably take them to the pathologist.

About an hour later, in a voice that could be heard all over Manhattan, a lab technician shouted to the keeper of records the good news that "Dr. Mandell's urine is negative for melanin." Several of my waiting room comrades immediately nodded reassuringly to me, acknowledging the favorable nature of that information.

About 30 minutes later, a man in a lab coat asked which one was Dr. Mandell. When I identified myself he said he was a pathologist and returned my slides. When I asked him what he thought about the slides, he formed a circle with his thumb and forefinger and extended the other three fingers and quickly disappeared. This was a sign of approval by a beer company at the time, and I was left to wonder if the pathologist meant by this gesture that the slides were well made, that he agreed with the diagnosis of previous pathologists, or that I didn't have cancer at all.

Sometime later when the waiting room occupants were breaking out the sandwiches and hard-boiled eggs, I was escorted to an examining room with no magazines to temper one's impatience for a 45-minute wait. Then I yielded 20 ml of blood to a phlebotomist and was examined by an oncology fellow and finally by the courteous and engaging clinic head himself accompanied by two foreign physicians.

The head of the clinic told me that he and his pathologist agreed with the diagnosis of malignant melanoma and agreed with my previous surgeons that I should have wider excision with removal of regional lymph nodes and skin grafts to cover the operative site. I could not follow his description of the surgical anatomy of the neck but pretended that I did. I didn't know if removal of regional nodes was standard for that site or if it meant that the surgeons had found palpable glands somewhere along the way. On the basis that what you don't know can't hurt you I didn't ask for any explanation. The foreign doctors nodded, seemingly in silent agreement with everything that was said. I wondered whether they spoke or understood English.

Things then moved rapidly. I was admitted to the New Haven Hospital and was worked up consecutively by medical student, intern, and assistant resident, all of them polite, tired, and slightly deferential to a colleague. At 8:00 p.m., someone, probably the surgery or anesthesia resident, insisted I be sent for a preop chest film despite my having had a normal one two weeks before. It was a busy afternoon and evening so I had little time to think about what was to come. The safety of the surgery caused little concern, but I couldn't help wondering if there were already a nest or two of melanoma cells hidden in a node beyond the surgeons' view.

Later that evening I heard two voices growing louder and then diminishing as two interns passed my half-opened door.

"What kind of a doctor is he?"

"Internist."

"Does he know what he has?"

"Yes."

"Jesus!"

I knew they were talking about me because I was the only doctor-patient on the floor.

Anesthesia, surgery, and postoperative care went smoothly and quickly. The nurses were wonderful. I hoped they thought I was a good patient, but if they did they never said so. I suppose I was just another patient coming through a busy unit. A friend of mine on the medical school faculty brought me *The New York Times* daily but slightly tainted his generosity by repeatedly informing me that he was paying for it himself and giving me a daily cumulative total of his expenses in my behalf. Too young to understand what was going on, my children occupied most of their visiting time raising and lowering my hospital bed with one of them in it.

Late each night when visitors had left, I talked at length with a patient in the room next to mine. At 27 she was dying of Hodgkin's disease and was well aware of her prognosis. Although I had passed the examinations put out by the American Board of Internal Medicine, she seemed to know a lot more about being sick and being a patient than I did. Maybe there should be boards in patient oncology. My wife and I said we would visit her at the rehab center she was going to after discharge, but we never got around to it. She died within the year.

Several days postop I suddenly grew tired of being in the hospital.

I wanted to go home and get back to work so I pestered my surgeon until he discharged me. At discharge he told me that if I were still alive in five years he might do some cosmetic work on the defect and scar. This remained a little joke between us that I enjoyed increasingly with each year of survival. After five or six years he seemed to have forgotten it, and I didn't remind him because I didn't think the esthetic improvement in my appearance would be worth the inconvenience of more surgery.

My surgeon suggested I go south and lie in the sun for a couple of weeks to convalesce. In the 1980s this seems like peculiar advice for a melanomatous subject. I agreed that his idea was excellent but instead I immediately returned to work.

The pinch grafts were still oozing when I went home and back to work but the dressing was held more or less in place by an ace bandage around my neck. My office nurse was nice enough to change the dressings so I wouldn't smell too bad, and, typically, I refused to discuss the reasons for the bulky neck dressing with anyone. I responded to unwelcome questions by feigning deafness.

In the 1980s we appear to see more melanoma survivors, probably because of an increased incidence of the disease and earlier excision, so it's easy to underestimate the dread such a diagnosis provoked 25 years ago. Although I read all the literature on the subject that I could get my hands on, for years I would never go to a conference or case review of melanoma. At these conferences there was always at least one doctor who had had a patient who was free of melanoma for so many years only to develop an explosion of metastases and die within weeks. When my patients had any kind of skin lesion, they were whisked off to surgeons for excisional biopsy with a speed that annoyed some and puzzled others.

In the years following my operation, insurance companies were not overjoyed to have me applying for life insurance. Their increased premiums made many policies prohibitive in cost so I remained "underinsured" during the time I needed life insurance most. By surviving I've had the last laugh, and instead of paying insurance premiums I used the money to buy airplane tickets to exciting places.

I think what I learned most was how nice it was to survive unblemished by metastases. Visions of metastases have never been far from my thoughts, and the ineffectiveness of chemotherapy and radiotherapy for melanoma mets has not been one of life's bright spots. Statements like "The mortality rate from malignant melanoma is increasing faster than that of any other cancer except lung cancer" from a 1985 American Cancer Society publication are not heartwarming. I chose not to discuss my illness with anyone other than a handful of intimate friends; getting this into the word processor has not been entirely easy.

At first my illness and surgery gave me more patience with patients who were frightened or who couldn't wait a reasonable time for laboratory and imaging reports to come back, but eventually that wore off, and I guess in the long run I was not more affable than before. For a while it made me better with people who acted in unpleasant ways or who seemed hostile on first meeting. It gave me pause to wonder if their behaviors were governed at least in part by something they weren't sharing with me. I did develop permanently more feeling and understanding for those who failed to get the same sort of support from their spouses that I did. Also, because my illness suggested I was mortal, I was led not to postpone pursuit of my hobbies of travel, reading, and writing. My main nonoccupational passion is chess and I realized that I would have to spend more time with that if I were to become an international grandmaster in this lifetime. (Twenty-five years later I still turn won middle games into lost end games.)

Living a met-free existence helps to put a lot of things in perspective. Trivia that might ordinarily consume you are easily set aside or even ignored. What people think of you becomes of little importance as long as you are convinced you are doing the right thing and as long as the few people in the world whose opinions are important to you agree. You don't become saintly or even necessarily a great guy, but you do learn to tune out a lot of unimportant matters.

I think I'm okay now because my doctors were good and because I have had the good luck so far to be immunologically sound. I've never had any mystical feeling that someone or something is looking over me with beneficence. There have never been any excursions into laughter therapy, odd diets, counseling, or psychological immunity enhancement. I have only thanks for the doctors and nurses who took such good care of me—I'm particularly grateful to my original surgeon, who was so disciplined that he sent an innocuous-looking lesion to the pathology laboratory when it would have been simpler just to have discarded it. Bravo for good training and good habits.

CHAPTER 32

MALIGNANT MELANOMA

NICHOLAS V. STEINER

When the dermatologist read me the pathology report over. the telephone, I was stunned. It was not unusual for Dan R. to call me, for during my 12 years as a practicing internist, I had referred most of my dermatology problems to him. As a rule, he didn't call unless something unusual turned up. Several days earlier, I had seen him for the removal of a small nodule from my popliteal fossa and then had put it out of my mind. Now, when my secretary told me that Dan was on the phone, I thought we would be talking about another patient, not about me. Instead he said, "I have the report on your lesion. It was a melanoma."

Through carelessness (or was it denial?) I had already delayed recognition of the problem. It had all begun one evening some weeks earlier when my wife first noticed the strange little growth behind my right knee as I stood at the bathroom sink. Surprised, I had glanced at it, then gone to bed, and by the next morning had forgotton about it. For one thing, its location made it an easy place to overlook. Assuming that I had taken care of it (after all, I was a physician), Inger put it out her mind, too. A few weeks went by before one evening, as I prepared for bed, the scene repeated itself. Inger suddenly cried, "It's still there!"

The next day I was in Dan's office. He was noncommittal about the lesion's appearance, and even later, I wasn't sure whether he had suspected the diagnosis at that moment. He was now calling to tell me what the pathologist had found: a nodular melanoma measuring 1.7 mm in depth.

Dan and I agreed upon my seeing Jack W., one of the senior surgeons at our hospital, and later that afternoon I was in Jack's office. After examining me, he recommended wide surgical excision and, because of its location, a split thickness skin graft to cover the defect.

DR. NICHOLAS STEINER is a 52-year-old physician who until the time of his retirement in 1984 practiced internal medicine in New York City.

In his opinion, there was no compelling evidence that a radical groin dissection would significantly affect the prognosis. I was just as happy to get by with a lesser procedure. Jack estimated that I would spend ten days in the hospital and another week at home before returning to work. I entered the hospital during the following week.

During my absence, a fellow internist/cardiologist with whom I shared the office took care of my practice. We had agreed beforehand to downplay to my patients the importance of my being hospitalized. They would be told that I was having a "minor procedure" followed by a little time off, and no one seemed to question this. Dealing with family members and fellow physicians, from whom I could not hide the facts, was obviously more difficult.

For Inger, this was the beginning of a time of deep worry. She had already heard of melanoma four years earlier when her good friend Ellen, a 29-year old flight attendant, had found a mole on her foot. When it turned out to be a melanoma, she was admitted to Memorial Sloan-Kettering Cancer Center. After additional work-up, she underwent excision and radical lymph node dissection, and when one of the nodes proved to be positive, she received regional perfusion with an antineoplastic agent.

Although Ellen recovered uneventfully, the illness sounded the death knell for her failing marriage. Several months after the surgery, she divorced her husband. In the four years that followed, she remarried, returned to work, and became a mother. To some, she appeared radiantly happy during those years—but to Inger, the uncertainty of the future hung like a dark cloud on the horizon. It was not surprising then, when I told Inger that I had melanoma but that I was "sure to be cured," her eyes filled with tears. I was 45 years old and believed that my best years lay ahead, but Inger was more realistic. She knew that as a 35-year-old woman with two young children and without an independent source of income, she faced an uncertain future. Believing that Inger's fears were exaggerated, members of my family expressed annoyance and asked that she pull herself together.

For my colleagues, melanoma denoted a refractory and relentless disease with a dismal prognosis. When many of these physicians encountered Inger on her daily visits to the hospital, their well-meant words of sympathy, the sad and worried expression in their eyes, and later on their averted looks unwittingly gave her the message all too clearly.

My own reactions to being in a hospital were unexpected. Family members, friends, and physicians who visited were surprised to be greeted by a relaxed, smiling, and uncharacteristically garrulous patient. They all admired my "courage." As I later reflected upon it, it was a clear case of optimism based on denial. My disease had surely been caught in time, I thought, and I would be as good as new when

I returned to work. In the meantime, happy to be relieved of the stresses of my practice, I read voraciously through a quantity of books which had been awaiting my attention since my previous vacation. Later on, I confess, I had difficulty remembering much of what I had read.

When colleagues visited, I did my best to allay whatever feelings of sadness, anxiety, or guilt I detected, reassuring them that all would be well. Relaxed in turn by my cheery manner, they tended to settle into their chairs and stayed far too long. One day I counted the colleagues who visited but lost count after the number reached 17. By the time the last visitor left, I had fallen into an exhausted sleep. Despite good intentions, physicians surprisingly often fail to give the colleague whom they are visiting the emotional support he needs at that moment. I have seen physicians unwittingly arouse guilt feelings in an ailing colleague because he has added to their work load. Needless to say, guilt is the last thing anyone needs while recovering from an illness. Whenever possible, it seems to me, discussions regarding shared patients and their problems should be avoided while a physician is ill.

During my hospitalization and convalescence at home, my income fell to virtually nil. Not enough time had elapsed for my disability insurance to take effect, and being in solo practice, I was paid only for those patients whom I actually saw. For a number of years, a small group of colleagues and I had cross-covered each other's practices during vacations. Since we had never made other arrangements in the event one of us became ill, the coverage that now took effect was the same as if I had been on vacation. Under this system, the "vacationing" physician paid the covering doctor for visits to his hospital patients while expecting to be reimbursed later by the patients or third-party insurance. The covering physician also kept whatever income he earned in the office. Belatedly, I realized that while this method had worked during vacations, it seemed less equitable when one was incapacitated because of illness. I was anxious to return to my practice, not just to relieve the burden of those who had covered me but because I needed to regenerate some income.

During a vacation later that spring, the white rectangular skin-graft donor sites on my thigh, just beyond the lower edge of my bathing trunks, attracted a few curious stares. In time, however, these faded and nearly disappeared, just as the memories and concerns over my illness did. I returned to the routine of my practice and life at home as if nothing had happened.

One evening at a dinner party three years later, a friend casually mentioned that Inger's friend Ellen hadn't been feeling well lately. Inger and I exchanged glances and later that evening, we called her. Ascribing her symptoms to "muscle pain," Ellen admitted that in recent days she needed her husband's help to get out of bed. Being a stoic and determined individual, she had continued to work as a flight attendant on transatlantic flights. She had not seen her surgeon in months and didn't have a primary physician. While I had no wish to fill that role, I suggested she come to my office the next morning.

When I saw Ellen, it was quite obvious that something was wrong, and I found her to have a left pleural effusion. She accepted my statement that the possibilities included infection, inflammation, and tumor, and agreed to enter the hospital for diagnostic tests. Initially, the answer eluded us. Routine tests were essentially normal, and the results of a thoracentesis and pleural biopsy were nonspecific. Then the CT scan gave us the answer we had feared: metastatic tumor masses in the pelvis, bones, and lungs.

Ellen returned to Memorial Sloan-Kettering, where a biopsy confirmed a recurrence of her melanoma; Inger's fears had been justified. Shattered by the news and the abysmal prognosis, Ellen and her husband eventually agreed to a course of cobalt therapy; but only after several months of alternative therapy including macrobiotic diet, intravenous vitamin C, and a faith healer proved ineffective. As Ellen's condition gradually worsened, many of her friends, apparently unable to deal with her situation, stopped seeing her. Others, including Inger, stood by and helped.

During the following week, I saw my internist and old friend Arthur A. There had been no special reason for seeing him; I was simply overdue for a medical checkup. Not having any symptoms, I relaxed as Arthur calmly proceeded through the physical examination. He had just finished examining my abdomen and was palpating my right groin. It seemed curious, I thought, that he should be lingering in one place for so long. At length he spoke: "I hate to tell you, Nick, but did you know that you have a couple of enlarged nodes here?" I was stunned. Within a second or two, the message had registered like a flashing neon light in my mind—the melanoma had recurred. I had metastatic cancer.

Arthur may have spoken as he concluded the examination but I heard nothing of what he said. I felt like the drowning person who sees his life passing before his eyes. At the end of this brief fantasy, I saw Inger and the children weeping at my funeral. Moments later, my thoughts were back in the examining room, hoping that I would soon awaken but knowing that this was no dream. Afterwards in Arthur's consultation room, we agreed upon my seeing Bob W., an excellent surgeon.

When I emerged from Arthur's office, the sidewalk seemed to be overflowing with people. As I looked at passersby engaged in lively conversation, I felt a mixture of sadness and anger at the injustice of my fate. Why me?

Later that afternoon, I sat in Bob W.'s office after he had confirmed the presence of the nodes in my groin. Indeed, I had to ask myself, how could I not have found them myself? Clearly, I hadn't been looking. Bob asked whether I wanted the surgery done at our hospital or elsewhere, perhaps at Memorial Sloan-Kettering. As I recalled my first operation, with the visits of so many colleagues and how painful it had been for Inger, I quickly decided against a repeat performance. The anonymity of being in another institution would provide the privacy I now needed. In addition, fearing for my practice, I figured that news of my illness would be less likely to leak out of a hospital where I wasn't known.

Not knowing any surgeons at Memorial, I asked Bob for a referral. The answer came from his younger associate, who had recently finished a year of training there. "There were many good surgeons there," he said, "but one man stands out. He has vast experience and, despite being extremely busy, he finds time to talk with and listen to his patients. His name is Dr. B." I called Dr. B. the same day and made an appointment to see him.

As I entered the outpatient department of Memorial Sloan-Kettering some days later, I couldn't help noticing the many people in the waiting area. Some appeared to be new patients carrying outside X-ray folders under their arms and wearing anxious expressions on their faces. Others, some of whom were visibly ill, were returning for follow-up care. Although appearing less anxious than the others, they had an air of resignation about them. Somehow I felt quite apart from all of them. Was it because I was a physician and knew what to expect, or was it simply that I did not yet think of myself as patient?

Dr. B. was just as he had been described—intelligent, likable, and straightforward in manner. After reviewing the findings, he told me that he planned to do a superficial radical groin dissection, and arranged admission.

Three days had passed since the realization in Arthur's office that I had recurrent cancer. Except for confiding in my sister, I had so far kept the news to myself. Inger was in Germany exhibiting her art work. The show meant a great deal to her. My mother was away for a week, to my relief. When I told her, I wanted to be able to add that appropriate steps were already taken. Similarly, I had delayed in calling Inger for I knew that my message would shatter the euphoria of her trip. That she was 4000 miles away didn't make my task any easier, but as soon as Dr. B. had outlined his plans, I called. When I reached her, she burst into tears, and I had to call back a few minutes later. This was without question the toughest phone call I have ever had to make.

It has been said that a serious illness either brings a married couple closer or tears them apart. Unfortunately, in the years preceding the onset of my illness, Inger and I had begun to drift apart and the bonds of our marriage had gradually weakened. Coming when it did, the illness actually held us together longer than otherwise might have been the case, for this was not a time to separate. But the strains inherent in an illness further intensified the divisions in our marriage. It was probably not coincidental that one of the most disagreeable scenes between us occurred on the evening before I entered the hospital.

The three weeks at Memorial Sloan-Kettering passed quickly, and in a strange way I even found myself feeling happy, much as I had at the time of my first operation three years earlier. How can such a reaction be explained? It would be some time before I understood, but eventually I saw that the hospital provided a refuge from stress and unpleasantness in my life.

During my postoperative convalescence at Memorial Sloan-Kettering, Ellen began coming to its outpatient department for radiation therapy. Her condition had been slowly worsening. One day she appeared at my bedside and, with a smile, reminded me of my visit to her several years earlier. It had been following a similar operation, on the same floor, perhaps in the same room. It is just as well that we don't know what the future will bring, I thought. Ellen had lost weight but was still a striking-looking woman. Determined to win the struggle with her disease, she carried her cane as if it were an adornment to her wardrobe, but when she left, I saw that she could not conceal a limp.

By the time I was discharged, Inger was regularly driving Ellen back and forth between home and hospital. She had begun to experience pain as well as weakness and needed help with stairs. In the eyes of my family, Inger's degree of involvement in Ellen's suffering was unnecessary and took away from time and energy that she could have given me. But I required virtually no care, and when Inger encouraged me to return to work as quickly as possible, I did so. Even in retrospect, this was in our best interest, for back at work I quickly returned to the old routine.

Ellen continued to follow a steady downhill course and within three months was dead. During her funeral, at which I was a pallbearer, I was aware of the stares of friends who knew that I carried the same disease within me. I suspected they were wondering how long it would be until they met at another funeral—mine.

As might be expected, this was a time when thoughts of the precariousness of my future and of my mortality often weighed upon me. I began to think twice before buying anything of value that I might not be able to use for very long. I turned down an opportunity to buy clothes for the following summer, not sure that I would be around to wear them. Despite having such thoughts, however, I was usually able to push them out of my mind simply by keeping busy. My practice continued to occupy most of my time and energy, and moments of real despair were few. Denial proved a useful defense mechanism.

On a routine visit with Dr. B. eight months later, he discovered another lymph node in my groin. With a sinking heart, I realized that I needed more surgery. Although I would miss only one week of work this time, I had to act quickly to rearrange my schedule. Not sure what to tell those patients who would question my absence, I mentioned needing "a small operation" to one of them, an elderly physician. Interrupting me, he said, "Never tell your patients that you are taking time off because of illness; tell them that you are going on vacation or to a meeting. They will gladly accept this and will remain your patient. No one wants a sick doctor." I knew at once that he was right and followed this advice thereafter.

When I returned for a follow-up visit one month after the operation, much to my dismay another lymph node had appeared. By now I knew that there was every reason to expect additional recurrences. It would be only a matter of time until I had to give up my practice. Despite the importance of this decision, it came easily to me, for there were no other options. Once I had so decided, the trick would be to find an acceptable buyer of the two assets in my practice—the office and the patients—without tipping my hand. I knew that if my patients learned of my illness before I had found a successor, many of them would seek out other physicians and, thereby, diminish the value of the practice. If I were to sell it to its best advantage, I would have to act at once and not—as a friend said—wait until I was negotiating from a hospital bed.

I began by notifying the colleague with whom I shared the office. Already having a busy practice, he had no wish to take on my patient load. He did, however, express interest in buying my shares of the cooperative in which our office was located. Finding someone to take care of my patients would be a more delicate matter. Cautiously putting out antennae, within a few weeks I learned of several interested young physicians. One in particular seemed promising. He was well trained, had been on the staff of our hospital for several years, and had a personality to which I felt my patients could easily relate. For a time he vacillated and, fearing that the deal might fall through, I had to perform a balancing act with the other interested parties. The arrangement was further complicated by my successor's having to come to a working agreement with my colleague in the office, and, finally, the board of the cooperative would have to give its blessing to the whole transaction.

For what seemed an interminable period of time, the negotiations dragged on without resolution. At one time or another, each physician and his attorney seemed to be ignoring or feuding with the others and, fearful that the talks would collapse, I found myself caught in between.

Several months later, when an agreement finally appeared imminent, I composed a carefully worded letter and mailed it to each patient. In it I informed them of my decision to leave practice but was deliberately vague about the reasons. A psychologist whom I had been consulting during this difficult time advised me not to dwell on cancer or a bad prognosis since my patients might become depressed enough not to return to the office. The letter also served as an introduction to my successor. This was important, not just for continuity of care but because, according to our agreement, his success with my patients would have a direct bearing on my subsequent income. The patients responded with a deluge of letters, telephone calls, and parting office visits. It was a busy and emotionally draining time, marked by much hugging and the shedding of tears, some of them mine.

Then, during these final days in practice, I received some unexpected bad news: A routine CT scan showed a new lesion—an abnormal lymph node in the pelvis. I needed another operation. With the concurrence of the two physicians and their attorneys, the closing was postponed, but plans for the take-over by my successor went forward. The day after he saw his first patients, I reentered Memorial Sloan-Kettering.

At surgery, the diseased lymph node was removed and, fortunately, my abdomen was found to be otherwise free of tumor. I breathed a deep sigh of relief. While convalescing, I made some telephone calls from my hospital bed, hoping to persuade members of the cooperative's board to accept the new arrangement in the office. At last, one month later, the closing took place. I was equally relieved that the surgery had gone well and that I no longer had to worry about the disposition of my practice. Hoping that my health would hold up, at the age of 50, I now looked forward to enjoying my "retirement."

In the 15 months that have passed since then, the pace and focus of my life have changed considerably. Fortunately, my disease has progressed at a far slower pace than might have been predicted. Six months after the pelvic surgery, yet another node appeared in the groin on the opposite side from the original lesion. It, too, was surgically removed, and in the nine months since then all has been quiet. I continue to be followed closely by Dr. L., an immunologist at Memorial Sloan-Kettering. Under the supervision of the latter, I have received several injections of an experimental vaccine grown from my own tumor cells. For what it is worth, I supplement my diet with vitamin C and E and selenium.

While I am able to forget about my illness much of the time, I do not delude myself that all is well. The main physical aftermath of the bilateral groin dissections has been lymphedema of both lower extremities, which is associated with variable degrees of discomfort. For the most part, the swelling is controlled with a custom-made waist-length elastic garment that must be worn continually except at night. The discomfort rarely requires use of an analgesic and can usually be relieved by lying down a while. This then becomes a good time for reading, writing, and reflection.

Having been away from medicine for more than a year, I am frequently asked whether I miss my practice. It is not a question that can be answered with a simple yes or no. I certainly miss the personal contact with those many patients and colleagues I enjoyed, and the pleasure of seeing patients get well again; these were the true rewards of medical practice. I do not miss the many stresses that had become ingrained into my daily life, nor do I miss having to contend with the growing list of problems (DRGs, spiraling malpractice premiums, etc.) which continue to erode the physician's way of life. Allowing for my health problems (I would obviously rather be healthy), I feel that the improved quality of my life makes up for much of what I left behind.

The biggest benefit of leaving practice has unquestionably been in having more time for leisure and the pursuit of interests for which there was previously insufficient time. Similarly, I have grown closer to my children than I had ever been during all those years when I was so preoccupied with my work. To say that all is well in my personal life, however, would be misleading. Since the seeds of marital discord were sown long before I became ill, it was unlikely that these problems would diminish in time. My wife and I have continued to drift further apart and at this time are facing a divorce. And yet, as unhappy as this prospect may appear, I view it as a not entirely negative development. For one thing, I anticipate spending time with my children in a happier environment than in the past. For another, I look forward to the freedom of a more independent life-style.

This has also been a time for reflection upon the meaning of my disease and its effects on my life. When I first realized that the melanoma had recurred, the words *Why me?* echoed through my mind just as they haunt other cancer victims. In vain, I sought a definable cause, something which I could blame. Perhaps being fair-skinned and freckled and having had more sun exposure in my youth than was good for me were risk factors. Even so, it still didn't explain why I developed cancer. "Why me?" remained an unanswered question. In time, however, other thoughts arose. Through my reading, I became aware of a growing body of evidence that points toward mental and emotional stress as being factors that predispose to cancer. The notion that chronic stress may cause selective impairment of the immune system and ultimately allow cancer to develop was particularly intriguing to me. And when I read the emotional profile of the typical cancer-prone individual in the book, *Getting Well Again*,[1] I was shocked to realize how much it resembled me. While my years of training made me skeptical of this approach to cancer, as time has passed, I am no longer so sure.

Finally, as I look back, it is strange to consider that for all the harm it has done, my illness freed me from a way of life which, despite its successes, was chronically stressful and often personally unsatisfying. The insight that emerged was attained at great cost but today I know better who I am. I know also that in spite of the uncertainty of the future, my life has become fulfilling in ways that I could never have imagined while in practice.

REFERENCES

1. O. Carl Simonton, Stephanie Mathews Simonton, and James L. Creighton, *Getting Well Again* (New York: New York, 1978).

CHAPTER 33

HODGKIN'S DISEASE

CHARLES S. KLEINMAN

Time was always the most valuable commodity. Passing from milestone to milestone. Striving for and meeting deadlines. Enjoying academic success and taking great pleasure in the pride that parents and then wife and even young children had in my academic and professional accomplishments. How could there be *time* for everything? The answer, it seemed, was to exert control. That is, by hard work, long hours, and steel will, one could control one's life. The rewards would eventually be forthcoming. For now we could postpone living because there would be plenty of time later. In the third and fourth decades of life it was natural to live for today. Professional accomplishment would, in turn, bring the material rewards that would make life more comfortable for us all and fulfill my need to be a successful provider. There certainly was no need and no time for looking back. After all, what lessons did the past hold, other than the "NYU lesson" that I learned almost 20 years earlier?

Success in elementary school in New York City was measured in grades and being skipped through the school years. Graduation from high school at 16 with college credits in mathematics and chemistry. Suddenly entering the "real world" of the premedical student. It seemed that everyone at NYU in September 1963 was a premedical student. As time passed, one at a time, classmates dropped science courses and started wearing three-piece suits. My "advisor" thought that it would be wise for me to continue advancing beyond my age peers. While my classmates from the first grade were planning for their high school junior prom, I was preparing for final examinations as a college freshman taking organic chemistry, quantitative analysis, differential equations, world history, and English composition. The result?—academic *disaster*. Grades that would return to haunt me as a 20-

DR. CHARLES KLEINMAN is a 39-year-old pediatric cardiologist in New Haven, Connecticut, and chief of pediatric cardiology at Yale University School of Medicine. He has a special interest in Hodgkin's disease.

year-old seeking admission to medical school. Grades in "key" premedical courses that would, understandably, overshadow the grades of the junior and senior years, grades that would overshadow strong board scores. Hence, the NYU lesson—don't let up for a moment. As a 16-year-old it seemed to be an either/or choice. Either take part in the newfound social world of the campus or grind. As a 16-year-old the choice was natural. I could always study later.

As a freshman in medical school (after a year of penitence in graduate school), the lesson was clear—work now, live later. After all, the competition would now consist of the successful premedical students. Retrospectively, there were more "real people" in that class than I would have predicted on the basis of the premedical students I had known in undergraduate school.

The "payoff" was coming—I obtained the position I hoped for, assistant professorship in pediatric cardiology at a top medical school. At the time, $28,000 per year seemed like a lot. The hours were worse than before. The NYU lesson was still loud and clear—apply yourself to your work. Establish yourself in a firm position—make yourself indispensable. During your "spare time," "moonlight" to pay off moving expenses that weren't quite covered by the university and to pay off bulging bank card debts. Since moonlighting was strictly forbidden by the university under penalty of dismissal, I obtained a position in New York City—far from the prying eyes of the university. After two years of working two jobs there was no longer an outstanding debt. After one more year the down payment was amassed, and we found our first dream house, a California contemporary in an apple orchard. My academic career was going beautifully. My work in prenatal cardiology was well received at national meetings and was being widely published. In April, Jessica and I would be attending our first international meeting, in Strasbourg. I quit my moonlighting job. Even my weight, the barometer by which those who know me best can gauge the stress I am under (they are inversely proportional) was under control. I was running about ten miles a day during which I reflected on the future. The present was satisfying—academic success, the European trip, a new home. My long-term goals were to attain professorship by the age of 40 and to direct a division of pediatric cardiology by 45 (I imagined myself returning triumphantly to the New York Hospital, the site of my years as a resident in my favorite part of my favorite city). My short term goal—to run in the Labor Day 20-km road race. All of these goals seemed attainable, if I remained in control of my career, and if this new respiratory allergy that was causing me to wheeze and cough after only four of five miles of running would subside after the unknown offending pollen was gone. I scratched from the road race owing to a nagging cough and a race-time outdoor temperature approaching 90° F.

The cough persisted. Our Friday morning cardiac surgery conference was uncomfortable for some of the participants because it was hard to hear the case presentations over the coughing. Rich M., a friend and colleague, leaned to me and suggested gently, but firmly, that I have a chest X-ray—after all, did I want to give some poor kid TB? I laughed but did promise to get an X-ray. After the conference I approached one of the X-ray technologists whom I knew and asked if she would take a chest X-ray of me, despite the fact that I did not have a patient identification number. She did so reluctantly and I awaited the developed film at the Xomat developer. When the unlabeled film emerged, I looked at both views and complimented the technician on an excellent practical joke. She had taught me not to impose on the X-ray techs anymore; now, where were *my* films? She convinced me that these were, indeed, my films. I know I was convinced, because I started to cry. The mediastinal mass was staring me in the face. The brassy cough and mediastinal mass reminded me of the slightly tender left supraclavicular node that I thought I had imagined one or two weeks earlier. My life—what was left of it—was collapsing around me. No one was there to break it to me gently; in fact, no one knew about it but me. How *dare* this happen? Why should Jessica not be showered with the things I had hoped the years would bring? Why should Ari and Josh not have a father to watch and help them grow? Thank God I have absolutely no sales resistance and during the previous three years had bought more life insurance than I could afford. Why hadn't anything been noted on my insurance physicals? Who was I kidding? They were probably moonlighting residents and academics who were having difficulty staying awake.

The next thought was not fear of dying, but rather that I was going to need a splenectomy and staging laparotomy. I had seen lots of Hodgkin's disease (I was sure this was Hodgkin's) while a resident rotating through the Sloan-Kettering Institute (I wonder if I caught this damned thing there?) and was always impressed that the patients looked pretty well when they were admitted for staging and always left looking ghastly. After wandering around for almost an hour contemplating discarding the offending X-rays, I found myself in Rich M.'s office. I placed the films on the viewbox in his office and looked at him with tears in my eyes. I watched his eyes dart about studying the X-rays and saw the tears well up in his eyes. This was not to be the last time I would bring my own X-rays to a radiologist friend (an unfair thing to do either to myself or to the friend) who would proceed to shed tears. This is an experience that our patients are spared. I have since joked with these two friends, telling them that when I write my memoirs they will be entitled "The Radiologist Cried."

Rich's first words were "Who is your physician?" My truthful reply was that in my three years on staff, I "hadn't had the time" to see a physician. An internist at the Health Plan was kind enough to see me that afternoon.

I drove to the Health Plan alone, carrying my own X-rays. Suddenly, I was not in control. I was seated in the unfamiliar waiting room, an "add on" patient who was lucky that this physician was kind enough to see him that day. I was scared to death and was naturally concerned about placing my well-being in the hands of a physician I knew little about. A brief inquiry prior to the drive to the Health Plan indicated that this fellow was the premier physician that the Health Plan had to offer. His reputation was excellent and his credentials impeccable, including completion of chief residency at that same top-ranked institution.

He was completely businesslike in our dealings. He was *not* going to allow me to be a consultant on my own case. I was patient now, not a physician. This is what I wanted to hear. The next thing I knew he was outlining a staging procedure which was to be preceded by a mediastinal exploration to biopsy the mass to establish a firm diagnosis. If there was anything that scared me more than splenectomy and abdominal exploration, it was thoracic surgery to be performed, not by one of my several friends on the university thoracic surgery staff but by another (albeit by reputation excellent) stranger who happened to be a cooperating surgeon with the Health Plan. At this point I demonstrated the presence of the supraclavicular lymph node and was scheduled to see a general surgeon, who would biopsy the node under local anesthesia. I was to return to see the surgeon at 4:00 p.m., but he was in surgery, and by 5:30 p.m. it was apparent that he would not be free to see me that day. Again, I was further diminished by this confounded disease. I had gone from being "in control" of my own destiny to being in the impotent position that many HMO patients must find themselves in. I didn't like it at all. I surely wasn't going to wait until Monday, so I took my X-rays and on Saturday morning posted myself outside surgical grand rounds awaiting Dr. C.

Dr. C. was known to me only by reputation as the finest general surgeon on the university staff. My friends all congratulated me on the good fortune to have been referred by the Health Plan to Dr. C. By Saturday morning I had convinced myself that if the Health Plan had referred me to someone else, I would have referred *myself* to Dr. C. He has been a great comfort to me and my family. He did not seem at all "put off" by my aggressiveness ("Excuse me, you didn't know me, but I am on the staff and I have this problem. . ."), and we went to his office where he examined me, confirmed the presence of the supraclavicular node, and explained that while he could biopsy it now, in the emergency room, it could not be evaluated for 48 hours by pathology anyway, and—he didn't have to complete the sentence. Anyone who has worked in a large hospital, even the very best, knows the advantages of having specimens hand-delivered directly to the physician or technician who will be processing them. I felt somewhat more at ease. Here was an excellent surgeon, a calming and gentle soul, a Southern gentleman with a bit of a drawl, self-assured without being self-impressed. Over his shoulder, on his wall, was a familiar and comforting sight—a residency certificate from the New York Hospital, identical to my own. I knew that I had found my physician.

That weekend was difficult. Our close friends, George L., a colleague who has been a friend since our fellowship days, and his fiancee, Sandy, Jessica, and I went to the movies to take our minds off my problems. This would have been a fine plan if we hadn't chosen to see *Ordinary People*, a movie about the heartaches that befall a family whose son dies tragically in a boating accident.

For the remainder of the weekend, Jessica had three rather than two children to tend to. At night I would stay awake, feeling in my underarms for night sweats, going into the kids' rooms to see them sleeping and to talk to them. I would go to the liquor cabinet to drink several ounces of vodka, *not* to drown my sorrows or seek a crutch but to check for the pain that supposedly accompanies alcohol ingestion in Hodgkin's patients. Lord knows what I would have done if the pain was there (it wasn't). Its absence and the alcohol itself were of little consolation. I held onto Jessica through the early morning hours and lamented the fact that if I were in any other profession I would *at least* have been able to hide behind my ignorance during that weekend in limbo. Perhaps I could have put at least an iota of credence in the statement by the internist: "Maybe it's sarcoid and not a lymphoma."

Monday I was on call for surgery. I expected to be paged in the morning to go to one-day surgery to be biopsied. In the meantime, I had had nothing by mouth since the previous midnight. I needed to feel in control. I told Jessica that she needn't come with me, that it was nothing. I went in for morning rounds in the ICU. They went faster than usual, since I heard nothing and said nothing during rounds. The call didn't come until late afternoon.

The biopsy went smoothly and hurt less than I thought it would. I had asked Dr. C. if he would stitch the wound and then let me carry the specimen to pathology myself. He laughed and said that he would take it. He was back in less than two minutes, explaining that the *chairman* of pediatrics was waiting outside the operating room to transport the specimen. I will never forget that kindness.

The next 48 hours were again filled with apprehension. By this time I realized that while this certainly was a lymphoma, it was not necessarily Hodgkin's and if you had to have something, the latter was probably "the best of the lot."

Forty-eight hours later I was called, not by my surgeon or internist, but by a friend, Hillel L., our pediatric cardiothoracic surgeon, whose wife was spending hour after hour with Jessica and the kids while I was going to the hospital each day. Hillel had "good news"—the biopsy showed nodular sclerosing Hodgkin's disease. A few minutes later he was in my office, three flights and two buildings removed from his own office. I was still holding the phone in my hand—I hadn't realized that he had hung up.

The next days were filled by tests, including nuclear scans, CAT scans (I learned that I can tolerate 48 cc of Renografin-76 intravenously without ill effect; the 49th cc makes me extremely nauseated, and the 50th makes me as sick as any of the cardiac catheterization patients who have vomited on our cath lab table), and lymphangiography. The last remains my least favorite procedure. Rich M. sat with me, reading *The New York Times*, throughout the two hours of the procedure. Dr. G., another radiologist on staff, interpreted the negative results to me and choked up when I thanked him for this kindness. Through the years, I thought that radiologists read X-rays, insulating themselves from the outside world, investing little or no emotion in patient care; yet when I was with them, it seemed that there was never a dry eye in the house.

Things were looking somewhat better. Yes, it was Hodgkin's disease, but I knew that from the moment I saw my own X-ray. At least my lymphangiogram and CAT scan suggested that the disease was confined to the lymphatic areas above the diaphragm, so that my disease "stage" was not beyond Stage II. This would carry a better prognosis than would Stage III or IV and might mean that I could avoid chemotherapy (which I feared more than I did the splenectomy that was coming).

Jessica and I made an appointment to meet with my newfound internist at the Health Plan in preparation for the splenectomy. It was Jessica's first meeting with him. When we arrived and introductions were completed, he informed me that he had been correct and the patient he had mentioned to me during our first encounter had, indeed, been proven, as he had suspected, to have malaria. Quite a diagnostic coup, but somewhat far afield from oncology. What occurred next I can only assume happens not infrequently in medicine, much to the discredit of our profession. My physician opened his copy of the University of Rochester manual, which is used as a standard text in medical oncology for medical students. He then quoted us the actuarial data on survival of the various stages of Hodgkin's disease. It bothered me somewhat that he was using, in 1980, the same edition of this manual that I had used as a medical student in 1970–1971. Even then, the figures for Stages I and II were quite good, while Stages III and IV were much less optimistic. The biggest differences between 1970–1971 and 1980 were in the survival of the two more advanced stages. I then asked the question I never should have asked. However, I was a frightened patient and lacked the retrospective vision that I now have. I asked, "What stage do you think I am?" Much to my surprise (I had asked the question already knowing about the negative lymphangiogram and CAT scan and hoped to reassure my wife), he said that he was pretty sure that I would be in Stage IV. To this day I cannot fathom his response. He based this on the presence of the "sentinel" left supraclavicular node, which usually presaged the finding of involvement below the diaphragm. Jessica was inconsolable, and I realized at that moment that that bastard was less informed about this disease than I was. I was making a conscious effort to avoid reading about Hodgkin's disease, but this was my physician—what was his excuse? Couldn't he have done *his* homework?

For the next two days I tried to call his office to speak with him. My calls were never answered. I still don't know whether the calls were ignored or his secretary never passed on the messages. Needless to say, I never saw this "hot shot" again but would not hesitate to do so if I ever get malaria.

The next question that arose was, perhaps, the most perplexing of all—how to tell my 70+-year-old parents about this matter. Never an easy assignment and more difficult still for someone who, at age 33, was still striving to please both of his parents with academic accomplishments, much as he did when he was bringing home report cards. Now I had to find a way to tell them that if all went well and the staging laparotomy was favorable, there was better than a 90% chance that their eldest son would be alive in five years. My wife and I decided that this would be the first time that I would not include my parents in all aspects of our lives. No, they didn't need to know, and they still don't know. It sounds terribly noble, but there is another side to this decision. My wife and I had enough to do to keep ourselves functioning, and we were straining our support system to the ultimate—we could not imagine undertaking the responsibility of providing emotional support for anyone else.

The last weekend before the laparotomy we spent with friends. We had dinner at Le Cygne and saw *Evita,* which starts with Eva Peron's death of cancer at the age of 33.

The day before my admission I learned another lesson in human nature from a fellow physician. My sister-in-law's employer, a well-known oncologist from New York, was kind enough to call to wish me luck and offer me a pep talk. He also inquired about the results of my lymphangiogram and CAT scan. When I told him that they were negative, he commented that he was sure that my physicians had a good reason for performing the splenectomy but, of course, I knew that if I were a patient at *his* hospital the splenectomy would not be done. Of course, as an otherwise healthy young male, I should be able to go through the splenectomy without difficulty. He offered a reference for me to read (I was in the medical library within moments) which was not a study on the accuracy of lymphangiography and CAT scan in staging of Hodgkin's disease but rather a study on the complications of splenectomy in a population of healthy adult males. Exactly what I didn't need! At the 11th hour there was a myriad of phone calls, including calls to friends and acquaintances in oncology in Boston, San Francisco, and New York, as well as discussion with my local physicians. In the end the splenectomy was performed, the spleen and paraaortic nodes were free of disease, and the convalescence was even less fun that I anticipated.

The radiotherapy was carried out under the direction of the director of therapeutic radiology, who treated me as a whole person. He answered my questions, anticipated others, and even suggested questions that I should have asked. His staff of technicians, physicists, nurses, and receptionists embody all that is good about modern medicine, from both a technical and a human viewpoint.

The radiotherapy was no picnic, but it was much easier to endure than I had predicted. The loss of hair was hard to take and even harder to explain to my parents. The abdominal treatments were administered at the end of each day, allowing me to break from work at 4:30 p.m. each day for radiotherapy. Thereafter, I had an hour to complete work and/or to return home before the hour of nausea hit. This way I was able to regain a modicum of control over my life despite this damned disease.

On the last day of my radiotherapy, I returned home to find that Jessica and our friends (one of whom was unflinchingly shouldering an even larger clinical burden than usual since I had been taken ill) had made a surprise party to celebrate the end of the radiotherapy. I was truly touched, but, unfortunately, walked through the front door at 5:30 p.m., the magical hour after the radiotherapy. I enjoyed the party even if I did not sip the champagne.

During the next two years there were two small bowel obstructions requiring prolonged hospitalization and, ultimately, reexplorations, one including a small bowel resection.

Each obstruction woke me from sleep at 11:00 p.m. On the first occasion there was no doubt in my mind about what was wrong. I woke Jessica and told her I was obstructed. We called the Health Plan. The triage nurse was dispassionate and even less efficient. After I described my history and symptoms (even embellishing them a bit with bilious vomiting, hoping that this would "trip the switch" to the diagnosis of bowel obstruction and earn a response), she was to get back to me to tell me whether to have my friend George (as always, available for us to lean on) drive me to the Health Plan or directly to the hospital emergency room. Twenty minutes later, swathed in towels to soak up my perspiration, we called back, only to be told that she had not yet had a chance to make the phone call. Needless to say, we went to the emergency room. The next time I obstructed, I called Dr. C. directly.

Two hours later, in my hospital room awaiting the arrival of the admitting resident who was to pass a long Canter tube via my nose to decompress my obstructed bowel, I finally asked the young floor nurse for the K-Y jelly and passed the tube myself (an exercise I would not do again and would not recommend to anyone else). That act marked my Declaration of Independence as a patient. I was no longer going to wait two hours for a resident, because I never made a patient in pain wait that long for a chance at relief.

Later in that hospitalization I heard two nurses in the hallway outside my room debating whether the patient in the next room needed more fluid or a diuretic to induce a large urine output. The poor devil was comatose from an inoperable brain tumor. His family and his physicians agreed he would not be resuscitated should he sustain a cardiac arrest. The nurses had called the neurosurgical resident, but he would not or could not respond within a reasonable time. A short time later there was a knock at my door, and the nurse asked if it was true that I was a staff cardiologist. I responded that I was a *pediatric* cardiologist and was told that that would do. Would I please examine my neighbor and render an opinion? I was, of course, reluctant to do so but was finally persuaded that I was the most available physician for the poor fellow. Transporting me to the bedside was not easy, what with the IV in my right arm and the Canter tube in my nose taped to my lip and forehead and pinned in a coil to my open-ended johnny. Two nurses under my arms helped me shuffle next door. I remember borrowing one of the nurses' stethoscopes and remember thinking that it was a good thing the poor guy was in a coma to be spared this bizarre sight. I don't remember whether I suggested fluid or diuretic. Forty-eight hours later he was dead. I don't think my ministrations altered his hospital course. I never did learn the identity of the neurosurgical resident who did not respond to the nurses' call—it's a good thing, too.

I was finally explored and the obstruction relieved. There were no private-duty nurses available, and this was one luxury that I learned to appreciate on the first night or two after surgery. The first eight-hour postop shift I received scrupulous private-duty nursing from Carl J., a physician friend and colleague from radiology, who spent the evening away from his family tending to me. He changed the soiled bedding that, to my chagrin, I kept vomiting on. He massaged my feet and back, held my hand, and baby-sat for eight hours. To me, this physician was the embodiment of humanity and gentility.

The future appears optimistic medically, now that I have been disease-free for five years and obstruction-free for two. My children are growing, my marriage is strong, we are outgrowing our first house, and my academic career seems to be thriving. I have gone through a second period of almost manic dedication to my work, in part trying to prove to myself that I can still perform at pre-Hodgkin's levels.

I have also gone through an earlier than usual midlife crisis—reassessing whether I've accomplished what I had hoped to and whether the future holds the promise of attaining my further goals. I think the answers are yes on both scores. I also have changed the form of those future goals. When I was about to undergo anesthesia on each of the three occasions during the past five years, my last thoughts were of my wife and kids—not of the NIH, my research projects, or of divisional directorships. These moments have helped me to recognize the true priorities in life.

The value of friendships has become even more evident; I will always appreciate the support that so many kind people offered while I was hospitalized. Even more important to our family was the unselfish support that some of our friends gave Jessica and our children. Their sensitivity to the needs of our children during this most difficult time made it possible for us to bear the emotional burden of living with a malignancy.

At the same time I have been changed as a physician. I have always thought that I had a large measure of compassion and empathy, but I found out that it is much easier to walk alongside a gurney than it is to lie on one.

I learned how easy it is to become a nameless, seemingly ignored entity, with explanation rarely offered unless demanded. I know of the need for each patient to have an advocate. In this regard, I have redoubled my efforts to communicate fully with patients and their parents. The patient in the hospital and his family often live from one visit to the next from their physician. There is no reason why there should not be communication daily, and more often if necessary.

Most families come to the hospital seeking efficient, professional care. They want to be cared for by people who are gentle, compassionate, and competent. They are not necessarily looking for a "buddy" who introduces him- or herself by first name, the way your waiter for the evening does at the local Steak and Brew.

Especially in pediatrics, but throughout medicine to some extent, the primary physician on a case not only is the care provider but should also assume the role of patient advocate. I now take this role more seriously than ever. One of my strongest advocates was Peter R., a pediatrician and pediatric anesthesiologist whom I requested to administer anesthesia to me.

I have become more outspoken in this regard as well. The patients and their parents have not minded at all, and at my institution it is not often necessary, but the occasional pediatrician or surgeon who doesn't take the time to communicate with parents or the occasional anesthesiologist who is cavalier in his treatment of patients in my presence hears about it. In the past I would have been more reticent about such things, but if the physician in charge doesn't stick up for his patient, then who will?

I have also learned that while patients and their families want to think their doctor is all-knowing and all-seeing, they also want him to be honest. Few people, especially physicians, like to admit when they don't know something, but better to admit that than pretend, because the distrust that the latter produces will undo the entire fabric of the physician–patient relationship and will leave the patient unfairly exposed and helpless.

During the months following the diagnosis of Hodgkin's, I wore the diagnosis on my sleeve. I felt that it was good for me and good for the children in oncology clinic for me to speak to newly diagnosed patients with Hodgkin's so I could tell them what to expect. It soon became clear to me that I was not ready to take on quite so heavy a burden as a regular habit. I, frankly, don't know enough about the disease to really counsel someone and am still vulnerable enough to imagine myself developing some of the complications that less fortunate patients develop.

Once, at Christmas time, I sat down with a courageous little 9-year-old with end-stage cardiomyopathy who waited in vain for the availability of a suitable heart for transplant. We spoke frankly of our fear of death and the need for hope. I think she supported me as much as I did her.

More recently I discussed my illness frankly with a 20-year-old with life-threatening arrhythmias. The side effect of the investigational antiarrhythmic agent became so severe that he decided he could no longer endure it. We discussed the issue of longevity versus quality of life, and I felt myself able to communicate at a different level than I could have a few years ago.

Even if all goes well, as appears likely, I will never be happy that my family and I have gone through the travail of the past five years. Nonetheless, much good has come out of this experience. I would like to think that eventually I would have reordered my priorities, placing family and humanism above some of the more tangible, yet less meaningful, goals that one may have in life.

I am learning that it is possible to live a life that is fulfilling, both professionally and personally, and that the ideal is to strike a balance between the two. There now seems to be time for both. Being in control of one's destiny need not preclude flexibility and should not require one to value one aspect of life over the other.

CHAPTER 34

CANCER OF SIGMOID

JAMES C. HAYES

We practicing physicians are frequently placed into the position of the bearer of bad news who gets punished for his honesty. There may be occasions when we are thanked by patients for telling them that their diagnosis is cancer, but more often we find that we have become enmeshed in the patient's new anger and depression. After dealing with this problem for a number of years with a number of patients, I began to wonder how I would accept the bad news when it came to me.

Two years ago I found the answer to that question. After a few episodes of crampy, left-sided abdominal obstructive-type pain, I arranged for a barium enema examination. Within minutes, my radiologist/colleague/friend advised me promptly, and in a matter-of-fact way, that there was a sigmoid lesion which was very likely carcinoma. Now I finally had a chance to see what my reaction would be.

There was none! I felt no dread, no panic, no fear. Psychologically, it wasn't as great a shock as hearing that my basement wall needed a $2000 repair. I went to lunch that day and then resumed seeing patients, thinking about my diagnosis only to the extent that I was considering how I would make time-off arrangements. The ensuing weekend passed with the usual social activities and minimal concerns.

What is this? I asked myself. Where is my reaction? Is my lack of reaction my reaction? Is this the denial that characterizes cancer psychology?

I didn't consider it denial. I knew perfectly well the facts associated with it, the possibility of metastatic disease, the need for surgery. I felt under my rib cage for the liver, not really expecting to feel it but prepared for the possibility, in a way that was characterized more by curiosity and detachment than by anxiety. I stood outside myself and peered in, wondering and interested, but no more than that. Hey, I

DR. JAMES HAYES is an internist and the medical director of the Pittsburgh Diagnostic Clinic. He is a clinician rather than an administrator and reports that he unmakes more diagnoses than he makes.

said, you're supposed to have some anxiety, be scared, worry a little. What's wrong with you? There was no reply and no glimmer of anxiety.

Of course, what we patients are most anxious about is the unknown. We are able to deal realistically with most events if we understand them. Our physician's knowledge makes that relatively simple. How easy it is for us to forget that patients require time to absorb what we tell them about their diseases. The facts are simple to us who understand them but so complicated and complex without our background and basis for comprehending them. There was only a little of the unknown for me, not enough to ring my alarm bell.

What I had to do was a task to be accomplished, something requiring arrangements in a practical sense, like going away on vacation or to a meeting. I don't even recall being annoyed about it. There was even a vacation sense of anticipation of knowing I would have a few weeks off, would be able to lie around the house and read some of the books that I had not been able to get to.

The events of the next few days were so simple I could hardly believe it. Almost between patients, I slipped into the bathroom and took an enema. No big deal. I saw some more patients, then walked to the proctologist's office. The procedure of flexible sigmoidoscopy and biopsy was simple, nontraumatic, and quick. My nonreactivity was maintained and I could have dozed on the proctoscopic table except that it was over so quickly. Waiting for the biopsy report didn't raise any hackles, possibly because there really wasn't any doubt anyway about the situation.

A day or two later, I walked into the hospital to my room, still wondering why the hell I was so passive, so calm. No anger. No guilt. No remorse. No fear.

The preoperative preparation included castor oil, which I had never taken unless it was given to me as a child and perhaps left some memory trace embedded in my psyche. The castor oil caused my first, and perhaps only, emotional reaction to the entire scene. Why the hell do we continue to use such anachronistic gook? I can't believe there isn't something equally effective and more acceptable. It is utterly absurd that we can install new joints, rocket to the stars, and devise a mechanical heart, and still use castor oil. If it is so essential, why can't our brilliant researchers isolate the active components and put them in capsules?

Well, at last I was acting like a real patient, upset and angry, and sure I could handle things better than the professionals. It is strange, though, that even now I retained my anger about the use of castor oil and resentment of those who insist on using it.

The lone bit of discomfiture didn't keep me awake. No sleeping pill was required, and I had no fear of tomorrow but still the idle detached curiosity about what it would feel like after the operation. Would the nausea last long? Would it hurt bad? Would there be liver metastases? Would I have a colostomy? Oh, well, go to sleep and don't worry about it. And I did.

In the morning, calm still prevailed. The nurse awakened me for premedication, and I promptly went back to sleep. I barely recall climbing onto the carriage, vaguely remember being pushed through the hall, and have no recollection at all of the operating room or the people in it.

A moment later I awakened in my room and looked around. My first sensation was paradoxical because it was really awareness of the absence of a sensation, namely, nausea. Hey, pretty good anesthesia. I don't remember that my abdomen hurt badly. The gastric tube was hardly even noticeable.

At the earliest possible time, I began to move. My anesthesiologist/colleague/friend had discussed this with me beforehand and emphasized it and encouraged it. Move! Sitting on the bedside wasn't necessarily easy and coughing was no fun, but they were accomplished about as well as could be expected. The absence of unnecessary compassion or concern from those around me clearly made it easier. Making little jokes about pain eases the tension more than anxious empathy.

My surgeon reported the good news (I guess). I cannot remember the details of what he said through the haze of that first day. Frankly, I didn't care that much at that point. What will be, will be. What if he hadn't been able to bring good news and had spoken of local extension or liver metastases? I think that I would have been equally apathetic about those matters at that point.

There was one curious and interesting postoperative occurrence. As an internist, I have always felt that the surgeons left gastric tubes in too long, but they always seem to worry about that dreaded ileus and the absence of peristalsis. The tube wasn't really all that bad, but I was happy when it was pulled on the second day. My idle curiosity and clinical detachment had returned by then, and so I wondered how long it would be before my paralyzed and traumatized bowel began to distend. Instead, I was startled to hear and feel the most astounding gut activity my professional life has ever experienced. It resounded throughout the room and into the hall and never really let up for many days. In fact, it continued in an attenuated form for many weeks postoperatively. My surgeon's explanation was that this reaction was just the bowel's physiological response to emptiness, but I don't buy that. For a patient who doesn't know or care, it might have been a reasonable enough explanation. But as an interested physician-patient with considerable awareness and interest in what was going on, I was intrigued by the lack of interest or even curiosity of the surgeons as to this phenomenon. Even now, I don't know if that occurrence is usual or unusual, ignored or acknowledged. It seems to be something that nobody knew or cared about, and since it obviously wasn't causing any problems, it needed no attention. My explanation? In a manner not disclosed to me, the surgery must interfere with the autonomic nervous system control of intestinal motility. But it never caused any cramps or diarrhea. Can someone out there enlighten me?

How quickly the recovery ensued! Stomach and bladder tubes came out quickly, IVs were discontinued in a few days, and a full tray was supplied more quickly than I imagined, even if I wasn't so hungry. The pain diminished, my legs became stronger, and walks in the hall were easier. Move! Blow up the pulmonary gadget. It must be time to get out of here now. I could do all this at home. So I was out in six days.

Home wasn't all that great for a while and the books remained mostly unread. But progress was relentless and so, on my 20th postoperative day, I felt strong enough to go to the country club, get in a cart, and catch up with my regular golfing friends to ride around and enjoy the warmth of a sunny afternoon. I caught up with them on the 15th hole and borrowed a club to try a few easy swings. Not bad! So, on the 16th tee, a par three, it seemed not too bad an idea to try a real swing with a real ball; so, I hit in on the green and sank the putt for a birdie.

I doubt if the surgeon would have approved of that, for reasons of tradition if no other. I didn't ask him. But I think that story must be an example of the basic principle of: Move!

Two years later, I remain free of recurrent cancer but cognizant of the statistics, which are favorable for my lesion. There are still no fears or anxiety but clinical awareness of the possibilities. I have answered the question posed in the beginning of this essay—namely, how will I react when the news comes? I think I am also prepared for the next phase of that scenario. But only time will tell.

The final points are that our knowledge as physicians should make us better patients, and that the unknown is the enemy. That imposes upon us the responsibility to transmit the utmost possible understanding to every patient, about every disease.

CHAPTER 35

MYCOSIS FUNGOIDES

"MOSES LLEWELLYN"

At age 13 I noticed that some areas of my skin were red, scaly, and constantly itching. When I was taken to the doctor my family was told that I had eczema. Steroid creams were prescribed but the lesions progressed without any relief. I saw another physician, who thought that something was wrong with my liver and ordered daily injections of vitamin B and liver extract.

Gradually the lesions became larger and then appeared on my buttocks, thigh, and forearm. In addition, inguinal nodes became prominent. When I was 22 years old I saw a dermatologist at a prominent institution who had been recommended by a nurse. During my visit he took biopsies from various sites and diagnosed *Parapsoriasis en plaques*. He was most informative and told me that there was no cure and recommended continued use of topical steroids. I experienced no pain but the lesions were, of course, unsightly.

I kept in touch with the dermatologist, and during one of our conversations he asked whether or not I would be willing to attend a dermatology conference with him to be one of the sample subjects, holding out the hope that someone might be able to offer new insight or suggestions. For me this was an act of desperation. I went to the conference and was examined in minute detail by some of the participants and scorned by others. Some treated me with respect but to others I was a specimen and treated just that way. No new therapy was recommended.

I continued with the topical steroids. My lymph nodes grew larger. I was near the completion of my first year of medical school when I contacted the dermatologist to inquire as to "the state of the art." He informed me that there was a dermatologist at Memorial Sloan-Kettering Cancer Center who wanted to try electron beam irradiation on patients diagnosed with *Parapsoriasis en plaques*.

"DR. MOSES LLEWELLYN" is currently a consulting cardiologist.

I agreed to see him and the inevitable skin biopsies were repeated. Axillary lymph nodes were now prominent. The biopsies were read at Memorial Hospital as *Parapsoriasis en plaques* and at Columbia University College of Physicians and Surgeons as "suggestive of *Mycosis fungoides.*"

Since there were differing pathologic interpretations, the decision was made to continue the steroids and repeat the biopsies in three months. I was now in the second year of medical school and returned as scheduled for the repeat biopsies. A few days later I was called by the dermatologist, who informed me that I had *Mycosis fungoides* and that therapy was possible. An appointment was set up for my next visit. Not knowing the pathophysiology and consequences of the disease, I was excited, to say the least. The excitement was short-lived. That afternoon I went to the library and read just about everything written on *Mycosis fungoides*.

Mycosis fungoides was first described in 1814 by a Frenchman, Alibert. It is a cutaneous T-cell lymphoma usually affecting white males age 40 to 60. After the diagnosis is made, progression is rapid, with death within six months to one year, but some survive up to five years. The various treatments use topical nitrogen mustard, leukophoresis, systemic chemotherapy, and electron beam irradiation. Of course, I became extremely depressed.

Because of the prominent lymphadenopathy, I was admitted to the hospital to have a lymphangiogram done—an excruciatingly painful procedure. This was my first contact with residents and clinical clerks who showed a total lack of concern for me as a person and a patient. I remember most vividly a group of persons entering the room. I recognized the resident who admitted me. There were no introductions. My case was presented and a lengthy discussion ensued. The gist of the conversation was that death was near. The covers were removed and they all drew near. I was something new, a freak show. The covers were left off and the discussion continued as they left the room.

I met with the dermatologist and the radiation oncologist, who explained what was being offered at their institution. They suggested total skin electron beam irradiation (TSEB) plus total nodal irradiation. Weekly treatments of TSEB were begun shortly after. The treatments were painless. I was very compliant initially but began to miss some appointments because I did not want to deal with the idea of being sick. In addition, my medical studies were neglected because of the preoccupation with my illness. "If I am going to die shortly, why do I need to continue medical school?"

I failed my microbiology course and simply was not prepared to handle failure. It felt as if my world was crumbling. That day I just wandered aimlessly around the medical complex. I was at the breaking point.

I sought the services of a psychologist who was there when I needed to talk or vent anger. No pharmacologic intervention was necessary. Before entering medical school I wanted to become a concert pianist, so I began the application process for admission to the Julliard School of Music. I was, however, in no frame of mind to devote the hours necessary for the audition.

My weekly treatments of TSEB were time-consuming. I was introduced to health care workers who were not psychologically prepared to deal with patients. Frequently I encountered technical staff who were gruff and most unpleasant. My doctors were nevertheless reassuring and available. As my treatments progressed I lost the hair from my body and the back of my head. My nails turned black and my skin a charcoal color. I could no longer sweat from my body and frequently had severe episodes of sweating from my forehead.

I completed the course of TSEB. Some areas of my body appeared not to have responded and localized irradiation was necessary. I decided to take a few weeks respite before starting the daily total nodal irradiation. My skin was marked and tattooed. My first treatment was, of course, painless. However, on my way home I began to feel extremely cold and nauseated. This was followed by episodes of vomiting and severe retching. These episodes were daily and at times lasted up to four hours posttherapy. I remember quite vividly walking around Central Park drinking as much water as was possible to help with the episodes of retching. Antiemetics were of little help.

This period of therapy was the worst. One afternoon after completing my therapy, I felt depressed and despondent. I was waiting for the train and, midst my episode of retching, the train was approaching in the distance. Suddenly I thought, "Why not throw yourself in front of the train?" I stepped to the edge of the platform. However, by some unknown force, I was pulled from the edge of the platform. I stood there crying and shaking.

I later contacted my psychologist. Her assistance was invaluable. At times, however, I felt that I was too dependent.

I failed my second year in medical school and had to repeat.

It has been eight years since the completion of the therapy. There are no signs of recurrence. There are, however, visible reminders. My skin is no longer erythematous, but there are radiodermatitis changes. I have lost the hair from my body as well as the ability to sweat from my body.

This process has been humbling. It took quite a long time to fully realize what was going on. I read everything, but it did not sink in. I am comfortable with myself and the disease. There is no longer the preoccupation with death. I now have a positive outlook and a desire to enjoy life—see new places, meet new people, and learn of other customs and cultures.

My interaction with patients has been an empathetic one. I have at times tried to relay my story to difficult and noncompliant patients to let them know that their inner turmoil is by no means unique to their situation. Very frequently it has helped. As a physician I have tried to spend the extra few minutes just to ask, "How are you doing? How are you dealing with your situation?" Frequently there is an outpouring of fear, uncertainty, and depression.

One of the difficulties during my illness was that I knew so much about the disease, more so than the layman, and this was terrifying. This is equally true for the patient who knows too little. This fear is frequently compounded when lengthy discussions, relevant to the disease involved but not necessarily to the specific patient, are made by us at the bedside.

CHAPTER 36

ACUTE MYELOGENOUS LEUKEMIA

JACK J. LEWIS

For almost 45 years, I've had two alcoholic drinks before dinner. In November 1985 there was a sudden change. I lost my taste for alcohol. At about the same time, the Southern California winter evenings seemed to me much colder. Neither the weatherman nor my wife agreed.

Around January 6, 1986, I began experiencing muscle aches. Two aspirin tablets gave relief. In my private practice of medicine, I saw a number of patients with "colds" or gastrointestinal cramps or muscle aches or combinations. My belief was that whatever viruses were causing these conditions were the cause of my symptoms. However, as time went on, I promised my wife that if I was not 100% better by the weekend of the eighteenth, I would see my internist.

On Monday morning, January 20, 1986, I felt well except for very slight muscle aches. After working a full day at my office, I went to see my internist, who is located next to a very large medical center.

He went through a systems review. There had been no change from four years previously when, because of some strange chest symptoms and a treadmill test with a 0.1-mm ST elevation at the end, thallium, technetium, and coronary angiogram tests had been performed; they were all negative. His thorough physical examination was clear. When the blood count was finished, he was shocked to find that my hemoglobin was 7.3 grams. He ordered immediate hospitalization and consultation with a hematologist-oncologist.

DR. JACK LEWIS at the time of his illness was a 65-year-old specialist in internal medicine at the Cedars-Sinai Medical Center, Los Angeles, and associate clinical professor of medicine at the University of Southern California. He was also a captain USNR-R. He received his A.B. in 1942 and his M.D. in 1946 from Stanford University and did his postgraduate work and residencies at Yale University (1947) and the University of Chicago (1948–1952). He was chief of medicine and director of research at the Atomic Bomb Casualty Commission at Hiroshima, 1953–1955. As this book went to print Dr. Jack Lewis began to suffer the final relapse of his disease. He remained at home, intellectually alert and spiritually courageous, until lapsing into coma two days before his death. Dr. Lewis died on the morning of June 15, 1987, in Los Angeles.

Later that evening, after the rigamarole of the admitting office, an iliac crest bone marrow smear and biopsy was performed. The diagnosis was acute myelogenous leukemia.

Speaking in a monotone, the oncologist advised me to follow the UCLA protocol of radical chemotherapy. This would consist of an induction course of thioguanine, ara-C; and daunorubicin, followed by two consolidation couses of the latter two drugs. During these courses, each of which would require about six weeks of hospitalization, I would have to have red blood cell and platelet units available for transfusion. Finding the donors and having them give blood designated for me would be our task. He went on, stating that I would be very sick and that the chance of remission would be 35 to 45%.

On an intellectual level I heard and understood what he was saying. My thoughts were: my God, my poor wife, my family, my patients, and my office staff. Here was a fellow doctor telling me that I had a fatal disease, and that if I spent more than four months in the hospital on poisonous drugs that, with luck, my chances of remission were a little bit better than 33%. The word *remission* was not defined.

We all agreed that some thought should go into the decision of whether I should have chemotherapy. My wife called my son and daughter-in-law in the San Francisco Bay area, my daughter in Chicago, and my physician brother in the Sacramento–Davis area. They were all at the hospital by the following day. Meanwhile, I called my receptionist and the office manager and told them to start canceling patients' appointments.

Over the next 24 hours I talked again with my internist, the oncologist, a psychiatrist, and friends, some of whom were physicians. The question was whether to embark on chemotherapy or whether to allow the disease to follow its natural course.

The same questions were raised with my family. My wife and daughter, who were very stunned and upset, said it was my decision and that they could not ask me to go through such a terrible treatment.

My son, distraught and crying that it was not fair, and my brother, deeply distressed, both wanted me to have the chemotherapy since it was the only chance for survival. I decided to go ahead.

I spent the day being transfused with washed red cells and platelets and had the first of several transfusion reactions of chills and high fevers.

While the hours of transfusions were going on, there was a great flurry of nonhospital activity. Obviously I was not going to see patients for a very long time; there were the economic factors: income dropping precipitously but rent, salaries, supplies, insurance premiums, and other expenses continuing. Social security and insurance forms had to be obtained and numerous blood and platelet transfusion donors found.

My physicians seemed to know very little about how a blood bank functions. It was my wife who had to learn and then teach us. Very early, the head of the blood bank came in and pontificated about replacing blood and getting designated donors. The blood bank was divided into two divisions, geographically separated and not communicating well. There is the blood donor area where blood is drawn and plateletpheresis is performed. Then there is the storage area where the cells are typed and stored. For plateletpheresis, the donors report for screening. A tube of blood is drawn. Forty-eight hours later the donor calls, and if the tests for hepatitis, AIDS, etc., are clear, an appointment for the pheresis is made. There are two machines for pheresis; on one, the platelets have to be transfused within 24 hours; on the other, the platelets are good for five days. The latter machine can be rather daunting. Though some leeway is allowed in scheduling, having blood drawn from one arm while the pheresed blood is returned in the other arm was a trial for many noble donors. With no help from the medical center, my wife always was able to have available for me two units of washed red cells and one platelet pack.

On Wednesday morning, January 22, I was taken to surgery and a Hickman catheter was placed in my left subclavian vein. That afternoon, chemotherapy was started. ara-C was given by intravenous drip, days one through seven, and daunorubicin by slow intravenous push daily on days five through seven. On day five, I had nausea, vomiting, diarrhea, and severe abdominal pains.

The story now becomes anecdotal. There are rare flashes of memory. On February 1, three days after finishing therapy, my temperature shot up to 106°F oral. All I can recall is begging for more blankets and the nurses replying that I was going to be put on a cooling blanket. Within the next 24 hours, antibacterial and antifungal agents were started. The weakness and fatigue were indescribable. I remember thinking, "I'm so tired I have to lie down," only to realize I *was* lying down. All my muscles were aching. I had complete loss of appetite; weight loss was rapid. On February 6, TPN through the Hickman precipitated pulmonary edema. The physicians told my wife that I might not come through the crisis and advised her to have my son and daughter return. Furosemide was pushed. There was a good response, and by the time my family arrived I was breathing fairly well with oxygen. I was pancytopenic and was being sustained by washed red cells and platelet transfusions. Mask and glove isolation procedures were carried out and no visitors except family were allowed. Ice chips, toothbrushes, raw fruits, vegetables, flowers, and toilet paper were forbidden. My son and daughter worked out a scheme where each would fly in on alternate weekends.

Improvement was starting, and now there was enough awareness for me to be distressed by dependency, particularly because I was so weak I had to have someone else doing my anal care following a bowel movement. On February 10, I was jaundiced and several liver function tests were abnormal, but scans and hepatitis investigations were clear. The soles of my feet and toes and the palmar surfaces of my hands and fingers felt like they were burned; over several days huge blisters appeared in these areas. The areas then began to slough. All of my hair was shedding. The skin of the palms, the soles, and the scrotum were clammy, not with sweat but with a sticky secretion. This was particularly bothersome in the scrotal area, where my scrotum would almost be glued to the inner aspects of my thighs.

Improvement continued, my white count slowly rising from 250 per cmm and the platelets from 20,000 per cmm. As sick as I was, I realized and was grateful for the superb team of nurses assigned to me. Another bone marrow aspiration and biopsy was performed. This led to a great deal of anxiety and apprehension while awaiting the outcome. If leukemic cells were still present, what further therapies, if any, were available? If clear, what was next? The oncologist reported that the bone marrow was clear. As soon as my white count rose over 3000 per cmm and my platelets over 75,000, and if my hemoglobin stayed over 8.0 grams per dl, I would be going home.

A few days before I was to go home, when I was obviously on the mend, the resident on the service asked if a medical student could take my history and do a limited examination. This was a great learning experience for the student and me. He was so terrified at having a physician for one of his first patients that he could barely take the history. His physical examination was pathetic. For my part, after almost three hours, I was exhausted. I realized that beginning students cannot start with complicated cases because they don't know what to ask. Their first dozen or so examinations should be performed on their young, healthy classmates.

There were some interesting parts to my history. I had not smoked. Two fraternal male first cousins died of malignant melanomas. Two fraternal female first cousins died of rheumatic heart disease before the antibiotic era.

On July 4, 1942, I was commissioned as an ensign H-VP just as I started medical school. Remaining in the Naval Reserve, I was assigned during the Korean War to the Atomic Bomb Casualty Commission in Hiroshima, Japan, where I examined victims of the atomic bomb. This was interrupted by duty in Tokyo during the Bikini hydrogen bomb test. I was the American doctor who examined the radiation-burned Japanese fisherman. With a hand Geiger counter I went over every portion of their fishing vessel and catch, which had been covered with radioactive ash. Did this have anything to do with my developing leukemia?

Improvement was slow but steady. Five weeks and one day after admission, I was discharged. During the last week or so of hospitalization and the weeks following, I tried to reflect on death and dying but seemed incapable. Instead, my fantasies would focus more on my funeral service: what wonderful things would be said about me, who would say them, what music would be played, who would be the pallbearers. Though these were fantasies, they did cause discussions within the family, so the thought was given to burial plots. I wished to be buried in the same Jewish cemetery where my parents, some relatives, and friends were placed. This led to my wife's buying plots for both of us. My son also taped the second movements of the Brahms double violin and cello concertos.

The first interhospitalization period was difficult. There was continuing fatigue and weakness, no appetite, hair coming out in patches, and skin flaking. The Hickman catheter needed meticulous care. I flushed it with heparin daily and changed the dressings three times a week or when it got wet from showering. None of my various schemes for keeping the dressing dry in the shower worked. I washed the perineal area with warm soap suds after defecating. This detailed attention to the dressings and personal hygiene was required by the constant possibility of infection.

Much time was given to disagreements with the overhead and disability insurance companies. Most were quite uncooperative. The office situation was in turmoil. There were many business matters needing resolution. My wife was placed in the position of making many decisions that were causing her anxiety and apprehension. The numerous problems and pressures on my wife greatly concerned me and kept me from a lot of hours of needed rest.

During this first recuperation period, my practice was sold. There was first a momentary period of relief that part of the huge financial burden was gone and that the buyer was a very fine, compassionate physician. The relief was quickly followed by a sensation of emptiness. Half a century of planning, training, and then practicing as a physician had come to an abrupt and stunning halt. This was dying in a different way but one I could more easily comprehend and be introspective about.

Friends and their children lent me great emotional support, and, practically, they were sources of erythrocyte and platelet transfusions. Meanwhile, I received cards and letters by the hundreds from patients telling how comforting and caring I had been when they needed me and what good medical treatment I gave them. Instead of making me feel better, these cards and letters made me feel sad.

My second hospitalization had its bad moments but was not as severe as the first. Again, there was hair loss, nausea, vomiting, severe blistering and sloughing of hand and foot skin, diarrhea, plus a new complication. This was horizontal splitting of the fingernails with peeling from the nailbed outward. This was particularly distressing because the uplifted peeling nail would catch on the bed clothes and pajamas and was painful.

The dose of ara-C was 3000 mg per m^2 dissolved in 250 ml given IV over a one-hour period every 12 hours. For some unknown reason, I was very apprehensive about this therapy. A schedule of 2:00 a.m. and 2:00 p.m. doses was arranged. During the day, I tried to immerse myself in a mystery or espionage paperback. At night, the sleeping medication had me in such a deep sleep that I would not awaken while the nurses gave the drug through the Hickman catheter.

After five weeks and three days, my second hospitalization was finished. At home the nail problem was helped to a great extent by my wife's suggestion of nail polish. In a thick layering, the nails would no longer catch on threads.

Having bought burial plots, my wife and I were discussing who I would want to officiate at the services. I had not been a member of any congregation. In going to weddings, funerals, bar mitzvahs, and high holy day services, I had listened to many rabbis and had not been impressed except by one. Through a friend, we had several meetings with this rabbi. These meetings were quite gratifying and were very similar to sessions in the hospital with the consulting liaison psychiatrist. After the third meeting, we were relieved and comforted by his offer to conduct the services if I should die in the near future. The illness did not make me more religious. It just seemed to hasten decisions that probably should have been made sooner.

The second interhospitalization period was much easier. My hair came in thicker and darker than previously. Because I was feeling better, I went out to theaters, concerts, restaurants, and friends' homes for dinners.

My blood counts were done every two weeks. They were still low, but the hematologist thought that within another two weeks I could go in for my second consolidation and last hospitalization. Alas, on going into the hospital, my counts were too low for therapy. However, a bone marrow was ordered. This was an ordeal; the doctor performing the task had to do it four times before getting enough bone for the biopsy. This was also the fourth bone marrow and, again, there was the anxiety and apprehension while awaiting the result, which showed that I was still in remission.

Having psyched myself for the last consolidation and hospitalization, I was frustrated and angry at being sent home to wait for my counts to rise.

Ten weeks later, I entered the hospital for what I hoped would be the last time. The same nursing team that had taken care of me on my three previous entries greeted me. I felt I was among old friends. In addition to the dosage change of ara-C, I was given prednisone orally and as a cream for hands and feet, prescribed in the hope that the blistering and peeling of skin would be eliminated. This regimen was successful.

The third course of treatment was as difficult as the previous courses. As the blood counts continued to drop, I received many erythrocyte and platelet transfusions, which were always available owing to my wife's efforts. In my second week of hospitalization, I awakened with an itch of my right calf. There appeared to be an insect bite, though this seemed illogical given the sealed, air-conditioned isolation confines. That night my temperature was 99.2 degrees and I was lethargic. Within 36 hours, there were muscle aches and fever and now on the right calf was about a centimeter-size black area surrounded by a raised erythematous tender 3-centimeter area. The infectious disease specialist cultured the lesion, blood, and urine. Antibiotics, clindamycin and gentamicin, were started through the Hickman. Within 48 hours, my temperature was 102 degress orally and the muscle and bone pains were very severe. Headaches were mild but constant and responded very well to acetaminophen. The cultures of the blood and skin grew out *S. aureus*. The clindamycin was stopped and vancomycin substituted. The Hickman catheter was removed as the possible source of infection. Small lesions were appearing, but on culture showed no bacterial growth. Hepacaths were inserted but all clotted in about 12 hours even though the platelet counts were below 40,000. As usual, I had no appetite and the weight loss of 13 pounds was obvious. Slowly, the fever diminished and the terrible muscle pains abated.

As the fifth week of hospitalization neared and I was getting better, I had two emotional feelings. One was of guilt. Discussions with the psychiatrist and the rabbi did not help in resolving this sensation, though the latter did draw the parallel to the Book of Job. The other feeling was of no longer belonging to my peer group. I felt somehow I was no longer to be one of the doctors going on rounds or attending lectures, that somehow I didn't deserve the privileges.

Finally, on August 22, after a total of 16 weeks in the hospital, four bone marrow biopsies, and numerous blood and platelet transfusions, I was allowed to go home.

The psychiatrist emphasized that I had to realize my life was changed. He said that I should do those things that would give me pleasure, that the reward of private practice was no more.

My first month at home was one of recuperation. I was forcing myself to eat more and regained my weight rapidly. Fatigue was an irritation. Every afternoon I would have to lie down. Insomnia was a problem. My first week home I took 0.50 mg of Halcion each night, the next week 0.25 mg of Halcion each night, the following week 0.25 mg, and then I stopped the medicine. The next five nights were difficult, with an average of three to four hours of sleep. Thereafter, I slept without any aid.

Other changes were occurring. My hair was regrowing at a much slower pace. I had no axillary and scant chest hair. Pubic hair was returning. The scalp hair grew to about 1 1/4 inches and then seemed to stop.

I have not awakened each day and marveled at the sunrise. There has not been a looking at a leaf or flower and suddenly having new insights into the wonders of nature. Yes, I have sat at the sea's edge and, as I have many times before, thought about the beauty and the power of the breaking surf and of all the millions of years past and to come that will see the phenomenon continue.

My last blood count showed 45,000 platelets, 2400 white cells and 10.7 grams of hemoglobin. I hope that by January 1987 these values will all be in the normal range. If so, then I will try to find a position that can use my 30 years of experience in the practice of internal medicine.

Looking back from this horrendous year, what would I advise? Be prepared for a catastrophe and hope it doesn't occur.

Have overhead and disability insurance, an agreement with doctors to cover in case of long incapacitation, a plan to sell or relinquish your practice.

Backup systems are a must. Family and friends are a source of love, caring, food, books, and blood.

Within the hospital, the nursing team was most important. They tried to make me as comfortable as possible, always tried to be encouraging, even in desperate situations, and showed unbelievable dedication. Next in importance was the internist. He and his associate were the only physicians who looked at me as a total human being. I wasn't just an infectious disease or a dermatological problem. I was a patient who was being assaulted with very poisonous substances, and, as a result, numerous organ systems were not functioning well. I would recommend that everyone have an internist before illness strikes.

Being at a medical center has advantages. Consultants of all types and the latest equipment are readily available. There is a large blood bank. When there are serious and not so serious emergencies, there is house staff at all times.

A last few notes. I have pondered many times whether I would have gone through this therapy knowing now what it is like. I can't honestly answer. It is easy to say now that I would not, but I'm not sure that this is the truth.

The day before I left the hospital for what I hoped was the last time, one of my doctors told me that he had never seen a patient do so well in this therapeutic regimen. I was aghast, and when I repeated this statement to the head of my nursing team, she confirmed his statement. I was still very dubious and told my wife. She agreed with them, having been on the oncology wing every day for 16 weeks. When I questioned that if I did so very well, what had the other patients on this regimen done, I was told that most had not survived the therapy.

I asked my oncologist what was the definition of remission, which was the "joyous" state I was in. The answer was that the bone marrow showed no leukemic cells. How long might this last? Perhaps months, perhaps years. Maybe a cure? Who knows? Was it worthwhile? Who knows?

CHAPTER 37

BENIGN GIANT CELL TUMOR OF SACRUM

RICHARD E. THOMPSON

The sciatic symptoms started in January 1983. I was terrified. Not of dying, not of physical pain, but of being incapacitated. As a traveling hospital consultant, I'm just as much in private practice as any "real" doctor. What if I had to take time off my busy schedule for an operation? What if the rehabilitation period stretched beyond a month or six weeks? What would happen to my family's economic security while I got rid of this "slipped disc"?

As it turned out, those were the *least* of my worries!

In February 1983, I stopped off in Georgia to see an orthopedist friend who had reconstructed my knee and in whom I had great confidence. He confirmed the bad news. I had a "disc." The good news was that I could continue to travel. As long as the symptoms were sensory and not motor (e.g., foot drop), I could hope for spontaneous resolution without surgery. The prescription: heat, Tylenol, bed rest when I could, and exercises.

For the next five months I continued to travel in the face of worsening symptoms, making two to four stops around the country each week. I fell into a routine of sleeping on motel room floors because the beds were too soft. I declined dinner invitations from clients because the pain would not allow me to sit at a table for more than a few minutes at a time.

On the road, orthopedists and neurosurgeons in my medical staff audiences offered advice: Had I considered chymopapain injections? Had I had a CT scan? Was I aware of the new theory that such symptoms might not be caused by disc displacement but by interruption of the blood supply to vertebral processes? "Why are you walking around? You should be operated on!" "For God's sakes, don't let anyone operate on you unless you get a foot drop!"

DR. RICHARD THOMPSON is a 52-year-old consultant on medical staff organizational affairs, including bylaws, peer review, Joint Commission accreditation, and paralegal issues. His most recent book is *THEORY I: End Your One-Minute Search for Excellence* (SENSS Publications, 1986).

At home, Joan vacated the master bedroom. I used the full dimensions of our queen-size bed, assuming the weird positions back patients learn, seeking some relief from the pain.

Finally, I determined to spend an entire week off the road and in bed, hoping for a "cure." The first week in July 1983 was selected as "healing week." But the experiment was a failure. Symptoms progressed to the point that I couldn't even stand. The pain "shot me down"—a new bizarre kind of pain in a disturbing new distribution in the perineum.

At the urging of all the contacts I'd made by now—physical therapists, a rehabilitation hospital, and my orthopedist friend in Georgia—I finally decided to have a work-up, *but* without interrupting my busy travel schedule again.

On August 9, 1983, while working with the Medical Executive Committee and the Credentials Committee of an upstate hospital, I accepted the offer of a neurologist, Dr. A., to squeeze me into the radiology department's busy CT scan schedule. He would then examine me thoroughly the next day after my business was concluded and before I left town.

I remember the exact moment when I began to fear the worst. It was during the CT scan when the radiology techs suddenly became solicitous and called a radiologist to see the scan that was unfolding before their eyes. At the conclusion of the scan, the radiologist asked several questions, was also solicitous, and suggested that I should get off my feet and be taken back to the meeting room in a wheelchair! I declined.

During my presentation to the Credentials Committee, I received a message from Dr. A. to come to his office immediately following the meeting.

"That's it," I thought. "It's bad news. I lost the battle to avoid surgery. I must have a whopping big disc displacement."

The CT scan Dr. A. mounted on the view box in his comfortable office was of *my* back! And it didn't show disc protrusion. Instead, where white bony sacrum should be, there was only blackness. (Copies of that CT scan are now in the "teaching files" of three hospitals!)

"Dick," said Dr. A., in a gentle manner that I will always appreciate, "you must catch the next plane back to Chicago. Forget tomorrow's meetings; forget your entire schedule for an indefinite time. Your entire sacrum has been replaced by some kind of tumor, and your symptoms are undoubtedly due to nerve root pressure or—worse—invasion."

I didn't shake, shout, or cry. I suppose I'd suspected the unbelievable truth. Me! Actually joining the list of medical school horror stories about people who ignore back pain, attributing it to noncorrectable causes while a tumor gains a foothold, grows, and eventually takes over vital structures.

As I thanked Dr. A. and shook his hand, I said, "Okay, but I'll be back to finish my work."

His reply: "I hope so, Dick, I hope so."

The next plane back to Chicago was not until the next day. Three or four concerned physicians offered to spend the evening with me—afraid I'd be depressed. I declined. I wanted to be alone.

I phoned Joan in South Carolina, where she, a consultant in her own right, was working with a client. I asked if she would return to Chicago the next morning. I told her the back thing was some kind of tumor. She received the news calmly.

But the next day, when she met me at the airport, she was in tears. "Don't be frightened," I offered lamely, scared to death myself—needing her desperately but not wanting to say so.

"Of *course* I'm frightened," Joan sobbed, "and I'm *angry*. I'm just *angry*! Why you? You're too good a man!"

We walked down the concourse, hand in hand, finally realizing, after 29 years of marriage, how much we really meant to each other.

The first job was to find a doctor.

Where should we start? Do you call an orthopedist because it's a bone tumor or a neurosurgeon because it's compressing nerve roots? An oncologist? An oncologist!?! My God, I'm a tumor patient! I might be a dead man already. Were we facing surgery, radiation therapy, chemotherapy, or all of the above? What would I be like after therapy? In a wheelchair? On crutches? Would I be able to travel at all? Would I have bowel and bladder control or ostomies? Would penile erection, which had gone entirely as nerve roots became involved, ever return?

I phoned my general internist and encountered my first disappointment with "the health care system." Even after the third call, and even flaunting my M.D. degree, I couldn't get the phone service or receptionist to contact my physician or give me an appointment for the next day. (Of course, the internist was horrified and embarrassed when he eventually found out what had taken place, but his apologies later didn't help Joan and me when we desperately needed help.)

Finally, I called an ophthalmologist. That's right. Dr. S. had been a good friend since we'd worked together on some bylaws and credentials issues a couple of years before. His response was immediate. Within a couple of hours, he had arranged for me to be hospitalized and seen by two senior staff members—an oncologist and a neurosurgeon.

Once admitted to the hospital, I continued to learn from the patient's perspective. There's a major difference between going to the hospital just long enough to make rounds and going to the hospital as a cancer patient! Word spread; a parade of house officers and medical students came to see the CT scan and, of course, to ask me to tell the story all over again. So this was what it felt like to be a "fascinoma"!

I also learned how simple words from a physician can strike absolute terror into the hearts of patients. A well-meaning internal medicine resident remarked offhand, as he pushed on my belly, that my liver seemed "a little enlarged." The fear of metastatic malignancy nearly turned me to jelly.

My first (of five) operation must have been a bloody mess. It was an emergency procedure because I blocked off during the myelogram and immediate decompression of the sacral nerve roots was necessary. A good biopsy was obtained, but resection of the tumor was impossible. Fortunately, this initial operation was performed by a careful neurosurgical team who preserved my neurological function intact.

Now, the wait for the "path report."

A couple of days later the good news came: *benign* giant cell tumor! A brief sigh of relief, but only brief. The bad news—the tumor's size and location infiltrating critical structures—remained. Decision time. How to try to eradicate such a large bloody lesion without causing permanent neurological damage?

I was that week's tumor conference case. The choices presented to me were the following:

- Radiation therapy. But tumors of this cell type generally do not respond, and complications of radiation therapy were possible.
- Incomplete resection. "Get what we can and get out." But that would be a repeat of the first operation and not likely to be very successful.
- Block resection. The likely result would be ostomies and a wheelchair.
- Referral to Sloan-Kettering Institute, New York Memorial Hospital, for "cryosurgery," a technique reportedly used on this type of tumor by one of the surgeons there.

I went home to recuperate from the first operation and to take a few days to decide which of the alternatives I'd go for. I added a fifth option. I called my orthopedist friend in Georgia who had a different recommendation, which I also considered.

Finally, I decided on the Sloan-Kettering route. My own physicians, primarily my neurosurgeon, in whom I had great confidence from the very beginning, could then follow me on a long-term basis.

During the next two or three days, Joan and I summarized and discussed our financial position. We were relieved to see that we could make it for two months—even three, if we had to. What would happen after that we had no idea. Our future would depend on my mobility or lack of it, after the tumor was treated.

On August 25, 1983, my son Greg drove Joan and me to O'Hare Airport. I remember telling Greg that I would probably not make it home for Labor Day but would surely be able to see the play he was to star in in October.

I was not to be finally dismissed from the hospital until January 7, 1984.

During the long routine admitting procedure at New York Memorial, I began to have second thoughts about going into a hospital where no one knew me personally. I longed for the shortcuts made possible by contacts developed through membership on a hospital medical staff—shortcuts that insulate physicians from having to learn what it's like to deal with "the system" as an outsider.

In my hospital room the parade of medical students and residents began again. I was reassured when the surgeon to whom I had been referred came in. He didn't seem to find my case unusual. In fact, as he viewed the CT scan we'd brought with us, he commented, "Oh. One of those."

I hadn't yet had one study—a femoral angiogram. It was ordered. I dreaded it, and I was right. In my case the angiogram was necessary to ascertain the tumor's blood supply prior to surgery. But the painful experience made me think about how many times around the country, every day, physicians can submit patients to pain and risk merely by casually inscribing "angiogram" on the order sheet.

A treatment plan was decided on:

- An initial operation would clear up residual drainage from the first operation, caused by the nature of the tumor.
- A 30-day course of radiation therapy would, I hoped, (a) decrease the vascularity of the tumor, so less bleeding would be encountered during subsequent surgery, and (b) decrease the size of the tumor and discourage it from growing further.
- A definitive operation would be performed to remove as much tumor as possible.

Then began the delays.

The radiation therapists couldn't see me for a week and couldn't start my 30 days of therapy for another week. In fact, hospital routine appeared to follow a three-day week: Tuesday, Wednesday, and Thursday. Nothing at all could be accomplished on weekends, of course. It seemed to take Monday to get cranked up again after the weekend, and Friday was wind-down time, in anticipation of the next weekend. Maybe that's the way all businesses are run these days.

Joan had to return home. Enter "Cousin Earl," memorable among several compassionate individuals to whom I owe a great deal. My first cousin Earl and his wife, Margaret, lived near New York; he had just retired from his position as one of the vice-presidents of American Airlines. Ironically, Earl had been a great help a few years earlier as a member of the advisory board to a Kellogg Foundation project that I directed, aimed at measuring and responding to the "expectations and perceptions" of hospitalized patients! With his usual intensity, Earl seemed to take on my illness as his new full-time work.

Earl and Margaret, John B., Barbara J., and a few other acquaintances and visitors, plus whatever tranquilizer the doctors had me on, kept me from being lonesome and discouraged to the point of depression. But I was not comfortable in the hospital. While many persons I encountered seemed caring and committed, there were some nursing shifts on which squabbling and turf-guarding appeared to take precedence over responding to patients' needs. I wonder if other bedridden patients experience the fear I felt, engendered by the realization that one is totally dependent on the actions of others.

I asked if my radiation therapy could be completed back in Chicago. After some discussion, it was agreed that that would be permissible and arrangements were begun.

Happy day! Saturday, September 17! I had a plane reservation to Chicago, detailed instructions and curious-looking maps of my body for the Radiation Therapy Department, and instructions (a) not to resume work and (b) to return at the conclusion of the radiation therapy for my "definitive" operation.

That morning, while I was dressing to catch the plane, and about the same time Joan was preparing to come to O'Hare Airport to meet me, my sacrum gave way—a pathologic fracture through tumor.

My discharge from the hospital was canceled, of course. The depth of my disappointment can't even be described.

The next two weeks were quite painful. For several days, during initial healing of the pelvic fracture, a bed scale hoist was used to get me from my bed to a pram so I could be wheeled down to radiation-therapy. There I was turned, rolled, and lifted onto the hard, narrow table by several (usually thoughtful) therapists. Then, after the treatment, back to the pram, and upstairs to be hoisted back into bed. I couldn't believe I was a helpless invalid! I was to remain absolutely bedridden for the next three months and partially so for a long convalescent period after that.

Near the end of the month of radiation treatments, I became concerned about a combination of new symptoms and about the feeling that my complaints about these new symptoms were not being heeded. I couldn't get one foot to work right. On two occasions, I didn't return a Fleet enema. I don't mean there was "no result." I mean my bowel didn't even respond to the stimulation! I dribbled some urine. And, of course, erection had been completely gone for nearly two months now.

I was frightened. I knew decompression surgery had been necessary previously; I knew symptoms were worsening; I wondered if I needed decompression again. I pushed, as politely as I could, for the definitive surgery.

On October 15, 1983, the operation took place. Scheduled for 8:00 a.m., the procedure began at noon and went on for several hours. Again, several units of blood were necessary. The cryosurgery technique expected by my referring physicians, by my family, and by me was not used. Apparently the tumor was too massive and bloody.

My family's primary memory of the day is that, in the evening, while awaiting my return from the recovery room, they left the hospital for supper and were refused reentry to the hospital by the security guard unless they could prove they were hospital employees. They finally persuaded the guard to contact the nursing unit and, after several minutes of frustration turning to panic and then anger, were finally allowed back into the hospital. (Security guards, telephone operators, admissions clerks, and cashiers are major contributory factors to favorable or unfavorable impressions of hospital care!)

The surgeon's report was "two cups of tumor removed—it's a good thing we went in. . . ." The pathology report apparently revealed good results of the radiation therapy, with only dead and dying tumor cells to be found. Good news.

But now the nightmare really begins.

I have no clear recollection of events from October 17 through about November 10. I do remember beginning to feel strange—"outside myself," I called it. I wondered if I had meningitis. I began having (I know now) some weird, hallucinatory thought content. The following portion of the story is hearsay from my family.

I did have meningitis, which at first wasn't recognized. It was misdiagnosed initially as "a psychotic reaction to his illness." My primary surgeon, by the way, had left the country for a time, leaving residents in training in charge of my case.

Events during this three-week period apparently included the following:

- The meningitis was recognized.
- Intrathecal therapy was necessary, through a cisternal approach. (I remember hallucinating about someone sticking a banana knife in my neck.)
- The neurosurgery service took over my case.
- An operation (the third at Memorial and fourth overall) was performed by a senior neurosurgeon to repair a hole that had been left in my dura.

For most of these three weeks, I was apparently in intensive care, hallucinating loudly much of the time. It's amazing to me that, during the ensuing months, I began to remember some of the hallucinatory content. For example, I recalled thinking that Joan and I had made an agreement: If the report from the "definitive operation" was malignancy after all, or if the operation was to leave me unable to lead a "quality life," then I was to be allowed to die. Somehow, part of my mind believed this is what had happened. There was never any such pact, although Joan and I have discussed, before and since, the possibility of a living will asking each to spare the other the indignities of futile life-support systems.

Two events may have contributed to saving my life:

1. A physician friend from the New York area visited on October 17 or so. Concerned by my appearance, he phoned a friend of his who is on the Memorial medical staff. Apparently this physician set the wheels in motion for accurate diagnosis and vigorous treatment of the meningitis. (So "shortcuts" set in motion by a physician friend played a role after all.)

2. Joan got mad. Prior to the accurate diagnosis, a neurologist was explaining the rationale for the misdiagnosis and Joan disagreed. The way she tells it, "He gave me a superior smirk, and I just couldn't control myself." For whatever reason, that neurologist became a key to my eventual recovery. Before I left the hospital, he presented me to the weekly neurology conference as a case of near-miraculous recovery from a state of coma. (Addendum: Three or four months later, back home, an item in *AMA News* caught my eye. The primary authority being cited in a legal case was the book *The Differential Diagnosis of Coma*, by Jerome Posner, M.D. and another author. Dr. Posner is the neurologist my wife challenged!)

For whatever reasons—probably a combination of effective treatment of the catastrophic complications and personal will—I finally "woke up" and became rational. My family declares that one factor was their insistence, and mine, that my doctors discontinue the drugs I was on. Apparently I expressed *my* objection by ripping out IV after IV.

I found myself weak, emaciated (50-pound weight loss), and completely bedfast. This was the beginning of several weeks of having to learn how to sit up in bed, how to take a few steps using a walker, and how to use the bathroom instead of soiling the bed. In general, a reenactment of the motor development of early infancy.

Finally, I was returned to Chicago, but not yet to my home. I had walked into Memorial Hospital on August 25, 1983. On November 15, 1983, I was carried out of the hospital on a pram, taken by ambulance to the airport, and flown home on a special stretcher arrangement available through at least some airlines. Four first-class seats are bought; the patient and stretcher take up two of the seats, attendants and paraphernalia the other two. Don't try flying this way if you're claustrophobic. But there was no other way. I still could not sit up more than a few minutes at a time.

On arrival at O'Hare, Joan and I were taken by ambulance directly to the hospital, where I was readmitted.

The subsequent two months in the hospital included rehabilitation (God bless physical therapists!) along with painful debridement of a large wound in my back which had refused to heal primarily after the fourth operation. A fifth operation was performed a week before Christmas by a plastic surgeon.

During this convalescent time, my "exercise walks" up and down the halls of the neurosurgery nursing unit took me by a closed door marked Pain Clinic. I was reminded that patients can easily mistake discomfort for pain and addict themselves to analgesics or even narcotics. To this day, I prefer to ignore discomfort rather than taking even a Tylenol or two. No way am I going to become an "impaired physician," hooked on pain-killers and/or alcohol.

I missed Christmas and New Year's at home. but on Saturday, January 7, 1984, I finally came back through the front door of my own home. On two canes, to be sure—but *walking*!

We estimate the total cost of this illness, almost all paid by insurance, to be in the range of $150,000. Of course, that's just the direct cost. No telling how much lost income during the time I was incapacitated. My surgeon's bill was paid promptly, but the insurance company insisted on auditing the pharmacy bill, which alone approximated $15,000. All those tranquilizers, I guess, plus the fact that I was on IV cephalosporin antibiotics for much of my stay in Memorial Hospital.

Gradually my business resumed and I got back on the road. My first speaking engagement after returning home was in January 1984, out in Libertyville, Illinois, only an hour from the house. Joan took me, I spoke sitting down, and I came right back home to bed. By March I was traveling alone again, taking wheelchairs to the airplanes and having rental cars brought around for me, since my quadriceps muscles weren't dependable enough to try those high bus steps. (Later, I learned that some rental car buses hydraulically "kneel" to accommodate elderly or lame individuals. Nice.) Of course, I was completely dependent on the skycaps and airline personnel, both for the wheelchairs and because there was no way I could carry a suitcase. Most skycaps, airline personnel, and fellow passengers were thoughtful. Only a few scurrying people here and there seemed to think, "If you can't move faster, you should stay at home."

At this writing, I've progressed from a light shoulder bag and two canes to only one cane and being able to carry a suitcase.

I don't know how long my mobility will last. Both calves and feet are constantly numb. When I'm tired, the left leg especially feels as though it could just quit moving at any moment. Follow-up CT scans continue to show no recurrence of tumor. I don't know why, but I'm very confident it will not recur. My fear is of getting "sat down" by the residual damage of the original tumor and its treatment. But I have no problems with bowel and bladder control. I have no foot drop. And, yes, erection and ejaculation are back!

I've written this account hoping that those who read it will (a) acknowledge and promptly attend to symptoms, rather than ignoring them (no one is indestructible); (b) attend to the "people needs" of patients and family members; and (c) be aware that physicians who are *disabled* are not necessarily *impaired*.

CHAPTER 38

SEMINOMA OF TESTICLE

HAROLD W. SCHELL

In 1948, at age 25, I developed bilateral mumps orchitis with most involvement on the left. Upon healing, the left testicle was atrophic.

I had been troubled with chronic back pain since the age of 20, but the pain became more bothersome in 1951 while I was serving on active duty as a naval physician at Parris Island, South Carolina. Lying in bed one night, I thought about the causes of back pain. When I came to "tumor–testicle," I discovered a 1.5-cm nodule in my atrophic left testis.

The following morning, the mass was confirmed by the chief of surgery at the U.S. Naval Hospital, Beaufort, South Carolina. Chest X-ray and intravenous pyelogram were normal. The verdict was: "It might be inflammatory; take an antibiotic and return in seven days." I left the hospital, drove a few miles, turned around, and returned to the surgeon and said, "Let's get on with it!"

The next morning, a left orchiectomy and excision of the spermatic cord were carried out under spinal anesthesia. Few words were spoken during the procedure. I became anxious that findings might be unfavorable. Postoperatively, I was told that no enlarged lymph nodes were identified, although one "normal" lymph node was resected from the inguinal canal.

Pathologists at Beaufort Naval Hospital reported, "Tumor of testis, mostly seminoma–Lymph node examination reveals no tumor." The microscopic slides were sent to the U.S. Naval Hospital in Bethesda, Maryland, for review and recommendations for further therapy.

On the scheduled day of discharge, I discovered a ¾-cm subcutaneous nodule in the left scrotum. The surgical chief thought it was a stitch problem, although he could not rule out "fast-growing tumor."

DR. HAROLD SCHELL is a retired superintendent and medical director of Uncas-on-Thames Hospital, the Connecticut State cancer facility.

Back in the operating room the same day, the benign nodule was removed under local anesthesia. I doubt the nodule would have been removed if I had not been a physician. I was discharged later that afternoon. The anesthesia had worn off, and the ride home to Walterboro, 50 miles away, was tough because of intense scrotal pain.

Bethesda Naval pathologists concurred with the diagnosis. The hospital tumor group recommended 250 KV radiation therapy to four anterior abdominal ports and three posterior ports administered over four to five weeks. The dose and port size were outlined in detail. Since the same therapy was available at Beaufort or Bethesda, I elected to remain near home.

The course of radiation therapy was exhausting and uncomfortable. Five days a week, my wife would drive me 50 miles to the hospital for treatment and 50 miles back home. Although I felt well in the morning, each treatment was followed by nausea, vomiting, and anorexia the rest of the day. I lost weight and drank lots of martinis.

The navy pronounced me cured and fit for active duty at the conclusion of radiation therapy, but I was devastated and despondent. No one told me there was a reasonably good chance for survival. I believed I was going to die soon. My wife, eight months pregnant, and our 3-year-old son would be left with little means. I felt I was shirking my duties by dying. Although I laughed a lot, it was hard to do so and was not genuine. I became jealous of my wife, imagining that she was already looking for another. Anger over my illness, the typical "Why me?" was present.

I had been raised as an involved Episcopalian but my teachings seemed somehow insufficient to help me. I needed to strengthen my belief in a higher being so I undertook a three-month study of religions of the world and decided to follow an unorganized faith with a private belief in God. Praying became important and helpful for me. This is still true.

Whether to block out my thoughts or to prove myself, I became more ambitious and was driven to function as well as I possibly could. I earned promotion to lieutenant, USNR, and became chief of the largest infirmary at Parris Island. Discharged from active duty in October 1952 (with my slides, X-ray films, and therapy reports), I returned to private practice in Connecticut. I was depressed and started to worry about the therapy I had received. The fear of dying persisted.

I consulted a local surgeon, a friend, for advice. He had the slides reviewed at the Armed Forces Institute of Pathology, where they agreed with the tumor histology. He then referred me to the chief of urology at Massachusetts General Hospital, who concluded that if a radical retroperitoneal dissection was not done, I would die. I wondered if his recommendation represented possible overtreatment because I was a physician. Several statements he made suggested to me he was running a series. After the visit, he sent me a letter telling me I would die without the operation. This was overwhelming, not only because this type of surgery had never been mentioned but because it reinforced my worst fears. I felt no anger over the situation but I had to face another decision to try to save my life. My local surgeon would not make the decision for me, saying that I would have to make up my own mind. I believe I wanted someone to make the decision for me.

Looking for help, I turned to the director of medical education at a Hartford, Connecticut, hospital. He was a special friend in whom I always had great confidence. The microscopic slides and all my records were reviewed. New chest films and intravenous pyelogram were normal (I developed hives during the second IVP). A meeting was arranged for me with the director of medical education and the chiefs of surgery, urology, radiology, and pathology in attendance. They agreed there was no absolute answer. However, with no evidence or recurrence in 18 months (May 1951–November 1952), they believed it was reasonable to evaluate chest films and IVPs every six months and avoid radical surgery at that time.

The decision, of course, was just what I wanted to hear. The fear of dying lessened somewhat but the nagging worry of what each six months might turn up still concerned me.

The first six-month studies were normal, but I developed generalized urticaria during the third IVP in spite of preprocedure IV antihistamine. Another problem.

At this time, May 1952, the director of medical education had a long talk with me. His advice was straightforward and succinct,. "No more intravenous pyelograms; check a yearly chest film. If symptoms develop, retrograde pyelography would be necessary. *Get along with your life!*" It was obvious to me that this physician was treating my despondence just as much as my resected tumor. His advice was sound—I have had no recurrence in 34 years.

Reflecting on this life experience, I am surprised that I can recall 34-year-old events in such detail. The period was filled with concerns about the other testicle, which had also been involved in the mumps inflammation and had been poorly shielded during radiation therapy. Would a second tumor develop requiring a second orchiectomy? As years went by, there always seemed to be some new occurrence that interfered with a rebound from my depression. I was unable to purchase life insurance until five years postop, and then only at the highest rates. A medical college radiotherapist declared that my radiation treatment had been totally worthless except perhaps to cause damage. Following radiation treatment, daily diarrhea persisted from 1951 to date. The diarrhea was studied with stool cultures, proctoscopy, mucosal biopsy, and small and large bowel X-ray films. All results were normal. My irritable bowel continues irritable. Study at another time concluded that chronic depression was present and proved intractable to antidepressant medication.

In spite of low spirits, increased ambition and drive continued. After a short time in private practice, I went to Boston for a year and completed my residency in internal medicine (1955), passed my boards in internal medicine, became a fellow of the American College of Physicians, and obtained a clinical faculty appointment at a major medical school.

In 1956, I accepted appointment as clinical director at a Connecticut hospital to develop a treatment program for the care of patients with advanced cancer. A state-of-the-art radiation therapy center was established. I instituted and became chief of a cancer chemotherapy clinic and a nuclear medicine department. I have had scientific papers published and worked with the American Cancer Society, getting the chance to teach a lot about cancer. There has been little time for introspection.

I firmly believe my illness and reaction to it contributed greatly to my attitude toward terminally ill patients. My ability to appreciate their concerns and understand their fears, whether expressed or not, helped enormously in management. Doctor-patient rapport seemed easy to establish. This aptitude gave me the opportunity to help a large number of patients and their families. It seems impossible that I involved myself in the care of over 12,000 patients who needed help when they were dying. Helping them has been very rewarding (self-serving?).

My family was not spared pain. In the early years after the illness, it was hard to hide my gloom and preoccupation with hopeless feelings. "How will my family get along?" The home was not often filled with laughter with a despondent dad present.

As the children grew up, they became more distant from me and closer to my wife. After all, it wasn't much fun being around a dispirited dad. I felt lonely and carried the burden of my concerns more or less alone. Prayer helped.

Fear of another pregnancy was a great concern to me. Because shielding of the remaining testicle during radiation therapy had been poor, the possibility of a deformed baby was ever present. As a result, marital sexual relations suffered greatly.

My father informed me and always believed that no one could be a "real" man with loss of half his function. This was a downer and hurt our father–son relationship.

In later years, it has been my lot to develop hypertension, myocardial infarction, diabetes mellitus (80 units insulin daily), severe diabetic neuropathy, and avascular necrosis of one hip.

My irritable bowel and dejection continues. My tumor is gone.

CHAPTER 39

RENAL CARCINOMA

HADLEY L. CONN, JR.

My hospitalization in 1971 taught me several important lessons, the most important of which is the error of being a hospital patient on or shortly after July 1. This date brings a concatenation of circumstances, a new group of interns, vacation time for a significant fraction of the hospital staff and faculty, and the Fourth of July holiday. It is better to beware the first of July than the Ides of March.

In addition, I also learned the danger of the contribution of past experience to an ideation that circumscribes freedom of thought. We emphasize the value of medical history but become susceptible to the mistake of giving it unquestioned primacy.

In late June of 1971, we were preparing for our family holiday on Nantucket scheduled to begin on the first of July. My wife was entertaining some of her college alumnae downstairs while I had sought refuge in a journal while lying in bed upstairs. My attention began to be drawn to an increasingly discomforting pain in my right costovertebral region, with some extension down toward the inguinal area. In a very short period the pain had fixed a message in my brain, renal colic. The danger of fixed ideation in this instance evolved from a similar episode in 1963.

On that earlier date, I was recuperating from one of those routine hospital operations and had celebrated my discharge of the next day by joining a colleague in undue praise to the talents of Bourbon county. When I awakened at 5:00 a.m. on the day of my discharge with classical and most intense pain of renal colic, I first felt a sense of disbelief and then a moment of truth. Hereupon, I learned two other verities about hospital care. First, the nurse did not at that hour respond immediately to my several insistent pulls on the bell cord. Pain and an-

DR. HADLEY CONN is a 65-year-old professor of medicine, chairman of medicine emeritus, and director of the Cardiovascular Institute at the Robert Wood Johnson School of Medicine. At the time of the events described, he was a professor of medicine at the University of Pennsylvania School of Medicine.

noyance became partners. When the nurse arrived and saw my plight she immediately returned with a sphygmomanometer and stethoscope, determined to take my pulse and blood pressure in spite of my insistent demands to call the surgical resident. She then alienated me further by insisting that I stop rolling around in the bed since she could not take my blood pressure or feel my pulse under those circumstances. I assure you doctors act just like other patients at this time, maybe worse since they have more insight. I have thought a lot about how to resolve this failure to communicate. There may not be an acceptable resolution to this "noise" in the communication system.

After what seemed to me a very long time, the resident appeared and administered an injection of morphine, for which I was exceedingly grateful. Both the pain of renal colic and its relief are dramatic events as experienced by the patient. The pain disappeared rather quickly and an emergency urogram performed on that Saturday morning showed no evidence of abnormality. My departure was not delayed. My surgeon was dubious about my version of the whole episode, at least until the following Monday, when the laboratory reported red cells in the Saturday urine specimen. Nevertheless, my mind was firmly imprinted with respect to the pain and its apparent etiology in my case.

Between 1963 and 1971 my health care was modified by institution of an antihypertensive regimen which resulted in slightly symptomatic hyperuricema as a consequence of the diuretic drug effects. Consequently, a uricosuric agent, Benemid, was added, further projecting a focus on the possibility of uric acid-induced renal colic. Zyloprim (Allopurinol) came later.

Back to the bedroom scene of 1971. The pain became worse although not unbearable. Remembering the virtues of hot water, I then took a very hot shower with minimal improvement, and a hot bath with similar outcome. A mental review of available narcotic agents turned up only one APC with codeine, quickly devoured. After an hour it was nearly midnight with little or no relief. Then began a call to nearby academic friends who, it turned out, likewise kept no narcotics at home. Another lesson: Keep at least two morphine tablets in injectable form in your medical bag even if you don't plan an active ambulatory practice.

Somehow I managed to agonize through the night until about 5:00 a.m., when I called a local physician acquaintance who happened to be the father of my son's current girlfriend. This engendered enough leverage so that he arrived somewhat reluctantly on a Saturday morning, July 1, at 7:00 to give me an injection of morphine. Given my 1963 experience, I confidently expected to have the entire episode behind me in a few hours. My hopes were at first fulfilled, relief of pain and the subsequent associated feeling of well-being. This lasted regrettably only a few hours. Now I was faced with the Saturday evening of July 1, of which I fortunately retain little memory.

By very early Sunday morning, I realized all was not as expected. Rather I was in such agony that I called another friend, chief of medicine at our local community hospital, and asked if he could arrange for me to have an injection of morphine in the emergency room in transit to our university hospital. I also called the latter to indicate that I was coming to the emergency room with a urologic problem. The modest bouncing of the car on the way to the community hospital produced some of the most severe agonizing pain that I have ever had. I soon learned another sobering lesson. The nurse on call would not give an injection of morphine until the doctor in question personally showed up in the emergency room and wrote an order for the medication. I was told to remain quiet, 1963 all over again, and be patient. Both were impossible. After another agonizing hour the doctor arrived and I was given an injection to prepare me for the 15-mile trip. From the outset this too was complete torture, and I would like to be able to offer some advice as to how to make ambulance trips under these circumstances more bearable.

Once in the university emergency room, I was on familiar ground and was recognized as someone to be believed rather than suspect as a possible malingerer or morphine addict. Pity the suspected one who has to wait still longer. Adequate narcotic was given and my only memory is being told that it would be necessary to perform a retrograde urogram. Following that I vaguely remember being told that it would be necessary to admit me to the hospital. This was Sunday, July 2.

What I did not know was that I had a large clot obstructing my right renal pelvis and that the force of the dye injection had perforated my ureter and extravasated the dye outside it. Even my doctors knew only the latter. So the doctor as patient seems particularly susceptible to the unexpected complications. Further verification of this axiom came from subsequent hypersensitivity and finally an outright anaphylactoid reaction to postoperative urograms.

What I hadn't been told was that the failure to visualize the renal pelvis was interpretated as a probable pelvic tumor, and that the chief of the service was away over the long holiday weekend, which was to include Monday and Tuesday, July 3 and 4. No one apparently gave much thought to the alleviation of my pain during this period, and order-writing and related decisions were delegated to the new intern with one day's experience. No doubt it was wise to withhold the proposed diagnosis from me but the arrangements for pain control were disastrous. Very shortly I became aware that the morphine dose (I never learned the amount) relieved my pain for only about 2 to 2 1/2 hours, after which I was urged by the nurse to take hot baths, or just "tough it out." All medical students have been taught to write for a given dose of morphine every four hours, or at greater intervals if possible. There seems to have been little or no discussion of the well-known fact that in many individuals the rate of metabolism is such that pain relief lasts three hours or less. Since 1971, I've been trying to promulgate this message widely without evident success. In any event, the nurse proved unsympathetic, so I asked to speak to the intern. Being new, he was overwhelmed by his duties and made an appearance after a few hours, promising that he would speak to the senior resident. The latter was taking calls from home and the intern apparently didn't consider this issue important enough to disturb him at home. My personal attempts to use the telephone in my room turned up the disconcerting fact that the assistant chief of the service and the chief of the service were enjoying the long July fourth vacation out of town and were unreachable by phone, or at least I was so informed. For the remainder of Sunday, Monday, and Tuesday, I dealt with the pain rather like a primeval animal full of distress, annoyance, and hostility, which endeared me to no one and didn't change any order on my chart. Even my suggestion that the narcotic dose be halved but given twice as often struck an unresponsive chord. If you haven't had renal colic for four or five days, you can't fully appreciate this paragraph.

It came as a great sense of relief to have my good and cherished friend, the chief of the service, finally appear on Wednesday morning and announce that I would shortly be taken to the operating room. Normally this would have resulted in a sense of anxiety and perhaps a flurry of questions. But now I was simply grateful that the matter of the pain was going to be resolved.

My next recollection was being back in my room with tubes attached to several orifices. The most restrictive and annoying one came out of what I presumed was a large hole in my back. However, an unbelievable sense of satisfaction came from the relief of the pain and from the fact that my wife and one of my patients, an internationally known portrait painter, were holding my hand and asking solicitious questions and giving great reassurance. It certainly was a sense of exceptional pleasure to have a world-famous man come to the recovery bed and to spend the afternoon with me simply because I was his friend and his doctor.

Thereafter, special-duty nurses were demanding this and that. The pulmonary therapist was demanding that I blow harder and harder into his bottle even if it resulted in ejecting my kidney through the massive wound that I perceived as extending from near my spine to near my inguinal area. There was no rest for the weary during the next

24 hours. I still haven't figured out whether these ministrations are necessary to recovery or whether it would be better to allow one to rest and to recover his strength. In my case, after more than four days of severe, almost relentless pain I certainly wanted to opt for the latter choice. But it was against the rules.

The next day brought me some unexpected news that was definitely memorable. The context of its delivery demonstrated still another problem in communication with patients. The assistant chief of the urology service very abruptly informed me that he and the clinical pathologist had looked at the sections of the material removed from my renal pelvis and a diagnosis of transitional cell carcinoma had been made. Therefore, he was planning to have me return to the operating room on the following day for a nephrectomy. Under most circumstances my response to this declaration would have been one of disbelief, alarm, and anxiety. My overriding feeling was one of exhaustion, so I could only mutter that I really didn't think I had the strength to have an operation the following day and that I would like to have the chief come to my room and discuss options with me.

The assistant chief always looked stern and businesslike, whereas the chief nearly always had a smile and a reassuring manner. Both were well known and highly talented academicians, but I always have preferred a smiling face and a little reassurance. Shortly thereafter, the chief appeared and said the material removed was principally a huge blood clot obstructing my renal pelvis, and only one small section had shown cells possibly indicating a tumor, and that he felt it would be wise to postpone any operation until further review of the histologic sections had been carried out. Naturally, this was an opinion with much greater appeal and a recommendation with which I readily agreed.

The rest of my hospital stay was for the most part uneventful, only to be terminated by an event that again proves the axiom that doctors as patients seem to get more than the usual complications. With the catheters removed the only worry was the basic cause of my problem, and a promise was exacted that I could leave the hospital ten days after the operation. On the afternoon of the ninth day I suddenly felt exceedingly flushed, I had a headache, and my temperature was found to be approximately 41°C. While a urine culture was obtained, I was told that if I felt well enough I could still depart the following morning. By discharge time I wanted to leave, although the urine culture was positive for *Pseudomonas*. At that time most of the effective drugs required intravenous administration, although one with greater potential toxicity could be given intramuscularly at home.

So home I went. My next-door physician-neighbor agreed to give me injections of the prescribed antibiotic. I immediately learned firsthand that this antibiotic causes extreme pain at the site of injection for several hours. After two or three days I was sure that the cure was worse than the disease. Only a few months later did I learn that my audioacuity for frequencies above 12,000 was nearly nil. Whether this was caused by the medication will remain a mystery. Certainly dogs will never get any sympathy from me about the pain or discomfort of high-frequency noises.

This stage of my illness could be characterized by relative euphoria in spite of the possibility of a dire prognosis. Anyone who hasn't been through four or five days of relentless pain, an operation, and a series of complications in association with diagnosis and therapy will probably not be able to appreciate the unbelievably happy feeling of returning to his preillness state. It is no wonder evolution gave us adrenal glands and CNS opioids to withstand tortures of this extended nature.

Whatever the ultimate histologic diagnosis, my mind had vigorously fixed on a resolve for a new awareness and appreciation of different aspects of the world. Up to the age of 50, my behavior had been a dedication to successive goals related to better teaching, better education, better patient care, academic advancement, and publication, combined with the desire to raise and educate in an elitist way a growing family of five children. Many of my wife's friends told me how little my life seemed dedicated to her happiness and satisfaction. Now I came to a different view of life, one that has been expressed in various ways by others upon learning that their life was likely to be significantly shortened as a result of a life-threatening illness. I promised myself that I would emphasize the smaller details of life, "to smell the roses," to enjoy vacations with my wife, and to stop believing that my actions would have a dramatic influence on the outcome of the world.

Some 14 years later, I'm still a strong adherent of this philosophy. It does seem, however, that as the sense of imminent demise recedes, one is in danger of recidivistic behavior. Much more conscious effort must be made to remind one of these valuable resolutions. It's probably not wise, on balance, to have a life-threatening illness every few years, but it almost certainly would lead us to a heightened awareness of our mortality and a greater determination to behave in a more charitable manner and take a much broader view of what is important.

The end of this tale is a little anticlimactic but predictable by those pathologists who frequently report on isolated, small pieces of human tissue. The Armed Forces Institute of Pathology confirmed the original diagnosis, with a diagnosis of Grade I transitional cell carcinoma. The chairman of pathology at one of our most renowned institutions compromised. He gave a histologic description compatible with transitional cell carcinoma, but concluded that the actual diagnosis and most definitely the management should be determined by the clinicians. The third consultant, a pathologist in New York City with wide experience in examining genitourinary tumors in dye workers, concluded, "I don't really know what the diagnosis is but I am convinced it is not a malignant neoplasm." The consequent uncertainties are faced each year by thousands of patients with a similar diagnostic conclusion—a familiar example being the patient given a diagnosis of carcinoma *in situ* in a colon polyp. Realism and denial in proper proportions are probably the ideal emotional response, however reached. It certainly helps to have a sympathetic and optimistic physician who nevertheless insists on the necessary follow-up studies without creating undue anxiety or financial burden. Fortunately, I had such a physician. Each passing year brings a greater level of confidence that this problem has been successfully dealt with and that the cause of my demise will come from some other source.

If this kind of unexpected and traumatic experience can significantly increase the level of humility and sense of greater humanity in a physician, the experience is probably salutory. Great physicians have said that the perfect physician would have experienced all the various disease entities known to man in order to understand them appropriately. The axiom has undoubtedly a tongue-in-cheek aspect. However, one hospitalization for a serious illness enhanced by a few unexpected complications, a firsthand experience of the foibles of nurses and house officers, and the relative inflexibility of hospital regulations provide a remarkable number of new and useful insights. Good judgment and wisdom can come from an appreciation of the dubious and even erroneous judgments of others as well as those one makes himself.

PART VI

CHRONIC DISEASES

CHAPTER 40

CHRONIC RENAL FAILURE AND HEMODIALYSIS

A. PETER LUNDIN

I am a nephrologist who is also a 20-year veteran of hemodialysis. I was a patient before I was a doctor. I am comfortable with both roles, and each has taught me ways to augment the other. Having a chronic illness has offered me a number of advantages in my medical practice. It has helped me to understand the thinking processes and motivations, fears and concerns of being a patient. I have learned to combine the patient's insights with the knowledge and technical skills of a physician. Being a patient has taught me to modify my approach to diagnosis and treatment of diseases in ways that stress prevention and minimize harm. Most important for the person with health problems is regaining some predictability in living. That is not possible with every illness, but it is certainly true for many of us who rely on hemodialysis to stay alive.

In the normal course of things, I should have been dead years ago. I was unlucky to have renal failure but lucky enough to have contracted uremia as the science of treating it was turning a corner. Twenty-two years ago none of my doctors expected me to survive more than a short time. Indeed, my escape back into life was a close one.

When I was only 19, our family doctor found protein in my urine. Further testing revealed that I had only one functional kidney and its function was less than half normal because of chronic glomerulonephritis. My family was informed, but since there was no medical treatment for my problem, they decided to keep me in the dark. As it turned out, this decision was fortunate since I continued planning for my future as if I had one. I hoped, in fact, to become a physician.

DR. A. PETER LUNDIN is 42 years old and is a practicing nephrologist in Brooklyn, New York. He is an associate professor of medicine at the State University of New York Health Science Center at Brooklyn. His primary interest is in caring for patients with chronic renal failure and those on hemodialysis.

Within a year or two of diagnosis I was getting up at night once or twice to urinate, and I had difficulty keeping up with friends physically. I could no longer play intramural basketball because of sheer exhaustion. By late fall of 1965, I was unable to climb a flight of stairs without resting to regain my breath. All this time I never sought answers about how I was feeling. Obviously, I was handling my symptoms with a lot of denial. I must have realized innately that something was terribly wrong but could not deal with it on a conscious level.

My most vivid memory of the days when I was "merely" a patient is of the renal clinic that I attended regularly at a nearby university medical center. There my blood pressures and weight would be dutifully recorded, and on each visit I would be seen by a different medical student (I assumed they were doctors) who always asked the same questions and was given the same answers. I even learned to provide answers for questions the current "doctor" had forgotten to ask. A physical exam followed, and then the clinic was over. The clinic always interfered with my classes, in particular a difficult lab which was hard to make up. I look back on that experience with annoyance for the considerable inconvenience it caused me with no apparent benefit. My clinic visits helped my family keep up-to-date on my deteriorating status, and I provided grist for the university's academic mill. But, for myself, I don't recall ever receiving any helpful advice or even information about my symptoms.

To my family and doctors, who knew the truth, school was only a means of occupying my mind and keeping my attention away from my failing health. My education seemed unimportant to them, but not to me. I was sustained only by goals, whatever their futility. The annoyance I still feel has taught me, indeed compels me, to respect all the patients' other needs in relation to the service I render them. I find it helpful to remember irksome events of my experience in order to avoid acting similarly toward others.

By early 1966, my mornings began with episodes of nausea and vomiting, and at night I was sleeping in a chair because I couldn't lie down without gasping for air. The straight A's I earned at midterm became B's by the finals. I could no longer go on and was admitted to the hospital, where a low-protein, salt-restricted diet led to remarkable improvement of my symptoms, but this was only temporary. The doctors felt that there was nothing else they could do for me. I had a terminal illness that was nearing its end. I might have been saved by a kidney transplant if I had had a suitable related donor, but I did not. At the time, the hospital did not do cadaveric transplants, and hemodialysis was available only to those awaiting a transplant. I vividly recall the sad look that came over the face of my intern when, asking why I was reading an organic chemistry textbook, he learned that I was preparing for the next quarter of premed. I think of him sometimes and wish he could know the results of all that studying.

Although there was little my physicians could do, my family sought alternatives. My father learned of an experimental maintenance hemodialysis program at the University of Washington in Seattle. Those were the days before dialysis was government-supported, and community-supported dialysis such as that in Seattle could be available only to a few worthy citizens. There were criteria for acceptance to the program. Being young, single, and unemployed, without family or social responsibilities, I did not meet many of them and, under usual circumstances, would not have been considered for acceptance even if I had been a Seattle resident. The University of Washington had, however, a program of remote home hemodialysis, and I was most fortunate to be accepted. My family was determined that I should have this opportunity, however uncertain my future. My father was willing and, fortunately, able to meet this considerable expense. I began hemodialysis in March 1966. Interestingly, to this day I remain unaware of most of the circumstances surrounding my entry into the Seattle program. Although most participants in the decision are still alive, I have never sought to clarify the events, perhaps because they are in some way too painful to relive.

After three months of training in home hemodialysis, I returned to home and school. I now encountered the most frustrating time of my life—the attempt to enter medical school. I had suitable grades, test scores, and recommendations for acceptance, but they were insufficient to overcome my being on hemodialysis. At that time, hemodialysis was considered by most physicians to be of only temporary benefit, and medical schools wanted candidates who would live long enough to justify the time and expense of training. I understand this intellectually, but emotionally I was devastated then and remain resentful even today. My goals and plans for the future, so necessary to keep me going, had come up against a stone wall. I had believed that most of life's obstacles I had faced until then were surmountable with a little extra effort, but the medical schools had refused to give me a chance. I truly believe that I would not be alive today if I had not been finally accepted at the Downstate Medical Center, whose head of nephrology had the courage and influence necessary to get me admitted. I now had the chance to prove myself and justify the faith this man had shown in me. I graduated *summa cum laude,* and in the eight years of medical school, internship, residency, and fellowship, kidney problems kept me out sick for only two weeks.

My transition from patient near death to dialysis patient to nephrologist with a medical problem (my choice of specialty should be understandable) has affected me profoundly, especially in my views toward life and living. Life has become exceptionally precious to me, and as the commercial says, "You only go around once." I know that kidney failure will shorten my life, but I want as long and as healthy a life as possible. That is what anyone wants. To accomplish this, a wise patient needs to seek out a competent and trustworthy physician.

I doubt I am an easy patient to care for—doctors seldom are, perhaps because we know too much, or think we do. I want a doctor who can put up with my foibles, listen to my symptoms, and make an objective decision. There are many doctors whom I admire but who may find me intimidating. A doctor caring for another physician may become self-conscious or fearful of being criticized for making an error. In the area of dialysis, while I would listen to the advice of someone I trusted, I think that over the past few years I have given myself the best advice. Should I develop nonrenal medical problems, however, I want a doctor to whom I can give total decision-making control.

A question I am sometimes asked (and which I sometimes have trouble with) is: How does one find a doctor to trust? My own choice is for an intelligent doctor who keeps up with the latest knowledge in his field, who pays attention to his patients when they speak and understands their needs, and who, if the cause of the problem is not obvious, will pursue the right explanation with bulldog tenacity. I want no doctor who shoots from the hip, who uses expediency or acts before having sufficient knowledge of the problem.

In short, my ideal doctor is careful, compassionate, and clearly attentive to the primary medical principle: "First, do no harm." Note: This essential advice to physicians is not "Find a cure" or "Save lives." These are admirable and desirable goals, but they may not be in the patient's best interest. We all know of patients who have come to grief because the physician has felt that he or she must do *something*. I am not speaking here of genuine life-or-death situations. Obviously, almost any risk is worth taking to save a life. I see among some of my colleagues, however, the urge at times to aggressively seek an answer or diagnosis regardless of its benefits or risk to the individual patient.

Before my illness I wished to be a surgeon, admiring their ability in cutting to the heart of the matter, achieving quick, frequently curative solutions to medical problems. I still admire this ability but am now aware that not everything can be cut out, or even cut into. My life has not been prolonged by short, swift, or incisive methods but by careful attention to my hemodialysis and cautious assessment of what might be happening to me. *First, do no harm.* The cornerstone of my survival has been my awareness of the necessity of first looking at the disadvantages of any treatment, medication, or regimen modification. A good scientist knows that a theory must hold up under testing, so he will look for its weak points. Negative scrutiny is essential since a medical hypothesis can never be proven, only disproven. Efficacious treatments can withstand every attempt to prove them false. Just so should a physician look at everything a treatment might do to a patient, the bad along with the good, and decide if the benefits outweigh the risks. I have tried with my own patients to use this technique that I use on myself.

My approach to long survival on dialysis has taught me a more cautious practice of medicine. Being on the receiving end of discomfort, inconvenience, pain, and even danger has made me think very carefully before inflicting procedures and tests on my own patients. I myself have undergone several cystoscopies, a cardiac catheterization, and liver and bone biopsies. Some were for diagnostic purposes; others, like the cardiac cath, were for research. At the time I agreed to them, I thought it was my duty as a patient to cooperate in research. I no longer think, however, that patients should participate in research that is potentially fatal. I find I can ask patients to submit to tests for research purposes only when I am willing to undergo the same ones myself. Invasive procedures for diagnostic purposes must fulfill the strict requirement of providing answers beneficial to the patient, not just for intellectual satisfaction for the physician. I can never forget patients who suffer harm, no matter how transitory, as a result of an unnecessary medical event or physician recommendation. Consequently, I take action only when diagnosis or treatment is essential.

I have learned to balance risks and benefits in everything I do for my health. The patient in me strives for a long, uncomplicated life. The physician looks for the best ways of avoiding problems. It is this balancing act that has led me to postpone getting a kidney transplant, which, to the uninitiated, should be the answer to all my health problems. The layperson (and, I am afraid, some doctors) sees transplants as safe, sure, and lifesaving; I know that they are not necessarily any of these things. True, a transplant would give me a much higher quality of life if it works and is uncomplicated. But one can also be worse for the experience. A failed transplant can be debilitating and even fatal. Right now dialysis represents to me surety, predictability, and a life within whose boundaries I can cope. I have not yet been willing to trade it for the wild card of a transplant. Oddly enough, many of my fellow patients see the logic of this much more than do many doctors, who cannot understand not going for a "cure."

As a patient, I have become aware of certain realities which I apply in being a doctor. While the healthy person tends to suffer through minor ailments with a minimum of fuss, the chronically ill have a tendency to give significance to almost every new bodily discomfort and pay them more attention than they may deserve. The physician to the chronically ill must maintain a high index of suspicion, refusing to dismiss complaints as imaginary lest he or she miss the first indication of a potentially serious complication and recurrent chronic symptoms. For minor problems, my advice and personal practice is to give it a day or two, and if the symptoms resolve, then there is probably nothing seriously wrong. It is important, though, to assure the patient of your alertness and concern. Caring for the chronically ill is often a difficult and trying task and, thus, unpleasant to many doctors. Dealing with these patients requires patience and sustained concern.

What I have gained most from being a patient is the ability to feel extremely comfortable with other patients, particularly those with a similar problem. We share an experience. They feel confident that when I say I understand what they are going through, they know it to be true. I am most relaxed speaking at their meetings about commonly shared problems. I am not put off when they are angry or depressed over what has happened to them. They are facing one of life's major traumas and are entitled to react accordingly. I have learned patience and understanding and have found myself willing to go the extra distance with the angry or noncompliant patient. The sick, hurting patient is entitled at times to be rude or angry dealing with medical professionals; the physician and the nurse are not. At times this is difficult. A normal reaction is to give back in kind. Understandably, one gets angry at the noncompliant patients who appear to be harming themselves despite the doctor's best efforts at advising or prescribing. I have learned, however, that patients never interpret this anger as a sign of the doctor's caring about them; quite the opposite is true. In most circumstances, being honest and straightforward with any patient and giving the sincere impression that you care will win them over. Sympathetic persistence on the doctor's part is often rewarded.

Not all patients like my style or the fact that I urge independence on my patients. I do not see dialysis as the end of life but as an opportunity to go on living. Being on dialysis *per se* need not make one disabled in the absence of other disabling conditions. The angry patient with renal failure who cannot adapt to the new circumstances of his life may reject me because I apparently do well where he feels he cannot. Other patients may prefer to remain totally dependent on the doctor for every medical decision or see being on dialysis as an opportunity to live off the system. Dependence on the physician or entitlements is useful when health problems are new and acute or become serious and when disabilities are real. But daily dietary decisions and taking of medication necessary to control high glucose levels and high blood pressure, or to prevent renal osteodystrophy, can best be carried out successfully by the knowledgeable patient. Getting back into the normal swing of life as far as possible is the best tonic for a chronic illness. In my opinion, only those patients who are able to manage chronic health abnormalities and the circumstances of a chronic illness requiring frequent adjustment can expect to minimize complications. Their survival depends on it. It is also apparent to me that the self-interest of a physician who deals with chronic patients lies in having it so. Patients who have neither the desire nor the intelligence to care for themselves require a great deal of constant attention if they are to do well. The alternative is to ignore them and their problems with the expected consequences. The busy physician cannot have time to attend to every patient's needs if much of his time is taken up by a few dependent patients with many or frequent complaints.

Like the dying individuals that they are, patients with renal failure need to go through several stages of adaptation before they come to an an acceptance of their fate. Unlike other dying patients, those with renal failure must adapt to a continued but substantially altered life. Depression, anger, bargaining, and denial come at different times and in different degrees to each patient. I wasn't told that I was dying, but my body must have sensed the fact of it. Denial was so overwhelming a defense for me that I don't recall experiencing depression, anger, or bargaining. Depression would have been a normal first response, but I remember the hospital days filled with conversations with patients who shared my room and time spent cheering up others with their problems. I don't recall being angry, thinking only of getting back to school and of the future. Depression and anger set in when my future seemed denied. The stages I missed I can see in my patients: depression on learning of kidney disease and later anger at the imposed restrictions and new circumstances of life. Anger may be directed at self, family, friends, or the doctors and nurses. I have learned that these stages are normal and not to be taken personally. In some ways, dialysis patients may be among the angriest of those with chronic illness. As their depression begins to resolve, they learn that dialysis can sustain their lives, yet this is the time they find themselves most dependent on the decisions of doctors and nurses. This is when the anger may manifest itself, often as noncompliance to diet, medications, and treatment regimens. To some degree I bypassed this anger of dependency because I went directly into a home training program where great independence from the medical staff was taught as a necessity. I do remember being angry when my doctor doubted that I was adhering to my diet because I was gaining more weight than prescribed. I recall the diet of those days as being the most protein- and sodium-restricted in my 20 years on dialysis. As it turned out, the gain was due to high levels of sodium in my dialysis solution, elevated as a consequence of the use of water softeners exchanging sodium for the high levels of calcium in our water. Investigation before accusation would have divined the causes of my difficulties.

This early stage of anger comes as the individual struggles to get back in control. Many dialysis patients find themselves in the position where control is almost totally in the hands of doctors and nurses and the only choices for independence are self-dialysis or getting a kidney transplant. Some patients also use noncompliance as a way of getting control, however detrimental to themselves it may seem. I have come to believe, however, that noncompliance is not the intention of a patient to harm himself but more likely due to a communication problem between himself and the doctor. In my own experience, for example, one of the first things I learned as a dialysis patient was that aluminum-containing phosphate binders are very constipating, but my doctor never got through to me why it was necessary to take them. So, not surprisingly, I didn't, and paid for it with a parathyroidectomy. Communication is not simply talking at another person, as not all health professionals realize.

Those patients who are taught or learn on their own to be independent with their dialysis usually resolve their anger. Such patients gain considerable knowledge in the management of their illness, and with time, they usually become interested in the politics and economics of renal health care delivery. Precisely for the purpose of gaining political influence, the National Association of Patients on Hemodialysis and Transplantation (NAPHT) was founded by patients in the late 1960s. It arose out of another level of patient anger seen almost exclusively in those with a stable chronic illness like renal failure. It is an organization whose purpose I empathize with wholeheartedly. It arose because something in the relationship between dialysis patients and caregivers was lacking. The interaction often seemed adversarial in nature. Many doctors are uncomfortable with patients who seem to know or want too much. The priesthood does not easily share its hard-earned knowledge with outsiders. Decision making in medicine represents power, and power determines economics. The economics of dialysis has become a most particular sore point between nephrologists and their patients, weakening the doctor–patient relationship. The delivery of dialysis is providing one of the models for proprietary medicine, and the anger seen in stable, well-dialyzed patients is not the anger of concern over health but the anger of injustice.

For me, standing astride both sides of the struggle, there may appear to be some risk of contradiction, but I feel I have avoided it. As a patient I have gained considerable knowledge of politics and economics and am often dismayed that many nephrologists appear to be more interested in retaining economic and political control than in issues of patient welfare such as quality care. As a physician I am happy to share control with my patients. I have come to realize that a knowledgeable participating patient is, in reality, the easiest one to care for. In successive stages of the patient's health care, I see myself as diagnosing, supporting, educating, advising, and assisting as they grow in knowledge and skill. It seems in my interest to do this if I wish to reduce the anxiety that comes with caring for those who require frequent attention. I would like to run a dialysis unit where the most self-maintained of dialysis patients are satisfied with the care.

All is not a bed of roses, however, since there are many patients who are unable to come to grips with their medical problems and the circumstances of their continued survival. They lack the insight to see the benefits to themselves of more independence, or they may be lacking in frustration tolerance. People with borderline personalities can get renal failure. Although these patients cannot follow my example or live up to my idea of an independent, cooperative patient, I have found within myself a degree of patience and tenderness dealing with them that I would never have developed had we not shared an illness. At the same time, I can empathize with physicians who have difficulty with such patients. Caring for patients who cannot resolve their depression or early stage of anger, who complain nonspecifically or chronically, or who fail to give a precise history of their symptoms can be an exhausting experience. A successful outcome with even these patients is a challenge that, I am happy to say, I retain the stamina to accept.

Hemodialysis has given me 20 years so far, and who knows how many more. I may even take a chance on that transplant one day. For the first ten years or so, my nose was mostly to the grindstone. My wife has encouraged me since then to stop and smell the flowers a bit. Dialysis can be a grind at times, but life is worth putting up with a great deal for. As a physician and as a human being, I hope that I never stop growing.

CHAPTER 41

DIABETES MELLITUS AND COMPLICATIONS OF PREGNANCY

"GWENDOLYN AUSTEN"

I seem to have been on the receiving end of medical care quite frequently, with time to reflect on the varied experiences. In general, I feel I have gained better insight and empathy in caring for others. I also feel that some doctors and other professionals are far more considerate to their colleagues than others.

I am a full-time consultant psychiatrist responsible for services to the elderly mentally ill. I am married with a small baby. I have lived with a chronic illness, diabetes mellitus Type I, for 30 years. It has taken much thought to say "lived with" rather than "suffered from"! I developed fulminating toxaemia at 27 weeks in my first pregnancy, which was terminated therapeutically in the interests of my health. In the subsequent pregnancy I threatened miscarriage from 20 weeks but delivered vaginally a live baby girl weighing only 750 g at 26 weeks. This was quite an achievement for an elderly diabetic mother and much more successful than would have been predicted.

DIABETES MELLITUS

Both my parents were doctors and had recognised the symptoms when I was 6. I had recovered from a fractured humerus but looked a thin, miserable child as recorded on family ciné films. In the early days I was on a "free" diet and insulin. In retrospect, this must have been a very haphazard arrangement and must have engendered great anxiety in my parents about my intake. One minor experience at a checkup that sticks in my mind as lack of sensitivity on the part of the staff was being sent along a corridor with a jar to pass a specimen and having to

"DR. GWENDOLYN AUSTEN" is a 36-year-old practicing full-time general psychiatrist with a special interest in the elderly mentally ill, working within the National Health Service in a small university town in England.

run the gauntlet of all the other waiting patients. This seemed humiliating to a young girl, and I refused to do it. It made me very sensitive to this aspect of care. I suspect most people endure this embarrassment. I was not taught how to look after myself until I was 12 and now think it is much better for children to learn early how to inject and regulate their diets. It makes them much more independent. At the stage when all young girls feel they need to diet, I was on a fairly large carbohydrate intake. I asked the consultant if I could reduce this, but he failed to see the psychological importance of the request and more or less told me not to be so silly. He could have saved a lot of problems if he had compromised, since I would not have done anything drastic, but instead that was the start of my subterfuge. From then I had one diet and insulin regime that I stuck to and another for the clinic appointment. Since I have qualified and understand a bit more of the psyche of the diabetologists from a medical point of view, I have been able to say when I am being driven into lying and to make them accept me as I am.

I have thought a lot about the normality aspect. On the one hand, we diabetics are urged to believe ourselves normal and to lead a normal life, but on the other hand, the restrictions imposed in order to do this are far from normal and, since these restrictions are permanent, it is very difficult to see oneself as normal. Because of the widespread fear of others, one is often avoided or at the very least, treated circumspectly and left in no doubt that one is abnormal. Public education has improved this to a great extent, but this does not always reach teachers, potential boyfriends or girlfriends, mothers of friends, and potential employers. At one time under the English employment laws, diabetics, however fit, were encouraged to register as disabled and to apply for the small proportion of jobs reserved for the disabled. Many were too proud to do this to get a job. It would have done nothing for morale to have considered myself disabled. For many years I, like many diabetics, tried to hide from people that I was diabetic. I feel that those who do not hide their illnesses probably enjoy ill health and make the most of it. I think, in developing relationships, it is understandable that one should want to be accepted without imposing conditions from the start. I can understand the concern if no one knew and I were to collapse, but if they do know they become anxious and overconcerned. For me, it goes against the grain to play up any ill health, and I have often deliberately continued what I was doing whilst going hypo rather than tell anyone. One gets to know one's limits, and I would tell someone if I knew I was reaching that limit.

I have experienced the whole range of insulins over the years: pork, beef, and human; soluble, isophane, and protamine zinc; twice- and thrice-daily injections and the continuous infusion pump. They all lead to insulin tumours fairly quickly, despite attempts to find insulin so refined that this does not happen. Because of the anaesthetic effect after repeated injection into the same site, any diabetic who follows the physician's advice to rotate sites must be either extremely obsessional or masochistic! I think the same applies to the diaries of blood sugar or urine tests done, perhaps four times a day, day in day out, week in week out, and year in year out. But then I have difficulty in remembering to log my mileage, and I should be equally motivated to do that. I used the continuous infusion pump during and after pregnancy. It certainly gives better control, but I do not think it is as marvellous as it is made out. Because it uses soluble insulin, any faults lead to more rapid changes in control so one has to be vigilant day and night. On occasions when I have not been able to correct a severe hypo through the night, I have been driven to pull the whole thing out. This is certainly not advisable but at least it gave me peace of mind for a while. This is rapidly followed by ketosis, which then has to be corrected. I did not find the pump satisfactory with the demanding job I do. The body image aspect is important. Although the pump is smaller now, it is attached night and day and can make sex a farce unless it is removed every time. Swimming, showers, and buying clothes become complicated. The pumps are highly technical but have basic weaknesses. The bottle can break. The cannula often separates from the pump with the stresses and strains on clothing. The cannulae break very easily and, amazingly, the cat once affectionately bit through one while sitting on my knee!

I have endured many and varied diabetologists, and my overall impression is that few of them are normal human beings. They seem to be obsessional and geared to treating glucose- and insulin-processing machines rather than people. There are big personality differences between them and many of their patients, as there are in most branches of medicine. Obsessionals are selected into medicine, but many patients cannot follow the same principles in life such as perseverance and delaying gratification (in diabetics this is presumably a longer life). Physicians often cannot accept what many patients feel; i.e., a lengthy neurotically preoccupied life is not as worthwhile as making the most of the present. To be fair, the high expectations of the physician do to a certain extent help to improve control, but the higher the expectations, the less likely the patient is to bother to try and achieve them. I have seen this so often in clinics—the fiddling of the records. On and off over the years I have been involved with children's camps and young diabetic groups, and it is noticeable that to a certain extent, attitudes are dictated by the expectations of the doctor but not always in the right direction. As an example of this, when I was struggling to achieve good control during my pregnancy and had done my utmost,

I was told that it was not good enough and I was heading for disaster. This was the final straw. I said that I did not wish to return as often, as my morale would suffer, but this was refused so I just rang back later and cancelled the next appointment. It never seemed to be good enough, and I had reached my limit. How often do patients default because we leave them no other way out? I find patronising doctors the most offensive—those who treat their adult patients as irritating, naughty children. The ability to listen and empathise pays dividends not only in the wish to improve one's control but also in the willingness to attend appointments. A sensitivity to the dynamics of the situation and all the cues during the interview needs to be taught to all aspiring diabetologists or, indeed, to all aspiring doctors. I find it offensive for someone to imply that he or she knows it all because he has experienced a deliberate hypo in laboratory conditions with all the safety and security that entails! Hypos come in many forms, but the environmental context is particularly important. Yet to experience the restrictions of a diabetic diet, even without the injections and hypos, for a few days can give only a minute insight. Although this development is praiseworthy, it also tends to make doctors rather arrogant in their assumption that they know it all.

Considering diabetes in the work situation "balance" (the logo of the British Diabetic Association) is all-important. I do not wish my illness to govern my life but prefer to feel that I am in control. Therefore, it follows that to deal with all the exigencies of a medical life, particularly as a junior doctor, one needs to compromise and accept less than excellent control at times. Between-meal snacks have always been a bone of contention since I have often stabilised myself without these. Ward rounds sometimes took all morning, and I had no intention of drawing attention to myself by shiftily taking biscuits from my pocket on the way round. Activity levels vary among all the different jobs within medicine and one needs to restabilise oneself each time.

I had been to boarding school from the age of 12 and found to my amazement that very few would even consider taking a diabetic. The school I attended agreed to give me a trial, and I suppose it must be to my credit that I did not cause much trouble and they have taken others since. I had to show my glucose tablets to the matron each morning so she knew I had them. This made me feel like a small child again. I was not allowed any of the puddings but had to walk through the dining room to get my special—fruit or cheese and biscuits. This was so boring after six years that now more often than not I go for all the wrong things when out to dinner and have to try and compensate afterwards. All this was before the excellent revolution in diabetic cookery and the labelling of proprietary foods with the carbohydrate content. If I had been able to eat as normally as a child as diabetic children of today, I am sure I would not have been as tempted to cheat on diet. Now that I am married, I find my husband is a curry enthusiast and the diabetes has to be adjusted to cope with this. I would never dream of asking him to give up his curries. At school I was not allowed to control my own insulin but had to make a special trip to the medical room twice a day. I felt very much the odd one out. It is important for those looking after diabetics to have a good understanding of the illness and to try to minimise these aspects. In my work I have found elderly diabetics in institutional settings being told, often wrongly, how to manage their illness when they have many more years of experience with the condition. Why do we feel we have to take this control over their lives out of the hands of patients? Only people who are not mentally or physically capable need those things done for them.

Independence has a high priority. It is very important to me to be able to recognise my own hypos and not be dependent on others. This is very important when driving and swimming for example. I have found on one insulin (isophane) I did not recognise the symptoms and very quickly changed myself back. Imagine being woken in the night by the labour ward and having a ludicrous conversation with them. On that occasion, fortunately, I had my husband there to sort me out. He had the courage of his convictions that I was in fact hypo as I argued long and hard and almost refused the glucose. The trend towards more patient control is excellent. It is important to be able, with the help of finger-prick blood sugars, to sort oneself out at home as it becomes obvious that every hospital admission counts against the diabetic with insurance companies. The fewer the people who know about my diabetic peccadillos, the better.

To illustrate both the lack of knowledge in a therapist and attitudes to patients as doctors, I will describe an experience on an orthopaedic ward. I had a fresh plaster on my leg—fortunately only for a torn ligament. When I asked the nurse, who was a student, for a diabetic diet, I was told not to be so demanding, and "Why can't it wait until tomorrow?" I asked to see the sister and heard the nurse shouting this request down the corridor in a voice calculated to make sure I did not. I finally used the only means that it seemed would get the desired result—I got out of bed and set off down the corridor in my barely dry plaster. After this I was taken seriously. It makes me wonder if all our patients' unreasonable behavior (as mine was) is unprovoked. It is frightening to think of the more restricting conditions such as traction in the midst of this ignorance.

Finally, a few words on the diabetologists' motto: "The patient is always to blame." This is perpetuated to the extent that the patient has to accept it, and this has led to a considerable delay on my part in picking up faults in the continuous infusion pump, such as broken cannulae. On the assumption that it is my fault, I have carried on trying to put in extra units rather than checking out the equipment first. Although there is certain potential for denial or self-deception, the experience of hypo is not tied to the absolute blood sugar level but depends on the rate of drop, etc., and it is irritating to be told that one cannot be hypo because the level is not appropriate. Self-deception comes and goes. It is worse when one is on a fixed intake and feels hungry. Fortunately, I have only been on a carbohydrate-controlled diet and would not be able to tolerate the control of protein, fat, and calories as some diabetics do. I think it is worst after the initial adjustment period when the lifelong nature of the illness sets in. Spoonfuls of favourite foods become bigger and slices of bread go from thin to thicker ones. At times of stress, diabetics can resort to food for comfort as anyone else might. I did this when working for my higher professional exams and went through a bulimic phase. I had a carbohydrate craving that was almost insatiable and nothing else would do.

To me, the "good" patients seem neurotic, obsessional, and preoccupied with their glucose metabolism. I feel I have achieved a great deal and managed to travel widely. I have a good career and family and feel fulfilled despite periods of less than good control and the disapproval of the physicians.

PREGNANCIES AND PROBLEMS

I conceived first at the age of 32 with an IUCD in situ. I had not, therefore, achieved the three months' exemplary control thought essential prior to conception. I embarked on a rapid improvement using the infusion pump and had some success. At 26 weeks I had a cold, following which I felt exhausted and weak, but thought no more of it. I had noticed that my normally slim ankles had become much more solid, but not having experienced pregnancy before, I assumed that this was normal at this stage. There was obviously denial, since I had done quite a bit of obstetrics and should have known. However, my consciousness may have been partly clouded, as it indubitably was soon after. I could not get to work the next day, which is exceptional for me. That night I had to sleep propped up, and when I got up to use the toilet next door I was breathless on returning. By the clinic visit next day I had headaches and had gained 6 kg in two weeks. There was pitting oedema over my abdomen, and I still had not realised how ill I was. Over the next three days I got worse and worse despite bed rest, analgesics, and methyldopa. All the staff showed the utmost concern and I was moved to a side room. All the other patients had been trying to reassure me about the outcome since some had been through similar experiences, but I think at that stage I did not believe them. As I got drowsier, the decision was made to induce labour. I had intramuscular hydralazine with such dramatic effects on my consciousness that I wondered if induction was really necessary and if I could not hold on a bit longer. At that stage I was glad to be consulted about the mode of delivery if a choice were possible and elected for an epidural if caesarean section became necessary. I had an epidural, which must have caused the anaesthetist some concern in view of the amount of oedema over my spine. I went on to vaginal delivery. The epidural allowed me to feel the baby's descent and contractions without pain, which was a marvellous experience while we still had hope. The foetal heartbeat was heard and recorded up to the moment of delivery and kept our hopes up.

I had made it quite clear that I did not want strenuous efforts made to keep the baby alive in view of my previous experience in paediatrics. Although there seems to have been little hope anyway, I did hear later of a friend in a similar position who had a baby who lived but has severe brain damage. Most of the time I am relieved that we did not have to experience this. From that moment on I have nothing but praise for the evident change in approach of obstetric staff to parents of stillbirths. The days of rushing the foetus up the corridor to the hospital incinerator have gone. Expecting this, I had determined to ask to see the baby and to arrange a funeral for her. Before I had the chance, the paediatrician gave us the baby to hold and we were so pleased. My husband would not have asked but feels now that he would have regretted it. All the staff gave us every oppportunity to grieve.

On the more humorous side, if there is one at these times, the delivery was before a change of shift so we had a second shift of nurses helping us to facilitate our grief. The people who had been involved were really the ones who could help because the second shift were not as able to empathize at that stage. In those circumstances most people probably do not know what they need, and it was helpful that the staff made the decision for us. We were also clear that we wished to bury the baby, which led to a series of brushes with insensitive bureaucrats. The hospital did all they could to help us through, although there was no sign of a minister at any stage. The event had to be labelled "therapeutic termination" rather than miscarriage, which, it was thought, would be distressing to us but which did not bother me so much because I was so preoccupied in ensuring that we got her buried. The hospital pays for burials after 28 weeks but we were a few days early. Again, this did not bother me as much as I might have expected. We got the necessary certificate and approached the undertaker. We discussed burial of a 27-week baby but did not realise that we meant very different things until he asked for the date of death. The church's approach seems hypocritical, since we hear everywhere else that life begins at conception but not when one wants to bury a 27-week foetus. I was appalled to find that the body was usually sneaked in with another "proper" burial. We achieved what we wanted with an effort and later bought the plot and erected a headstone, which has been a great source of comfort to us. I would have felt terrible later if the body had just disappeared. I now also appreciate when patients say they prefer to have their relatives buried so that they have a visible memorial.

To get back to the medical sequelae—I stayed in my side room in the antenatal ward but found this so distressing that I got myself discharged long before I was fit. It was impossible to avoid the other patients and they did not know what to say. I had a massive diuresis and spent a lot of time waiting for the toilet, to pass litres at a time. I lost 10 kg in four or five days. I had acute epigastric pain going through to the back during the night but got no relief. It was implied that it was anxiety, and diazepam was prescribed with no effect. It seemed to me that in view of the massive and rapid changes in my body a physical cause was quite likely. I felt the interest in me had waned and there was less understanding. No one took the pain seriously and I had little sleep. The duty consultant next day had no bedside manner and said something to the effect that these things happen and walked away! The convalescent period was difficult, and I felt a lot worse than I must have looked. The headaches lasted three weeks, and I was not really up to making rational decisions about my health. My GP tended not to make authoritative decisions but to ask my opinion when I felt least able to give it. The eight weeks after the termination were the worst because I was not physically fit enough to do much so had too much time to think about it. All the part-knitted baby clothes went into storage. I found it difficult to read with the headaches. Having to attend the antenatal clinic for my postnatal examination was distressing. I did not want to be near pregnant women and babies more often than necessary, and that was not necessary, just administratively convenient. I did not even have the midwife visiting to check me since they are only required to do this after 28 weeks. I certainly felt in need of their visits.

During the second pregnancy I was anxious and probably overcompensated for this in my efforts to get to the end reasonably calmly. After all, I had been reassured that it should not happen again. We therefore went on a skiing holiday at 12 weeks. I was determined only to exercise gently. Unfortunately, I had the first small bleed then, which responded to self-prescribed bed rest. In the light of later events, I still wonder if the holiday was the cause of the problems, despite assurances to the contrary. From 20 weeks I had three more bleeds and three admissions to hospital. The first time was minor and admission not essential, but I elected to go in knowing I would find it difficult to be inactive at home. The next two bleeds were bigger and I felt sure that I had lost the baby. The uterus was as hard as a rock but opiates relaxed it and me. From then on I had gentle contractions regularly, which were disconcerting. The final bleed during the night was alarming. I got up to pass urine and lost a lot of fresh blood. I went back to bed and froze. I can now understand fears of exsanguination. The ambulance ride was rough and made worse by the ambulanceman, a union man who, knowing I was a doctor, quizzed me about local facilities. I did not feel I should have to be on my guard at this time. On admission I was in the labour ward. It is distressing to hear live babies being born but knowing that your prognosis is poor. The staff were very kind. In retrospect, one never loses hope, and it is this which keeps one going as in terminal illness. The cruellest thing the staff could have done would have been to demolish that hope completely.

While in the antenatal ward I was treated more or less like every other patient, with deference to my knowledge where appropriate. In some circumstances this attitude of treating one as the other patients are treated seems to be offensive, so I think it is the way in which it is done that is important. If all patients are treated with proper respect one does not wish special treatment. It depends on the therapists' countertransference and inbuilt grievances.

When labour finally began it was hours before I realised it, and it did seem as if the staff shared this denial. From 4:00 a.m. I experienced lower abdominal pains as opposed to the central abdominal contractions I had had up until then. Urinary tract infection was suggested first. I had minor analgesics first and finally pethidine, which still did not alert me. Despite the euphoria, I knew instantly when the waters broke. If I had realised I was in labour I would not have accepted the pethidine in view of the risk to the baby. My husband was sent for and fortunately worked just around the corner. He was told that the foetal heart could not be heard but I was not told. This may explain why he took so long to accept it when she lived. Events progressed very rapidly and the second stage started (over the lunch hour, of course) before the anaesthetist arrived for the epidural. I had not had antenatal classes yet so the only experience I had to draw on was my experience of obstetrics. I might well have panicked so a few essential aspects need to be taught early in pregnancy—i.e., familiarity with the labour ward procedure and equipment. I grabbed the gas mask thrust at me and, remembering the instructions, I breathed in deeply. Encouraged by the nice effect, I carried on desperately until I passed out. Coming around, I had no idea of the time and assumed it must all be over until I heard my husband say that I had delivered two "omelette-sized clots" and the baby was on the way and breech. She was alive and weighed 750 g, so part of the large retinue disappeared to the special care nursery. I do not remember much worry or elation because too much else was going on. Ironically the placenta was retained and manual removal was tried and failed. I had to brace myself (plus gas) while a painful attempt was made to remove it, in vain. I was next rushed off to a theatre and remember sitting up and vomiting just as the anaesthetic was to be given. I am still not sure if this was physiological or psychological, but I am sure there was ample cause for both. I did not have much time to think of the baby at this stage but had sent my husband to see her and report back. One of the thoughts that went through my mind during the delivery was whether the pain experienced before I got the gas would have been proportionately greater for a term baby. I hope not.

I came to hearing the paediatrician giving my husband the "50-50 chance," "take each day at a time," and "mustn't be too hopeful" routine. Surprisingly this was never done for me. Perhaps I was supposed to use my medical knowledge and common sense—at such an emotional time! With this second pregnancy I could not, again, say that I did not want too active intervention. By this stage we desperately wanted a live baby. During the last admission a paediatrician had been called to explain to me the outlook and the improvement in knowledge and skill in the two years since the last pregnancy. This did seem helpful. I was not able to see the baby until ten hours after she was born since I had so many intravenous infusions up that it was difficult to move, and I also had a severe hypo. I appreciated the polaroid photos brought to me, although the first were so poor that it was difficult to recognise a baby at all. Those photos rarely left me over the next few weeks when we did not have our baby at home to show people. When I was reduced to one infusion I was wheeled around to see her. In retrospect, we had a very false impression of her size. We knew she was tiny, but she didn't seem so tiny. When we had occasion recently to see a tiny baby in the unit, she seemed the same size as ours had been but was, in fact, twice the size. When I first saw her I remember saying that I must not allow myself to get too involved just yet, which seemed to surprise the staff. I still think it was an essential protective instinct.

We were fortunate that the signs were good from the start. She was a very active baby when so many were so very flat. I will mention some of the emotions associated with the special care nursery from a user's point of view. The attitude of the staff is the most important at this difficult time. Roughness and haste tears at your heart when the object is your tiny child. All the incubator watchers develop a preoccupation with the gadgets and dials so that even I, who should have known better, found myself judging the baby's condition by the dials rather than her clinical condition.

After a while you realise the periods of apparent apnoea or asystole are likely to be loose connections. I wonder how it might affect the baby in later years being exposed to constant beeps and buzzes. One has to keep reminding oneself that these babies are not as delicate as one might think but are probably the tough ones to have survived at all. Another aspect is the way parents sit by the incubators for hours largely ignoring others but dying to talk. It appears as if there is some taboo on sharing their anxieties and experiences, although when they do it helps a lot. As support groups help in so many areas of life, I think it would help these parents who are under such strain. Informal coffee sessions to discuss common problems and for the staff to help less formally with the emotional aspects would be very useful. It was helpful to know that other babies had been through the same and thrived.

After two weeks, when she was on only a minimum number of monitors, we were allowed to have her out for a cuddle, but it felt very strange. There was no weight to feel and she nearly disappeared through my arms! It was marvellous to hold her as often as possible. The only special treatment we had was probably fuller explanations. We had only one worrying period and that was when the patent ductus arteriosus was picked up on routine screening at two weeks. Indomethacin failed and led to a gastric bleed and ileus. I was very concerned when fluid deprivation was tried as her oxygen dependence was increasing. I could not see how she could progress and put weight on. I felt great relief when surgery was suggested and carried out quickly despite the risks, which seemed smaller than with conservative treatment. Watching her bouncing about in the ambulance as we travelled between hospitals was traumatic. It seemed as cruel as it did to see her wracked with hiccoughs with a large fresh chest wound. She never looked back after this. The level of background anxiety seems inversely proportional to the time survived. Because she has so few major problems I feel we have been able to treat her as a normal baby, and I surprise myself by how much I have blotted out of that period.

Only once did I feel there was emotional insensitivity. We moved to a nursery nearer home and one of the nurses obviously felt there were some emotions that needed to be explored and discussed. She was completely insensitive to the fact that six weeks after the birth I had already been through this, and her timing was wrong. She also failed to pick up that at that moment I wanted to be alone with the baby. Sensitivity to cues is important in staff if they are going to broach the emotional issues. In both units less than 100% honesty was instantly obvious. I knew straight away at the time of the PDA when the staff were covering up because they became shifty and anxious and discrepancies were let slip. When the baby had apnoeas at a later stage, I recognised them and did not appreciate excuses like the colour of the windows, etc. At these times she often needed a knock to recover. At discharge we were sent home with an apnoea mattress to keep the staff happy. I did not feel we needed it since it only happened when it was feeding time and I was with her anyway. One other point from the first nursery was the twice-weekly brain scans for research purposes mainly. I was very keen to watch this and discuss it. There were two very small subventricular hemorrhages, which spontaneously resolved. I was unable to tell my husband about these as it seemed too much at that stage. That was a mistake.

SUMMARY

I do seem to have experienced a lot of ill health and been on the receiving end of a lot of medical care. I could not cover it all. These are the things that come most readily to mind. In general, most doctors and nurses seem to treat a doctor differently, either with special consideration or else taking out previous grievances on them. On the whole, I feel there needs to be a lot more emphasis on psychological awareness of situations and interactions and emphasis on the patient as a person with dignity. I like to think I have some awareness of the defences I use and which I feel are mostly protective. I feel that only with minor problems is it reasonable or sensible to allow the professional who is a patient much say in the decisions. It created more confidence when I was ill to be dealt with authoritatively. People seemed to assume that my abilities were better than they really were. Finally—empathy, the most important aspect in its influence on my practice. Overall, I think it is a great help, providing one's experiences and associated emotions are properly worked through and in perspective. In my dealings with the bereaved (especially parents), I am sure it has helped my ability to empathise, but in the early days it did seem rather cruel to have to deal with such patients. I never tell patients if I have been through a similar experience because I believe one should not need to. It would also put the patient in a special position which would not necessarily be helpful. The patient needs to see his or her doctor as an unbiased professional who understands.

PART VII

ACUTE AND/OR SELF-LIMITED DISEASES

CHAPTER 42

ANAPHYLAXIS

BARBARA YOUNG

Several years ago an illness almost ended my life. The early symptoms were dramatic, but it was not recognised then as a potentially fatal condition. My illness was brought on by a habit, common among doctors, of treating my own minor complaints. I suffer from recurrent sinusitis, which usually clears quickly with a short course of antibiotics. During a particularly prolonged attack, I prescribed a short course of ampicillin for myself. I took the first dose in a pub where I had gone with a friend for a meal and washed it down with a beer. As we sat there drinking our beer and waiting for our food, I began to feel unwell. The first symptoms were dizziness and a sensation of light-headedness, soon followed by profuse sweating and a churning nauseated feeling in my epigastrium. I sat there for what seemed like a long time, fighting to retain consciousness and to appear normal. Objects on the other side of the room swam in and out of focus and the furniture and even the floor seemed to be bucking and rearing. The food arrived and I tried to eat, telling myself that the symptoms were due to hunger, but soon, I'm not quite sure how, I found myself lying on the floor in the middle of the pub with an anxious and fascinated crowd of onlookers staring down at me from a great height.

Soon I felt even worse. My head was spinning as I tried to raise it to vomit into a bowl that had appeared from nowhere. My abdomen was wracked with great spasms of pain, and I desperately wanted to open my bowels. Trying to get up only made things worse, much worse. My hands, feet, and mouth were numb and tingling. The crowd grew larger. Someone called an ambulance. I felt quite sure that I was suffering from an anaphylactic reaction to the ampicillin and kept

DR. BARBARA YOUNG is a 31-year-old immunologist who trained in medicine at the Universities of St. Andrews and Cambridge, taking a Ph.D. in immunology from Cambridge along the way. She recently attained membership of the Royal College of Physicians and plans to complete her training in clinical immunology in Newcastle, NSW, Australia, where she will settle with her Australian husband. She has a special interest in the cellular interactions in the immune response.

repeating over and over to my friend, who was a medical student, "Tell them to bring adrenalin, one part in a thousand, given subcutaneously."

I remained conscious, seeing the crowd of faces above me and hearing statements like "Oh, she's had a stroke. My aunt was just like that when she had a stroke. She never recovered, poor dear!" and "She's drunk, and at this time of day too. It's disgusting!" and "It's a very bad sign when they feel sick like that." I wanted to explain what I thought was happening, but I was too exhausted to try or even to care very much. At the back of my mind I was very glad they didn't know I was a doctor, lying there writhing around on the floor of a pub, retching and raving about adrenalin with my clothes half undone.

The ambulance arrived, and I was loaded onto a stretcher, still completely unable to help myself. The ambulance seemed to crawl all the way to the hospital. I think I dozed a little on the journey. When I arrived I had begun to feel a little better except for the spasms of abdominal pain, which were even stronger. I was wheeled through casualty into a side room. The nurses recognised me and were very sympathetic. I demanded to use the toilet and after a while a commode was trundled into the room. The nurses left me alone for a few minutes, and I put it to good use. The resulting action had all the violence and vigour of a tropical storm. The pains stopped, and I felt better.

Soon the casualty doctor arrived, and I was embarrassed to find I was slightly acquainted with him, having met him at a few hospital social functions. I told him what had happened. He was obviously puzzled and referred me to the on-call medical registrar, whom I knew quite well. We went through the whole story again. He was quite sure my collapse was not due to anaphylaxis but to the combination of a vasodilator (ampicillin) and an osmotic load (the beer), both taken in a warm environment, with the superimposed effects of hyperventilation. I felt thoroughly embarrassed. "A typical hysterical female doctor" seemed to me to be the foremost thought in all their minds. I sneaked off home feeling very ashamed of myself and extremely tired but convinced that I was not allergic to penicillin.

Eight months passed, during which time I moved to another city, another hospital, and another job. My collapse was so far forgotten that when I developed another attack of sinusitis, I once again prescribed a course of ampicillin for myself. This may seem like a rather obscure expression of a death wish. The thought did cross my mind that there was a possibility that I was allergic to ampicillin, but I briskly told myself to stop overdramatising things and blithely swallowed the first capsule. Luckily for me I took it in the presence of another doctor and even told her what it was. Half an hour later I began to feel slightly breathless and looked down to see that my forearms were very flushed. My head began to swim and I slumped into a nearby vacant chair. Feeling more faint by the second, I put my head between my knees and from that position rolled gently onto the floor. The course of events was much faster this time. Someone was kneeling beside me asking me what was the matter but already I was incapable of speech or even very much in the way of breathing. If I had felt ill the first time, this was ten times worse. My head felt as if it was on a roller coaster, swooping, spinning, buzzing, bursting. My mouth and hands were numb and tingling. Waves of nausea swept over me, and the spasms of abdominal pain left me weak and trembling. This time I was in no doubt as to the cause of the trouble, but I could no more speak than I could fly at that instant.

All this took place in the sister's office on the ward. There were five other doctors in the room with me, all just newly qualified and with no idea what to do. This being the case, they obviously decided to pretend nothing was happening and went about their ordinary business. As I lay on the floor I had a worm's eye view of their legs and feet as they stepped over me. I idly wondered if anyone was going to do anything or if they were just going to let me die there. Luckily for me, my boss paid an unscheduled visit to the ward just then. He was told that I'd not been feeling well and that I'd taken some ampicillin. He knelt down beside me and rolled me over onto my back. I lay there helplessly staring up at his face, gasped, "I can't breathe," and drifted thankfully into unconsciousness as I heard him shout for adrenalin. I was vaguely comforted that someone knew what to do. I came round again briefly as I felt him try to pick me up off the floor, thought, "Heavens, he'll get a hernia!" and went off again.

As described to me later, the next stage in this episode would have been extremely funny if it hadn't been so extremely frightening. The office was tiny and the doorway was partially blocked by the ward drug trolley, which was chained and padlocked to the wall just outside. Trying to get one limp body out of that room filled with six other bodies rigid with fear was difficult enough, but there were also several nurses running around in circles trying to find the keys to the intravenous drugs cupboard. I was hauled like a sack of coal into the corridor and heaved onto a wheelchair. One of the juniors, who must be all of five feet tall, set off down the corridor at a flat gallop, but my rubber-soled shoes acted as a braking mechanism on the tiled floor and my legs got buckled up under the chair, needing to be disentangled time and again. Nobody had enough coordination to put down the chair's footrest and put my feet on it.

I woke again as they heaved me onto a bed. My clothes were partially dragged off, and I felt the prick of a needle in my leg and the sting of the adrenalin injection. I sprawled there on the bed with my skirt hitched up round my waist, my blouse undone, and about ten of my colleagues standing there, open-mouthed, gazing at me. A few had gathered their wits enough to act, but the room was so full they were tripping over each other. Someone was trying to put in an intravenous line with little success. I wanted to use my left hand to point out a good vein on my right, but I could neither move nor speak. Another prodded repeatedly with a needle to stab my radial artery. A third took my blood pressure, obviously with an unsatisfactory result. A look of sheer horror spread over her face and she gave way to a more senior doctor, who had equal success. He was succeeded by yet another pumping away frantically on the sphygmomanometer.

I can vividly remember my feelings throughout this stage. First and foremost, my attention was occupied by physical sensations. My hands and feet were numb. I still felt very sick and dizzy but gradually the need to open my bowels took precedence over everything else. The waves of colic were frequent and severe. Breathing was a significant problem. It seemed that no air could get past my throat. I felt as if my larynx had been filled up with concrete. I didn't desperately want to breathe anyway but I heard a voice over and over telling me, "Breathe, Barbara. Come on. Take another breath in—and out. That's it. And again, breathe in—and out." It seemed easiest to do as I was told, so I breathed.

Another part of my mind watched the proceedings in a disinterested way. I was sure I was dying, but I felt quite calm and unconcerned. I think I was even surprised how simple it all was. I could notice that my hands were blue, my clothes all over the place, that needles were penetrating my skin repeatedly. Everyone looked frantic with worry, and I felt vaguely sorry I was causing them so much distress. I hasten to add that I saw no vision of the pearly gates or, as one friend later remarked was much more likely, I saw no little red-clad imps with cloven hooves and long-handled forks.

The power of speech gradually returned, and I demanded to use the toilet so persistently between waves of pain that the ward sister herded everyone out and produced a bedpan. She and my diminutive colleague, who had pushed the wheelchair, hoisted me onto it. I promptly fell off. The second attempt was more successful, and I managed to stay more or less upright while I used it, my two helpers, one on either side, propping me up with their shoulders. This time the result was enough to fertilize half of China and two reserve bedpans had to be rushed in. With returning blood pressure came normal inhibitions. I was mortified to have to open my bowels in the presence of two work colleagues and later to be washed by them. However, the pain had by this time subsided. I felt a little better and able to talk.

Meanwhile, the others had been holding a meeting in the corridor outside and had nominated one doctor to take charge of the situation. The differential diagnosis at that point was a ruptured ectopic pregnancy, a major pulmonary embolus (I'd been wearing an ankle bandage following a slight injury), and anaphylactic shock. Once I'd told my tale and been examined, there seemed little doubt. By this time I was beginning to feel the effects of intravenous hydrocortisone, an antihistamine, and a colloid plasma expander and felt better by the minute but terribly weak and tired. I was transferred in a wheelchair to a room on the female ward and a 12-lead electrocardiogram was done. I was still too groggy to notice that suddenly all the doctors but one disappeared. I later discovered that the ECG showed changes of a large myocardial infarction and that they had all rushed off to find a cardiologist. Then all the symptoms came back with a vengeance. Further intravenous doses of hydrocortisone, antihistamine, and even adrenalin soon brought them under control but also brought on violent vomiting. I was told I continued to vomit for about half an hour, although it seemed to be much longer. As soon as it settled, I was, much to my surprise, bundled into an ambulance, driven to the other end of the hospital, and admitted to the coronary care unit. A further ECG was done immediately and our senior cardiologist hurried over from his outpatient clinic to see me. Thankfully the second ECG had returned to normal. Everyone was at great pains to reassure me, but I felt so weak and unwell that I didn't feel afraid at all. I just didn't care.

This was the compliant phase of my illness. I was quite happy to have my blood pressure measured hourly, my pulse taken, my monitor watched. The rest of the afternoon included an echocardiogram and an isotope perfusion scan of the lungs. The injection of the isotope made me feel warm and flushed and was quite frightening, for it felt like the very early symptoms that had preceded my collapse. Both investigations were normal. After three hours I still had not passed any urine and my doctors had started to scare me by talking of urinary catheters. That was too much for me. I demanded to be allowed out of bed to get on the toilet and tried to pass urine. The two units of plasma expander I'd been given had done their work. Initially I managed a tiny trickle of fluid but soon it was a raging torrent. I used the commode approximately hourly for the next 36 hours, passing huge volumes of urine.

My boss dropped in to see me in midafternoon to find me sitting up in bed reading a textbook of anatomy which I'd appropriated from the small stock of books on the coronary care unit. I was planning to take a postgraduate exam during the next few weeks, and I was determined not to lose any study time. I think he thought I was mad. I probably was. Looking back, this was the beginning of the difficult phase of my illness. I became a very awkward patient. My boss wanted to ring my parents to tell them what had happened, but I refused to divulge their phone number. I couldn't bear the idea of any more people fussing and fretting over me.

The first two nights on coronary care were a nightmare. I could not sleep at all. The realization of how nearly dead I had been slowly percolated through my brain, accompanied by the worry that there might be some serious damage to my heart. I sat there wide awake watching the bips on my bedside cardiac monitor. I was convinced that if I took my eyes off it, it would stop. I felt as if the monitor was driving my heart rather than vice versa. Even if I'd been able to relax, sleep would have been impossible. The ward was just as noisy at night as during the day. Nurses' feet clattered up and down the corridor all night. New patients were admitted to the adjacent beds, the doctors discussing the symptoms and signs in such audible tones that I felt like joining in. The rest of the night was occupied by writing down a full account of the episode. After all, I reasoned, I might as well get a publication out of it.

The following day my blood pressure topped 100 mm Hg for the first time. As I felt better, the disadvantages of being in hospital became increasingly important to me. Everybody was extremely kind, but nobody seemed to consider that I might mind if they pushed the curtains aside and walked in while I was using the commode or washing. The noise was constant and the regular checks of pulse, blood pressure, and temperature disrupted every attempt to doze off. Each person who had been present at the initial collapse came to visit me during the first 24 hours. They all told me I'd given them the worst fright of their lives. Each one gave his or her account of the episode, frightening me a good deal more than I had been at the time. They obviously needed to get it off their chests and to apologise for not realising immediately what was amiss. I think they were shocked to realise that they'd almost let me die in front of their very eyes. One said she thought I was playing a trick on them and another sheepishly admitted he'd thought I was looking for a contact lens on the floor. I was wearing my glasses at the time!

The second night in hospital was made hideous by the cries of a very sick patient along the corridor. "I'm dying, I'm dying, I'm going to die," he cried out all night, over and over, until I felt like shouting back, "Well, for goodness sake, get on with it and be quiet."

He stopped crying about 4:00 in the morning. Perhaps he died. I never found out. I dozed off after a while, only to be rudely jolted back to wakefulness by some quite melodious but totally unwelcome singing in the corridor outside. One of the night nurses was adding her mite to the dawn chorus as she got ready the teacups and bedpans for the early morning rounds. She woke me up in this way at around 5:00 every morning of my stay in hospital, and neither heavy hints nor downright rudeness on my part could persuade her to stop. I was exhausted, but I couldn't sleep. My temper did not improve. On subsequent nights I reluctantly submitted to the use of a mild hypnotic, which gave me a sound and much appreciated sleep until our vocalist started up each morning to sing her welcome to the dawn.

In general, though, the nurses were wonderful. I was surprised to find they were so much more important to me in hospital than the doctors. From the very beginning they looked after me and attended to my needs in a quiet practical way which made me feel pathetically grateful. They were always willing to provide cups of tea when I couldn't sleep or just to sit by my bed and chat as I came to terms with my brush with death. The doctors were much less important to me. They flitted in and out, taking blood, examining me, and puzzling over the aetiology of my reaction to the ampicillin. I didn't care in the least, I just wanted to feel well again, or at least comfortable. I repaid all the nurses' kindness by being their worse patient. I was cross, impatient, rude, and tearful. Received wisdom has it that taking steroids makes the patient feel well or even euphoric. They certainly did not have that effect on me. I don't know whether it was the illness itself or the drugs, but I felt awful for the whole of the week I spent in hospital. With some reluctance I allowed my parents to be told what had happened. As I expected, my mother travelled down from Scotland the following day. For her trouble she also received her full share of ill-humour. I argued with her constantly. I demanded books to study and then couldn't concentrate. I wanted company and then complained that no one would leave me alone. I wouldn't eat. I couldn't sleep. The truth was that I felt so wretchedly ill that I took it out on anyone who came within firing range.

After two days I was moved into a single room, which was a marked improvement from my point of view. I was still attached to a cardiac monitor which gave a read-out on a screen in the sister's office. One afternoon I left my mother sitting in my room flicking through a magazine while I went to the toilet. A few minutes later four nurses stampeded into the room and frightened my poor mother half to death. They obviously expected to find me collapsed on the floor. My mother told them where I was and they tore along the corridor to the toilet. Meanwhile, I was sitting in there going about my business as one does in such a place. The increased intraabdominal pressure had induced a bradycardia and this was what had caused the panic among the nursing staff.

The reason I was kept in hospital so long and continued to be monitored was that two days after the initial collapse my ECG showed a prolonged QT interval, which persisted for several days. After many blood tests, many ECGs, and much discussion, the experts decided that I must have antibodies to ampicillin that cross-reacted with some element of my myocardium and caused delayed repolarization. I had fully adopted the role of patient by this time and took none of my usual interest in their discussions. All my natural curiosity was submerged in a desire to feel less ill. In addition, I think I began to deny my illness quite early on. I kept insisting I was well when it was perfectly obvious I wasn't. I kept telling everyone I was going to get up, dress, and go back to work. I was appalled when I was told I couldn't go back to work for at least three weeks.

Looking back on this whole experience I can see that it has made a marked difference in my behaviour towards my own patients in hospital. Having been overemotional, tearful, unreasonable, bad-tempered, and generally unbearable myself, I can understand why ill people exhibit that sort of behaviour in hospital. Before I was ill myself I found this sort of thing very irritating, but now it increases my sympathy. I understand that they are no more like that in health than I am. I think this helps me enormously to establish a relationship with my patients and get their confidence. I often find myself sitting on a patient's bed telling them I know just how they're feeling. I can appreciate the lack of privacy, the noise, the difficulty sleeping, the helplessness they feel. I understand their feelings of guilt about being away from work or not being at home with their children. I understand how irritating the hospital routine can be, how unappetising the food, how tiring it all is.

I must apologise for the prominence of descriptions of bodily functions in this account, but it would be impossible to describe my illness without giving these events the importance they had for me at the time. During the acute phase I was completely overwhelmed by the physical sensations I experienced. They were much more important to me than the convenience of the doctors and the efficiency of the running of the ward. It's easy for a doctor to forget that patients are in hospital because they feel ill and that's much more important to them than the fact that the doctor wants to examine them right at this minute. The doctor is concerned about discovering a treatable cause of jaundice, but the patient is far more worried by the fact that he itches all over and it's driving him mad. It's also easy to forget that patients are people and not just the mitral stenosis in the corner bed. For instance, the consultant cardiologist who looked after me was very pleasant, kind, and concerned. I liked him very much. However, before his ward round, a nurse would come into my room, help me off with my nightdress, and sit me upright in bed. Then I had to sit there and wait. As soon as the consultant, three or four junior staff, several medical students, a senior nurse, and Uncle Tom Cobley and all had filed into my room, the bedclothes were pulled back so that I was naked to the waist. Meanwhile they all stood around discussing me as if I weren't there. Eventually the consultant approached the bed and examined me and I was allowed to cover myself again. I don't think I'm particularly shy about my body, but I found this very embarrassing. How must it feel to the non-medically trained patient?

At last I was allowed home. Maintaining my denial that I was ill, I would not allow my mother to come to the hospital to collect me. I drove myself home in my own car, which had been sitting in the hospital car-park all week. I arrived home exhausted. The peace and quiet in my flat was marvellous. I had my first really good sleep for a week. I was still taking oral prednisolone for about two more weeks and continued to feel very odd and emotional. At times I felt almost depersonalised, as if I had no contact with the real world and real people at all. I felt as if the air around me had solidified and cocooned me. People spoke to me, but I couldn't seem to understand what they said. Framing a reply was too much of an effort. As the prednisolone dosage was gradually reduced, these effects wore off. I saw my consultant twice in outpatients. The ECG had returned to normal, and my heart was pronounced to have suffered no long-term effects from the experience. I went back to work.

It was a long time before my anxiety went away. For several months I had a blossoming cardiac neurosis which I admitted to no one. After all, I didn't want people to think I was being silly. I monitored my own pulse very closely and lay awake many nights waiting for my heart to stop. I still do occasionally. The doubts about the possibility of permanent damage to my heart I push to the back of my mind as much as possible, but I do wonder whether the truth was bent a little when they told me that no harm had been done. I wonder whether anybody really knows. That way lies madness, so I just don't think about it.

I don't think that being so close to death has changed my life in any other way. Of course, I still dine out on the story. Told with a certain slant to other doctors, it can be hilariously funny. People who nearly die are supposed to see their whole life flash in front of their eyes in an instant and as a result are often said to have undergone a fundamental change in personality or in their outlook on life. I can detect no such change in myself. I am merely very frightened of contact with any form of penicillin.

CHAPTER 43

VIRAL HEPATITIS

KENNETH W. BARWICK

My reasons for choosing medicine as a profession were not really different from those of many young men and women of my age and generation. We had attended college during the late 1960s, and even those of us who were not directly involved in the campus protests across the nation were affected by the political and social climate that pervaded the university campuses. It was a wonderful time to be a college student. Given the strength of our numbers and the visible response in other segments of American society, we on the campuses were convinced that it was a new age. We felt that principles of fairness and equality, sustained by growing concepts of tolerance, compassion, and fundamental human love, would transform our society and create a community wherein all would be treated with respect and dignity.

During the first weeks of my initial year as a medical student at the University of Florida, an article appeared in the local newspaper describing the "new breed" of students entering medical school. The author claimed that we were less motivated by the opportunity for financial gain, and were more concerned with the alleviation of human suffering. In those early days we did not know each other, and perhaps that helped many of us to believe that we would, in fact, be different. Between classes and in the first-year student lounge, most of us spoke of becoming primary care clinicians. A form of general practice had recently been redesigned and named "family practice," and we learned that several university and private hospitals throughout the nation were offering three-year training programs leading to certification as a family practitioner. Several of us decided early that this would be our choice.

DR. KENNETH BARWICK is a 39-year-old anatomic pathologist who is a member of the Department of Pathology at Yale University School of Medicine. He and his wife, Georgia, have two daughters and live in New Haven.

Near the completion of the basic sciences portion of our curriculum, I began to investigate opportunities of medical student electives in clinics serving indigent or impoverished populations. I learned of a small clinic in one of the poorest counties in the United States—Lee County, Arkansas—and immediately applied to spend time there. The eight weeks I spent in Lee County were among the most revealing and unsettling days of my life. For generations, blacks had picked cotton in the flat farm fields bordering the Mississippi River. A few years before, automation had visited Lee County in the form of mechanical cotton pickers. The already poor farm workers were ground into poverty. One day each week I left the clinic and went with the visiting nurse to assist in follow-up care for patients who had been previously treated at the facility. My own background from the lower middle class in the southeast United States had acquainted me with poverty and inadequate housing facilities. I was not prepared, however, to find whole families living in crudely constructed lean-tos consisting of pieces of tin nailed to boards, which were nailed in turn to the trunks of trees for support. For several families, the earth formed the floor of these shacks. A common disease of the children was impetigo, and we often lifted barelegged children from the ground to wash layers of dirt from the crusted sores. It was February, and the air was chill.

In the clinic, even as a Southerner, I had trouble making myself understood to the patients. It seemed at times that the language they spoke was something other than English. More significantly, I was convinced that my simple instructions regarding schedules for taking pills, not to mention basic principles of hygiene and nutrition, were not proving meaningful to the people who visited the clinic. I spent many minutes with each patient trying to be certain that my instructions were understood. They were a polite, even gracious, people, and it would occur to me later that they had exercised great tolerance in listening to my painstaking explanations. As the weeks went by, I felt deep inadequacies in my capacity to understand the life-styles of the members of that community. I sensed that I was incapable of relating to them in any terms that they would find meaningful to their way of life. At the completion of my term, I felt disoriented but even more determined to learn how to deliver primary health care. I was surprised and flattered when my tutor informed me at my departure that he felt I had interacted with my patients better than anyone who had previously visited the clinic.

During the final weeks of my fourth year as a medical student, I served as a student intern on the medical floors under the supervision of the house staff. It was an exhilirating, if fatiguing, time. I admitted patients in rotation with the medical interns and spent every third night in the hospital busily engaged in the endless duties of the medical intern. Becoming an active part of the fine-tuned house staff machinery that ran our medical floor was a happy experience, and at times I felt giddy with its importance. I experienced for the first time that special job of one who is so fortunate as to find himself completely immersed in an activity that seems necessary and right.

The Interns and Residents Match Program placed me in a medical internship within a prestigious eastern medical center. My high level of anxiety was increased when I learned that I would begin my year in the coronary care unit. After the first few days, however, I recognized that I was in the now-familiar world of house officer, under the supervision of highly capable senior residents, and I settled into the routine. The hours were grueling, and I learned for the first time that fatigue can actually be painful, and that a sleep-deprived body aches and protests when asked to continue movement. Nonetheless, I had the comfort of my fellow interns, and to this day I have never again experienced the intense camaraderie such as that of first-year house officers engaged in such a strenuous pursuit. It was good.

After the first several weeks, however, I noticed that the fatigue began to change its character. It did not go away, certainly not after the few hours of random sleep that I occasionally got in the hospital, nor even after the deep and heavy sleep of the night following my 36-hour shift. I would awake feeling the same sense of heaviness and exhaustion that had forced me into bed the previous evening, often before having dinner. I had completed the coronary care unit rotation and was temporarily gladdened when the head nurse told me at my departure that she felt that my bedside manner with patients was unusually kind. My new rotation was the emergency room, where we served 24-hour shifts, followed immediately by a day in medical clinic. My fatigue deepened and my appetite waned. Gradually I began to develop an aversion for certain types of food and became intensely nauseated at the sight or smell of them.

My attitude toward my patients began to change. I found myself easily irritated by them, and often angered. In medical clinic, it was only with great effort that I could listen impassively after 24 hours in the emergency room to the complaints of minor aches and pains of clinic patients. At times I wanted to scream at them and tell them of the great sense of fatigue that I felt and of the dull pain that throbbed in every joint of my body. Fortunately, I never did.

In the emergency room late one Saturday night, I was called to see an agitated patient who had been brought in by the local police. As I approached him, he swore at me and spat on my white coat. The heavy reek of whiskey struck my face, inducing profound nausea, and I hastily grabbed a basin and vomited into it. Seeing my distress, a veteran emergency room nurse took control of the situation and sent me to the bathroom to recuperate and clean my clothes. For the next several days, I had to be very certain not to allow myself to experience certain odors, especially tobacco and coffee.

Early one morning in medical clinic, I sat almost dazed as the nurses reported to work with cheerful greetings. Their delicately perfumed fragrances contrasted sharply with the sticky mustiness I sensed about myself after 24 hours of intense activity. I had always been thin and was surprised to learn that I had dropped 17 pounds from my usual weight. The leaden, aching body that carried me about at times did not seem to be mine. I arose to see my first patient, who was a late-middle-aged heavy black woman in for a checkup for her diabetes mellitus and hypertension. After her examination, I sat wearily instructing her about her medications and about fluid and salt restrictions. I detected a look of subtle amusement on her face and something of a twinkle in her eye as she listened to my labored monologue. I suddenly realized that this woman possessed a sense of life and its hardships that could never be known to me. The logic and worth of a low-fat salt-free diet might make sense to someone of my own socioeconomic class, but not to this large woman who undoubtedly had to feed her family with an income less than adequate to do it. I was temporarily embarrassed to realize that I was speaking to her of values that she could not fully share, and thoughts of the Arkansas population raced back to my mind. This was short-lived, however, as my own fatigue and depression pushed these thoughts away, and I finished with her and went on to my next patient.

My fatigue increased, along with a growing sense of weakness, and I pushed myself through my daily activities only by the sense of discipline I had developed during my years of college and medical school. More disconcerting was my deepening depression and emerging self-doubt. Fatigue and discontent were also evident in my fellow interns as we approached the midpoint of our year, and I initially felt that what was happening to me was happening to all of us. Soon, however, I began to doubt my capacities and to wonder if I had the strength and resolve to become a physician. I realized only with dull concern that my humanitarian concepts had lost their fervor, and that, indeed, I felt cynical at times about the petty complaints of my patients. I had been on a liquid diet for many days owing to my almost continuous nausea, and I began to suspect I was experiencing the early phases of an emotional collapse. After struggling with this humiliating concept for several days, I finally made an appointment with my chief resident.

The medical chief resident was an immensely likable young man who had the enviable quality of listening so intently that you believed he existed only for you as you spoke to him. He reassured me that my work had been good and that he doubted I was nearing emotional collapse. It was evident that my story had concerned him, however, and he scheduled me to see the departmental chairman.

My weeks of fatigue and emotional exhaustion had depleted my defenses, and I poured out my worst fears to the departmental chairman. I related my intense disappointment with myself. I had thought I would be readily capable of enduring the hardships of an internship. I told him my self-doubts had grown to the point that I did not trust myself with the care of patients. He pulled my file and seemed to indicate that he, too, was surprised that I was having such difficulties, in that my letters of recommendation were so strong from my medical school faculty. He recommended that I see a close friend of his who was a psychiatrist, and he set up an appointment for me. The psychiatrist was a warm individual who demonstrated obvious concern as he questioned me, first about my problems in the internship and then about my early life. In a subsequent meeting with the chairman of medicine, I learned that he felt I might be having some difficulty resolving problems of a separate identity from my parents.

I continued my duties as a medical intern but informed both my chief resident and my chairman that I no longer felt confident that I could stay in the program, and that I was going to look for alternatives. I learned that the Department of Pathology was short of house officers and made an appointment with the department chairman to discuss the possibility of transfer. Near midyear, I had been on call Friday night, which allowed me to be off duty Saturday night and then only to go on rounds Sunday morning, giving me all of Sunday afternoon off. I was sitting in a state of depression, near despair, when my wife called from Florida. She had remained there for two semesters to complete her own training prior to graduation. She immediately sensed the defeat in my voice and, over my protests, told me that she would fly to see me the following day. Monday afternoon I arranged for one of my fellow interns to cover for two hours while I went to the airport. When we met in bright sunshine outside the terminal, her first words were "My God—your eyes are yellow!" I was momentarily stunned, and then felt a flood of relief. An immediate trip to the clinical laboratories quickly confirmed that my serum transaminases and bilirubin were greatly elevated. In a few days I would learn that my serum was also positive for hepatitis B surface antigen.

My emotions for the remainder of the Monday afternoon and evening were a combination of joy and relief, which found their expressions as periodic episodes of spontaneous chuckling. I felt redeemed.

I was to learn, however, that I was incapable of immediate healing. After the giddiness of learning that my symptoms could be attributed to organic and not emotional disease subsided, I still found strong residual self-doubt. I could not be sure that my incapacities could be attributed solely to viral hepatitis. I had been offered a position on the pathology house staff, and I was reluctant to give it up.

Years later the emotions I recall as being most profound were loneliness and a strong sense of failure. Far more powerful than my physical symptoms after the first weeks of my illness, the sense that I had failed, that I wasn't good enough to be a physician, burned in my mind. I also felt alone, isolated from anyone who understood and could share my sense of pain and failure. I needed to make several important decisions, and I realized I was not capable of calculated thought. Fortunately, my wife listened and nursed me.

At the time of my diagnosis, my appetite had begun to return, and I was holding down some solid foods. I was relieved of my duties only for a week, after which time I felt strong enough to work in the medical clinic for three weeks and then return full time to the medical floors. The chairman of medicine called and expressed congratulations that my condition had been diagnosed and his assumption that I would remain in the internship program. I could not assure him that I would. In a conversation with my chief resident, I learned that there was some embarrassment in the Department of Medicine that I had worked for weeks with classic signs and symptoms of viral hepatitis that had not been noted. A letter from the dean of student affairs at Florida, from whom I had requested transcripts for my new application, expressed some surprise at what had happened and underscored his confidence in me. I was still not reassured.

I began my training in pathology with the assurance from my medical chief resident that I could return to the medical program and complete my training if I so desired. I soon learned, however, that I enjoyed pathology and that I had some small aptitude for it. I remain a pathologist today.

In the years after transferring to pathology, I had many recurrent episodes of confusion and doubt about my illness and the decision I made consequent to it. More than a decade later, many of these uncertainties persist. I have often felt cheated and enraged that a choice that I had dreamed of and had worked for had been so affected by an illness. The physical and emotional effects of the disease at so tumultuous a time of my life so delicately intertwined themselves that I have no hope of ever knowing what occurred during that internship year and how the year would have progressed without the episode of hepatitis. A nagging suspicion that if I had been of stronger character I would not have been so affected by the infection has often haunted me. I have often been struck with the utter silliness of something so profound as my career discipline being affected by something I could not control.

I must make one thing clear. The discipline of pathology is a proud and honorable one, and I feel fortunate to be able to play such a crucial role in day-to-day patient management and patient care. It is a good thing that I have become a pathologist, but the decision was not one that I made prospectively with forethought and deliberation. It was a decision forced upon me by an aberrancy in my health and attendant emotional fatigue.

I am, today, a teacher who has chosen to involve himself heavily in resident and medical student instruction and training. There have been numerous occasions during my tenure as a chief resident and attending pathologist that I have counseled or comforted a student in some form of emotional or physical distress. I do not do it wisely, or even with appropriate training, but I do offer a certain insight gained from my own struggle with a serious illness. My attitude and outlook have been altered by this episode in ways I cannot define. I think I am better for it. I am certainly different. Whichever, it was not of my own choosing.

CHAPTER 44

TUBERCULOSIS

RONALD J. KARPICK

One pretty spring afternoon in 1967, the chief medical resident flipped up a chest X-ray for my review. As the junior assistant resident (JAR) on the male medical ward at Duke Medical Center, I thought he was introducing a new patient. The differential diagnosis of a soft left-upper-lobe infiltrate was fairly straightforward, but when I inquired about the person's history, the chief resident only knew his name. It was mine. I had only a recalcitrant cough and the usual fatigue of a medical resident, so at the age of 26 the significant differential was tuberculosis or mycoplasmal pneumonia. Neither was serious, but nonetheless, I had to become a patient. My emotional high was abruptly terminated. The JAR year was nearly completed. I had an excellent rapport with my house staff, students, and nurses. I enjoyed the responsibility of patient care and teaching. This all changed within a few minutes when I had to leave the floor without completing the patient work-ups or student teaching of the day. The chief resident's word was law; I was crushed. Tears were in my eyes as I told the interns that I had to leave for what I felt would be a long time.

The next day the chief resident visited me in my apartment. We talked some more, and he examined me, drew some blood, and gave me a sputum cup, together with an IM shot of penicillin G. I did not think the latter was indicated and I don't think he did either, but we did not discuss it. My world had been shattered; I was no longer in charge. On the following day I was told to enter the hospital. Until the admitting clerk asked, I had given no thought to the name of my attending private physician. I chose Dr. M., an older, soft-spoken clinician who had had tuberculosis and who I felt would be pragmatic and empathetic. However, I was embarrassed, during teaching rounds, when Dr. S., a very fine chest physician, went to sign my chart and

DR. RONALD KARPICK is a 46-year-old practicing pulmonologist in Alexandria, Virginia. He is actively involved in all phases of pulmonary care and is happily married with two children.

was told he was not the attending physician. There was no malice intended and no political motivation. It was simply that there could be only one attending physician; nonetheless, I was embarrassed. It was good being in the hospital. A bachelor with no prior ties to the Durham community, I considered the hospital to be my home and support system. The tests were run quickly, including a five-hour glucose tolerance test, which I suspect was performed on my chief's urging, in an attempt to understand my tendency to become irritable toward the end of morning teaching rounds. My admitting intern quickly found the acid-fast bacilli in my sputum and was delighted to see them within macrophages. Since my tuberculin skin test had been positive while I was in college, the discussion arose as to whether my present disease was a reactivation or was related to my work-up several months before of a veteran with poorly controlled diabetes, fever, and pulmonary infiltrates. Since phage typing was not yet available, we will never know, although I think my disease was due to that recent exposure. When the diagnosis was established, the next step was to go for definitive therapy at a TB sanitarium. There was no sanitarium near my parents' home in Buffalo, New York, so I decided to go to Gravely Sanitarium, associated with the University of North Carolina in Chapel Hill. Leaving Duke University Hospital was painful. Tears of sadness welled up in my eyes and heart as I went back to pick up my microscope, lab equipment, and books, and to say good-bye to the nurses, interns, students, and a few of the patients. They all knew my diagnosis. They all knew I would be away from the hospital and program for a while, but no one knew how long or how the disease would affect me. I felt well. I had slept, rested, and eaten. I had even been allowed to complete all my charts, but I was stripped of all my duties and responsibilities. I left the hospital alone, no longer in charge of my life.

Since it was only a short drive to Chapel Hill, I stopped at a music store and purchased a guitar and a beginner's lesson book. I knew there was going to be a lot of free time, much more than I had had for the past two years. There was no directive from my training program with regard to how I should spend my hospitalization time, but I knew I would have a place in the same program when I was again healthy. Gravely was a small two-story brick building behind Memorial Hospital. The admission procedure was pleasant. I knew that the Durham tuberculosis expert was going to be my doctor. I had spoken to him on the phone about several patients and knew from my fellow house staff that he had had a thoracoplasty for tuberculosis as a young man and was regarded as a low-key, knowledgeable man. It was surprising to learn that a local woman's club was going to help pay for my hospitalization, and I wondered why my own school was not, and I still don't know. My room on the second floor was near the nurses' station with a view of the rear hospital grounds with picnic tables and a horseshoe pit. There was no doubt that I was a patient. There was a copy of the rules and regulations, an obligatory rest hour after lunch, work-up by a harried intern (who would rather be playing cards), standing at the doorway during morning resident rounds, and attendance at the monthly patient care conferences. There were all those isoniazid and *para*-aminosalicylic acid pills and the irritating streptomycin shots. There was the induced sputum and the threat of gastric lavage. Several of the pulmonary medicine staff of UNC would drop by to talk, but most of my early time was spent reading a huge backlog of journals and trying to coax a few notes out of the guitar. I soon became bored, however, and tried to help in the education of the UNC house staff that rotated through Gravely. They were not interested. Our backgrounds were different. My previous JAR was intense and demanded facts and knowledge. I expected to work hard (five out of seven nights), whereas the UNC house staff seemed to be more relaxed and laid-back, and worked only every other night. I turned my educational efforts next toward my fellow patients. They were a bit more receptive. But after about six weeks of informal discussion groups, they too became saturated. By this time I was comfortable in my role as a patient and didn't feel as acutely the need to control my environment, although I still felt apart from my fellow patients because of my Northern blue-collar socioeconomic and educational background. However, I came to enjoy being with them and made several friends. We worked on ceramics, table tennis, and horseshoes, and they even tried to help me with the guitar, but to no avail. There were some fine people at Gravely. Joe S., a black high school student with a tuberculous pleural effusion, was amazing with the guitar. He picked it up quite naturally although he had never taken a lesson or read a manual. Johnny M. was a redheaded adolescent with tuberculous meningitis who was very ill when he entered the hospital but quickly became a regular hellion. Stan T. was a good old Southern boy with an avid interest in his recently acquired Ford, his guitar, and leather work. Linda S. was a nurse with tuberculosis. She became a special person. We talked long hours about our experiences and joked quite a bit. She got me out of my serious side. We even had a contest as to who could get an ever-growing list of notes attached to the other's room door without being discovered. As a diversion, it became fun for a lot of people. We developed a healthy friendship, which never had the same quality after we were out in the pressured world of work and worries. A number of other people filled out my experience at Gravely. They were all different, all good people.

At the end of my three-month hospitalization, I knew the staff. My fellow patients and I had learned how to get a pizza brought in and where the special hiding places were in the bamboo stand next to the hospital. I had found a new home. My experience at Gravely was a good, wholesome one—one that opened many aspects of life for me. However, leaving the hospital was the occasion for happiness. I got back the freedom to leave the hospital grounds, the freedom of being able to walk around without a mask, the freedom of my own life. There was no great party. I just said good-bye to the nurses and friends and packed up my pile of collected memories, including a carved leather wallet from Stan and a ceramic Buddha from Linda. The staff gave me large bottles of INH and PAS, and I returned to my Durham apartment. That was the end of my rest, since the fellowship in pulmonary medicine had been decided upon while I was a patient. The lung had taken on a new fascination, and after I talked with a pulmonologist at Gravely and two others at Duke, it became apparent that lung diseases were more interesting to me than cardiac diseases, and they still continue to be such to this day.

I am healthy now, although there is still a faint scar in my left upper lobe. There is no disability. My illness left no other scars. I was distraught to have to vacate my Long Ward JAR position, but I did get deferred from the military draft and did get to enjoy the navy after my fellowship was completed. I learned to adjust to a new society, to be more at ease with myself, but not to be lax. I think I still was an intense pulmonary fellow. I still pushed my students and house staff but was more aware of their humanness, their need to be recognized as people with feeling and emotions. When I see patients in my practice, I continue to be aware of the frailty of both of us and how quickly the roles of patient and physician can be reversed.

I try not to hospitalize people, not because of DRGs but because of the hospital's impact on their lives. I can appreciate the loss of control, the dehumanization, the cost. I don't usually discuss my personal history with patients, but if they appear to be having a particular problem adjusting, I will tell them about my positive tuberculin skin test, my taking of medicines for 24 months, and the fact that I have a scar on my lung. Rarely will I talk of my hospitalization. I am not ashamed of it; it is just a part of my personal past life. It is educational to have an illness programmed into our lives so that we can experience being a patient and can hope to develop an empathy with our patients.

CHAPTER 45

TRAUMA

BARRY L. ZARET

That day in March, now more than three years ago, began like most others in the all too frenetic pace of the academic physician. It had snowed the night before. As I arose at 5:30 a.m. and prepared for my usual morning jog, I noticed a significant white covering on the lawn. However, once I was out on the road, the conditions were deceptively benign. The footing was good; I can remember commenting on this observation to myself as I traversed the course of my usual five-mile route. Upon returning I quickly showered and packed my overnight suitcase. This particular day would be more hectic than most. Arrive at the Medical Center at 8:00 a.m., conduct a teaching conference from 8:00 to 9:00 a.m., check on the progress of ongoing research in the laboratory from 9:00 to 10:00 a.m., make abbreviated rounds with my fellow on the cardiology consultation service, and then drive to LaGuardia Airport in New York and catch the shuttle to Washington, D.C. The afternoon was to be spent in Washington visiting a friend and reviewing aspects of his newly formed cardiology program at his medical center and then participating in an evening conference followed by dinner. The day should end at approximately 11:00 p.m. I would stay over in Washington and then catch an early air shuttle back to New York and then drive back to New Haven.

These plans were well in place and formulated with a certain ease that came from the substantial experience of "being on the circuit" and of combining the many facets of academic medical life. After saying good-bye to wife and children, I left the house at the usual time in the

DR. BARRY ZARET currently is Robert W. Berliner Professor of Internal Medicine, Professor of Diagnostic Radiology, and chief of the Section of Cardiology, Yale University School of Medicine and Yale-New Haven Medical Center. He has been at Yale since 1973, at which time he joined the faculty following completion of clinical and research training and military obligation. Dr. Zaret maintains an active interest in clinical cardiology as well as active research interests in cardiac imaging, ventricular performance, and myocardial metabolism.

usual manner. The initial portion of the somewhat boring and repetitive everyday seven-mile route to the Medical Center seemed fine despite the white covering on the road. However, as I continued, a certain uneasiness came upon me. Driving conditions were not that good. Furthermore, the car, which already had manifested a certain lack of stability under braking conditions, once again seemed less than sure-footed beneath me. Approximately two miles from home, on a downhill, a yellow school bus emerged suddenly and unexpectedly from a side street. I applied the brakes. The car suddenly began to skid out of control, heading leftward into the opposite lane. Thereafter, there was blackness, a blur, amnesia.

After what I now know was only minutes, I awakened. The well-organized academician suddenly found himself cerebrally fogged, lying in the passenger rather than the driver's seat, facing north instead of south, conscious of excruciating pain in the neck, aware of warm blood trickling ever so slowly down from behind one ear, finding it difficult to breathe because of an intense stabbing pain in the left chest that would abruptly crescendo with each inspiration. While in this fogged and clouded state, I found myself once again the physician, and with this, stupor was replaced by panic. A single thought burned through my mind during that lifetime of several seconds: Had I become a quadriplegic? Then, consciously, systematically, reflexly, and again attempting to gain control, I moved the digits of each extremity in sequence, first the lower and then the upper. With the movement of each extremity's digits, a new sense of partial relief approached. When it was clear that all four extremities were moving I lay still, now content to await help.

It may have been minutes, perhaps longer, but capable help soon arrived. By this time panic of being amnesic, even if only for a few moments, was upon me. This was balanced by the immediate desire to assume the pose of physician, even while the totally debilitated patient. My first remarks to those around me still remain. I immediately identified myself as a physician and then, as if I could reverse my current role, I indicated to them the need to fix my neck in a firm and stable position and not to move me until this had been done. Thereafter, conversation was brief. They caringly removed me from my totally demolished automobile and informed me that my car had skidded into another lane and had been hit by an oncoming car, but that, fortunately, the other driver was not seriously injured. The ambulance arrived. Again, seeking to establish my medical presence, I indicated that I was on the full-time staff of Yale-New Haven and that was the institution I wished to be taken to rather than to the other large community hospital in New Haven. Finally, as only an academician could do, I indicated that my suitcase containing only clothing could for now remain in the demolished car; however, my briefcase containing my all too precious slides, the basis of present and future lectures, should be removed and accompany me in the ambulance to the hospital.

During the ambulance ride, accompanied by the rhythm of a blaring siren, I confronted my own mortality seriously for the first time. I was not paralyzed and thanked God for that. I prayed; who could predict what other injuries were before me? In the emergency room I was immediately among friends and colleagues. They had been alerted to my impending arrival and were ready. A caravan of specialists met me and each addressed the specific problem relevant to his area of expertise: X-rays and more X-rays, blood samples, urine samples, arterial blood gases, and then neurologist, neurosurgeons, orthopedic surgeons, general surgeons, radiologists, cardiothoracic surgeons. Through the fog I recognized both the need to tell the story again and again, and the pain associated with doing it. The realization was soon apparent: there was something seriously wrong. Diagnoses: a large pneumohemothorax, multiple rib fractures, shattered scapula, concussion, assorted lacerations and abrasions. At a minimum, a chest tube would be necessary. Everything else appeared to check out well. Then, placement of the tube. No one can teach how sensitive the pleura are. As the tube was positioned (and it took several punctures before it was positioned adequately), a thunderous blast of pain vibrated through my body, beginning in the left chest and then spreading both caudad and cephalad. Could this be me? Why wasn't the tube positioned well on the first attempt?

Finally it was in place. The pain was over for the moment. Again, I felt the need to relay medical information to those caring for me. I informed them that I had run this morning and that joggers frequently have microscopic hematuria. They should keep this in mind before assuming I had trauma of the genitourinary system. And then there was humor: Who amongst the house staff would perform the rectal exam on the chief of cardiology? Would it be the more senior female resident or the junior male intern? I tried to assure them that at that moment this very liberated chief of cardiology was all in favor of affirmative action.

After what must have been hours, the patient was ready for movement from emergency room to the intensive care unit. The chest tube was in place, nasal oxygen was running, the intravenous lines were patent and sustaining. I ached and hurt as never before. For the first time this doctor was a patient. My wife was at my side, and I felt secure. Even at this moment I wondered how I would react as a patient. Over the years, I had cared for a substantial number of physicians, medically related personnel, and their families. I had had the opportunity of firsthand view of how complex, difficult, and frustrating the care of physicians can be. Would I be one of those frustrating patients? The answer in part came all too soon.

Because of the chest trauma and outside possibility of cardiac contusion, I was placed on a cardiac monitor. I could hear the refreshing cadence of my own heartbeat during the transfer to the intensive care unit. And now I was to be moved to a hospital bed in a somewhat secluded private room at the back of the surgical intensive care unit. The movement from stretcher to bed was difficult and filled with intense pain. I was aware of perspiration on my forehead and a sudden feeling of weakness and dizziness. And then the cadence on the monitor slowed; my heart rate slowed. It was immediately clear that this was a vagal reaction, presumably in response to the associated pain. My mind raced and immediately focused on the image of one of my colleagues, one of the grand elder statesmen of our Department of Medicine who only last month had been hospitalized with a myocardial infarction. I had taken part in his care; during this illness profound sinus bradycardia had developed and required the institution of atropine to maintain his heart rate. Administration of this medication had resulted in complicating urinary retention and need for a Foley catheter. The whole scene reproduced itself vividly before my eyes in those seconds as I blurted out to my nurses (who already knew me) that they knew I was a cardiologist and that I was sure this was a vagal episode. I asked them to please raise my legs to increase venous return and under no circumstances to give me atropine. At that moment I am sure they smiled knowingly and categorized me appropriately, just as I had categorized tens of physician-patients in the past. Fortunately, both the diagnosis and the patient-nurse interaction were good. The heart rate increased quickly, the vagal episode passed, and no medication was required. However, it was clear that this doctor, no matter how much he professed to want to, could not be the ideal patient. The dissociation of physician-hours in medicine applied to others and patient-hours in medicine applied to me could not be made. As I lay there in the intensive care unit I tried to inform those caring for me that I had an extremely high tolerance for pain and really did not want analgesia. If it was absolutely required, I really wanted only the minimal dose. Again, I am sure they smiled knowingly and agreed, at least temporarily. The low-dosage analgesia lasted for all of one cycle. As the pain became more and more intense, it was clear that this doctor-patient could not and would not attempt to dictate therapy.

The next few days remain a blur, even at this moment. There was the endless stream of colleagues, fellows, house staff wishing to see me and offer their good wishes, doing constant battle with the nurse lions at the gate determined to let me, even if I was chief of cardiology, get the appropriate rest and recuperation entitled to me under any system. The time passed slowly, and I remained dazed and perhaps under the influence of the analgesia I was receiving. I tried to read, would soon forget, and then try the same material again. I would try to sleep knowing that it was extremely difficult to move. All of the little things that we take so for granted when treating patients piled one on another to provide discomfort, annoyance, and pain. Sitting upright for a chest X-ray was pain. Obtaining venous blood samples was pain. An arterial puncture to measure blood gas concentrations was pain. I inappropriately grew to fear and hate a lovely gentle woman with a lilting West Indian accent who approached me every morning with her wonderfully antiseptic venipuncture set and numerous tubes, all of which would have to be filled with blood from my vein. I longed for the time when I could take a deep breath without pain, when I could turn on my side without pain, and when I could reach forward and shake the hands of my guests without pain.

After two days of hospitalization I remained in the intensive care unit. The chest tube had been removed a bit too early and had to be reinserted when the lung collapsed once more. Thus, unexpectedly, I approached my first Sabbath as a patient, still in our intensive care unit and probably at my psychological and emotional nadir. I faced this day of joy, rest, and spiritual replenishment as a pained, anxious, and depressed individual. That Friday evening, my wife and three sons brought our family Sabbath dinner to the hospital so that we could share that very important moment together. In the sterility and intensity of this very intense intensive care unit, we greeted the Sabbath together as we would do in the warmth of our own home; we offered our prayers over wine and challah and together ate the meal specially prepared at home for the evening. With the curtains closed, we raised our glasses and sang together over the bubbling noise emanating from the chest tube. My voice cracked and my eyes filled, but at that moment, above all others, I knew I would get well.

Thereafter, recovery continued, albeit often at the pace of Sandburg's "little cat feet." I left the intensive care unit, the tube was removed, and rehabilitation began. It was ironic that I found myself on the surgical floor where I had been rounding daily prior to the accident. Many of the patients I had been seeing were now far more advanced in their recovery than I was. The doctor suddenly found himself being rounded upon by his own patients. One of my favorites was a young woman whom I had followed through a complicated pregnancy during which pulmonary edema was the initial presentation of mitral stenosis. She had just had a mitral commissurotomy. She recovered quickly and now was almost ready to leave. She came to see me every day, checking on my progress, providing moral support, and doing what every good physician should do. We compared notes and suddenly there was a new bond between us that was different from the traditional health care bond; we shared this eagerly.

During those final days in the hospital, I noted for the first time a sense of intimidation amongst house staff and nurses caring for me. The dominant medical center physician was regaining strength and, therefore, must be treated differently. In this manner, there would be both gentleness and overindulgence and, perhaps in certain instances, neglect. Neglect arose not consciously but rather from a belief that the dominant physician-patient figure would not need routine medical care, such as physical rehabilitation, to the extent that the everyday patient would.

I left the hospital to continue recovery at home. Follow-up medical visits were few and I was soon on my own. Before long I was walking and then jogging and pushing perhaps harder than I should have. I had vowed that following this experience I would alter my life a bit and no longer push as hard. I adhered to that vow, perhaps for as long as a year. Thereafter, as I probably knew all along, I returned pretty much to my old ways.

The events of that week in March remain with me, still very close to the cerebral surface. One cannot adequately describe the near-death experience. One cannot put into words those few microseconds during which one does not know whether the remaining portion of a lifetime will be spent in a state of paralysis. Facing one's mortality, facing one's frailty and fragility is traumatic, yet healthy and important. It allows you to alter the intellectual, emotional, and physical forces that mold our singular universe into a more effective whole. You learn a lot about yourself, about life, and about death. I have learned these things in a manner that can only bring a knowing nod from the individual with a comparable experience. As a person I have grown and emerged perhaps a stronger individual.

On a personal level, my religious beliefs have been strengthened. A trend toward increasing religious commitment was clearly evident prior to this experience. Nevertheless, the experience itself helped crystallize many thoughts concerning religion, tradition, and the meaningfulness of my beliefs. Behind the curtains of the intensive care unit on that Sabbath evening, I saw the emotional and intellectual link to the generations established in the most classical and traditional of terms. From this position there would be no bending, and there has not been.

On a professional basis, this illness has had a substantial impact upon me. Throughout the years in medicine, from internship onward, I had always considered myself a sensitive physician. I could communicate with my patients, sense their needs, and attempt to meet them. My experience taught me how less than perfect those perceptions were. I suspect that in order to be an ideally sensitive physician, a treater of patients, one must experience at least some form of illness and undergo some degree of medical care. It is only then that our antennae can pick up and respond to the multitude of signals patients are sending us on a daily basis. These signals center not so much upon our well-tuned abilities as diagnosticians or therapists, but rather upon our abilities as uniquely sensitive and caring human beings. Do we recognize the anxiety associated with making a decision concerning, for example, surgery? On medical grounds the decision may be obvious. Are we sufficiently sensitive to what this means to the patient? Do we conceptualize the fear of illness in the patient sitting before us in our office? Can we assuage that fear in a medically sound but nevertheless sensitive manner? Do we realize the discomfort the hospitalized patient experiences while going through the most mundane of medical manipulations such as a venipunture or a chest X-ray? I have asked myself these questions over and over again. My answer is that frequently we are not sensitive to these issues. Our antennae are insensitive, nonspecific, and lacking in precision. Being a patient brings these thoughts and these signals forward and allows one to internalize, to make formal and concrete an awareness and response that makes the physician far more capable of dealing with the patient before him. I have seen this in myself as I now meet and deal with patients about to undergo cardiac surgery and other cardiac procedures. I can talk about the pain, the difficulties, and the subsequent joy of being able to sneeze or cough without being racked by a multitude of painful stimuli. There is no doubt that this experience has made me a better physician.

How do we teach this aspect of medical care? Heightened sensitivity comes only within the context of experience. Can the surrogate experience of some be transmitted effectively to many? This, of course, is a challenge of the current volume.

CHAPTER 46

ECTOPIC PREGNANCY AND COMPLICATIONS OF PREGNANCY

"DR. SUSAN PAT"

A mountain-climbing expedition to the top of Mount Athabasca was the most euphoric experience I had indulged in until the birth of my first child. My past had been blessed with good health and strong endurance. Activities such as hiking and backpacking were regular occurrences. In essence, there had been no major health problems in my life until my husband and I began family planning.

At the age of 19 I had achieved a Bachelor of Science; at 23, a degree in medicine; at 25, I had received a certification in family practice; at 28, I had finished my fellowship in psychiatry. Such a track record of academic accomplishments would indicate an anaclastic personality. Some people would call it stubborn and slightly obsessive. Also, throughout these youthful years I had had only minor health problems such as tonsillitis, a broken ankle, and occasional episodes of severe sinusitis. My life had been well planned. From the age of 4 I had wanted to become a physician and from 13 I had wanted to become a psychiatrist. All my academic endeavors were channeled along these lines. However, marriage and family were also important issues to me and were in the major plan. In my thoughts I had hoped to be married at the age of 30 and to have four children by the age of 35. This seems to be a very unrealistic plan with my present perspective, but at that time anything was possible.

In my last year of psychiatry residency, at the age of 28, I was found to have an abnormal Pap smear. Visits to the cancer clinic were necessary, and eventually all was determined to be fine as long as this situation was watched carefully. I was not afraid of cancer or any sinister problems. I was more afraid that a hysterectomy would be necessary and would defeat any plans of having children.

"DR. SUSAN PAT" is a 35-year-old practicing psychiatrist in Alberta, Canada, and a part-time faculty member of the University of Calgary Medical School. She has a special interest in child psychiatry and psychiatric concerns of the mentally handicapped.

Immediately I experienced a strong urge to complete my residency, although I was being encouraged to do further training in child psychiatry in a centre in the United States. I decided it was time to get on with the other plans for my life. I was involved with a fellow who had wanted to get married for several years. We had known each other for about 12 years at the time. We agreed that marriage was a good idea and we both wanted children very much.

The next year I began my private practice in psychiatry, setting up a child psychiatry inpatient unit in the children's hospital in my city, and began consulting to the various agencies dealing with mentally handicapped people. In April 1981, now married and homeowners, we decided it was time to start planning a family. I discontinued birth control pills. My past menstrual history was normal. I had had regular cycles since the age of 12, with no spotting and no history of infections. On August 10, 1981, I had some spotting. It was dark brown in colour and most unusual. We had planned on hiking that day and I found I was very tired and unable to truly enjoy the 12-mile hike. The spotting continued and then became an extremely heavy period. Two weeks later I realized that I must have been having a miscarriage. I was terribly distraught at this possibility. It would have been about six weeks after conception that the heavy bleeding started. I attended an obstetrician-gynaecologist who had seen me when I had the trouble with the Pap smear. She mainly specialized in people with cancer but did a small practice of obstetrics. Most of the female physicians I know in the city attend this woman for their obstetrical and gynaecological care. I felt very comfortable with her and with her call group of obstetricians. She also thought I had had a miscarriage and found a pregnancy test to be negative. An ultrasound did not show a pregnancy. She advised me to return to see her if the spotting continued and she would do a D&C. In the true form of physicians, I was terrified of having a general anesthetic. I did not want to have a D&C. The spotting continued but I did not go back to see her. I did not feel well for several months and attributed the spotting and the not feeling well to overwork.

On November 6, 1981, almost three months after the initial incidence of spotting, while shopping I doubled over in abdominal pain. My husband and I went home. I did not seek any physician's help at that time and continued to deny that there was a problem. The next day I was at a conference on hypnotherapy in the city. Again, I experienced terrible abdominal pain and left the meeting to faint in the washroom. A friend and colleague found me there and called an ambulance. The hospital to which I was taken left me in emergency for four hours. During that time one extremely painful pelvic examination was done. It was apparent that there was an inflammatory or acute process occurring in my abdomen; also, I was hypotensive. I strongly denied there was any possibility of pregnancy and insisted that I must have appendicitis. They waited overnight to see how things were developing. In the morning, on getting out of bed, I fainted and was rushed to surgery within 15 minutes. They found a ruptured tubal pregnancy in the right tube and removed it. On returning to the nursing unit, I began to experience pain from the abdominal incision. The night before I had a very bad reaction to Demerol with immediate vomiting, which lasted six hours and was not relieved by Dramamine. I never wanted to see Demerol again. The nurses gave me no choice; they stated that I must receive either Demerol or nothing. Apparently there was no resident or other physician who could write an order for morphine. I received the Demerol injection, being in such a vulnerable situation and in terrible pain, and began vomiting again for six hours, which only aggravated the pain of the incision. My opinion of nurses dropped dramatically. At midnight, 18 hours after surgery, I had not voided. The nurse on duty had never catheterized anyone. I offered her instructions. It was hard to believe I was in a university hospital.

The next day I was served a clear fluid diet, which included gelatin with a chunk of glass in it. It did not appeal to my appetite. Next they gave me Talwin for pain relief. This caused the most bizarre auditory and visual hallucinations. I was aware that I was hallucinating and realised the drug would wear off. I had been consulted as a resident on several people who had such experiences with Talwin. After this I decided I would rather live with the pain. About five days after this surgery, I was discharged home. My husband, who is not experienced in medicine, was very distressed by all that had happened.

I had had a tubal pregnancy and lost it. I was very depressed about this situation and felt as though I had failed in having a baby. I felt as though I would never get pregnant and this was a terrible loss. The loss did not subside until I did get pregnant again in March of 1982. This time I did not rely on my own judgment about anything. I kept a very close contact with the same obstetrician. I was very tense throughout the pregnancy, hoping that everything would go well. Even minor things like the baby's not growing very much in a two-week interval would upset me terribly, and I wondered if things were going okay. Because of my dreadful experience with the hospital on the previous occasion, I went to a hypnotherapist with a very good reputation to calm my anxiety about being in the hospital and to use hypnosis for pain control. Near the end of the pregnancy I experienced some signs of toxemia with a slight rise in blood pressure and a great deal of swelling. The obstetrician decided to induce the baby. The induction went uneventfully, and six and a half hours later our son was born. It was a marvelous experience. Even a few minutes after the delivery, I said I would willingly have another baby. Our child was healthy. It was quite a radical adjustment to become a parent and to deal with the fatigue one experiences with an infant. We were both so enthralled with our child that we wanted another one. I did not go on birth control, and because I had only one functional tube, it took longer to get pregnant. About the time of our son's first birthday, I became pregnant again. Again, I went for immediate care to the same obstetrician and was followed along very carefully. Ultrasounds were done to make sure the pregnancy was in the correct place. With the second pregnancy, I felt quite at ease and casual. I knew more of what to expect with a child and what to expect with my own level of endurance throughout the pregnancy. It was uneventful. Again I became slightly toxic in the last two weeks of pregnancy. Again I was induced. The day I went in for induction, the personnel in the labour and delivery suite were extremely busy. The membranes were ruptured and Prostaglandin gel applied to the cervix. I was to be put on a Syntocinon drip. The nurses were so busy that this drip did not start until 3:00 p.m. I was already in labour but there was nothing dramatic happening in the cervix. At 3:00 o'clock they began the Syntocinon drip. The nurse turned it up very quickly. At 3:28 p.m., I delivered that baby in bed. This was less than a half-hour delivery. The cervix was not completely dilated and tore. I did no pushing; the contractions pushed the baby out. There was a terrible mess and I had a lot of bleeding. They took me to the delivery room to repair the tears. The baby was in perfect condition. This was an experience I would not want to repeat. It was very frightening for both me and my husband. I had no control over what was happening. Nobody seemed to make the connection that the Syntocinon pump should be turned off.

On my return home, everything was fine. Three weeks after the baby was born, I had a postpartum haemorrhage and my husband took me to the hospital. A D&C was necessary and was done by the obstetrician on call. He was the newest member of the call group and seemed quite insecure about having a female physician-patient. I again went home after only an overnight stay. My health never did seem to pick up. I continued to feel tired and thought I must be going through a postpartum depression. The baby was healthy and easy to care for. I continued to work part time and have the nanny care for the children when I was away.

About eight months later, I found that I was exhausted all the time, I had stopped breast feeding and had had no resumption of menstrual cycles. I felt puffy, bloated, and tired, and on one occasion, I fell asleep while I was driving. This was most unusual for me. When I went to my family doctor, she found that I was anaemic. This was very interesting considering I was eating a good diet and had had no menstruation for almost one and a half years. She suggested iron pills. A pregnancy test was negative. A few days later I developed severe low abdominal pain, similar to the kind I had had when the tubal pregnancy ruptured. I went to the obstetrician, who examined me and found a mass in my left lower abdominal quadrant. She scheduled me for an ultrasound and scheduled me again for a pregnancy test. The pregnancy test was negative. The ultrasound showed a mass 4 cm × 6 cm in the left fallopian tube. The same day I was put in the hospital to have a laparotomy. On laparotomy the obstetrician thought I had another tubal pregnancy. I was devastated at losing another baby. Five days after the surgery, the pathology report showed no evidence of a pregnancy. The mass in the tube was blood-filled and had shown recent rupture. Several pathologists looked at it and did not know what it was. The obstetrician commented that "it was curious" and that "it could only happen to a doctor." I was intensely angry. One of the strong possibilities for this mass was a complication from the D&C done seven months earlier. Perhaps that physician perforated the uterus and caused this blood-filled mass in the tube.

It is now five months after this last surgery. We have celebrated the first birthday of our daughter. In recalling the events of the many obstetrical complications that I have had, I am filled with a great sadness and an intense anger. I realise that medical care was given sincerely by the individuals treating me. It seems that the problems occurred in spite of this. I have great anger about the induction being so rapid and all the complications that followed, as well as the complications to the complications. At first this anger was so intense that it came out in unusual places. I would get angry at my husband for things that were totally inappropriate. Now, as I look back on it, I find it hard to find a starting place for where the complications occurred. Perhaps the starting place was leaving family planning to such a late stage in my life. My goal of having four children may never be realised. The only way I could have further children is through *in vitro* fertilization. Throughout these problems I continued to work 30 hours per week. I have a very supportive and happy marriage. After three pregnancies and three bouts of surgery in four years, I feel an extreme sense of vulnerability. My life had really been untouched by physical illness until the complications with pregnancy.

In medical school I was taught that people have a range of feelings and that you can always relate to the feelings of another person. I could not have understood the sense of loss, grief, anger, and joy of the experiences of having my two children and all the obstetrical complications. It was worth it. It has left me more sensitive to others who may have gone through similar situations. It has emphasized to me my human vulnerability. It has made the defense of intellectualization and learning about medicine much less dependable.

CHAPTER 47

HEMORRHOIDECTOMY

WILLIAM B. OBER

In 1972, at the age of 52, I underwent a hemorrhoidectomy. Would you like to see my operation? *Mes fesses*!

The question sounds like a vulgar invitation to indecent exposure and voyeurism, but if the late Lyndon Johnson could expose his cholecystectomy incision to the TV cameras, what is so outré about looking at the site of a hemorrhoidectomy? Yet in this age when frontal nudity is commonplace, images of the anorectal region are taboo, except, of course, in pornographic displays of buggery and anilingus. Modesty, therefore, permits me only to tell you about my hemorrhoidectomy, not to display it as Coriolanus's opponents showed their wounds.

I first developed hemorrhoids in my late 20s. At first they were only a minor inconvenience, a bit painful on defecation, palpable when I explored the region digitally, and productive of an occasional spot of blood. But pathologists aren't bothered by a small amount of blood, and I was able to tolerate it as one of the ills the flesh is heir to. As the years went by, my hemorrhoids became larger. By my mid-40s they were circumferential. They were also more painful, especially if my stool was overly large or too firm. From an occasional nuisance they became a frequent source of pain, especially when one or another of the varices would undergo thrombosis. Bleeding on evacuation became more frequent and more profuse, and scarcely a week would pass that I did not have two or three days of pain and bleeding.

Matters got worse and worse; more than half my bowel movements were major events, and I knew that the time for surgery was at

DR. WILLIAM OBER, a 67-year-old pathologist, is director emeritus of the Department of Pathology at Hackensack Medical Center, Hackensack, New Jersey, and an assistant medical examiner of Bergen County. He formerly practiced pathology at Knickerbocker Hospital and the Beth Israel Medical Center in New York City and was on the faculty of Columbia University College of Physicians and Surgeons, Albert Einstein College of Medicine, New York Medical College, and the Mount Sinai School of Medicine. He writes essays on medicine and literature and on medicine and the humanities.

hand. Ordinary measures and precautions that I had been practicing for two decades no longer provided relief. I consulted a surgeon on the staff of my own hospital, a close friend and a fine pianist, a man with a delicate touch. Do I hear someone recall at this moment Dean Acheson's comment on being informed that Alger Hiss was suspected of espionage, "I shall never turn my back on a friend"? Well, I did.

Actually, my surgeon was a good choice. He was sympathetic. He examined me gently. His sigmoidoscopy—that was in the days before fiberoptic instruments—was not an ordeal. He arranged for a barium enema with the chief of our radiology service. That examination was well done, with minimal discomfort and a negative report. Even evacuating the barium and flatus had the charm of an unusual color and sound, a synaesthetic experience. I was scheduled for surgery.

The afternoon I was admitted, the only private room available was on the floor given over chiefly to male urology. It was unwritten hospital policy that except in cases of emergency, a staff member was always given a private room. As I surveyed my neighbors, I noticed that they were mostly men somewhat older than I, each wearing a blue-and-white pin-striped bathrobe, each carrying a plastic bag somewhat like an attaché case with a plastic tube running under the robe. These were, of course, postprostatectomy patients, and I wondered if perhaps the admissions office was trying to tell me something—the shape of things to come. However, I passed a comfortable night without apprehension, without sedation. I thought of the company of distinguished hemorrhoid sufferers of the past—Dean Swift, Karl Marx, Wagner, Chekhov—and I congratulated myself that my operation would take place in 1972 with safer anesthetics, better analgesics, and antibiotics. Indeed, the anesthesiologist, an agreeable young lady, had visited me, and when I told her that I had had an episode of myocardial ischemia a year ago, she said, "Don't worry, we'll breathe for you."

Morning came, and soon a nurse entered with preoperative medication, some intramuscular Valium. I made no protest as she stabbed my buttock. In a few minutes I was on a stretcher being wheeled to the operating theater. My surgeon was there to greet me and, as the aides rolled me over, he gave me an encouraging pat on the bottom. The anesthesiologist gave me some intravenous Pentothal for induction, and I was out like a light. I don't think I counted beyond four. The operation began a couple of minutes after 8:00 a.m. and surgery was completed by 8:40 a.m.

I woke up in the recovery room at about 1:30 p.m. At first I was disoriented, and I knew it. I struggled to move my left arm and saw that it was strapped to a board and an IV was running. "What the devil do I need that for? I can take fluids by mouth" was the thought

I phrased subvocally. However, the nurses were kind. One asked me, "How are you feeling?" I replied, "A bit groggy—dazed." She told me my vital signs were stable, and I nodded my thanks. Soon I was taken by stretcher to my room. It was, by then, about 2:00 p.m.

My good wife was waiting for me, properly sympathetic, and she engaged me in desultory conversation interrupted only by my dozing off from time to time. I was in no great pain, not yet. Gradually, I became aware of a desire to urinate, but the uneasy thought occurred to me that I couldn't. I had absolutely no desire to be catheterized. The hours passed and the pressure in my bladder became uncomfortable. I was anxious for my wife to leave so I could cope with the problem in my own fashion, but she loyally stayed on until about 5:30 p.m., leaving only when I told her, "Darling, I'll be very uneasy thinking about your driving home in the dark." She kissed me good-bye, and as soon as I felt she was safely down the corridor and on an elevator, I cautiously got out of bed for the first time.

I found my bed slippers and went into the toilet. I lifted the edge of the cotton hospital "johnny" I had been given, lifted the seat, and tried to void. I braced myself with one hand on the wall, the other lifting my gown, and strained and strained. After about five minutes, I succeeded in passing about a tablespoon of clear fluid, but I was exhausted by the effort and returned to my bed panting. The door to my room was open, and at this juncture, Dr. T. poked his nose through the door. "Oh, Doctor Ober," he said, "what have they done to you? I didn't know you were here."

At this point I must explain who Dr. T. is. He had come to our New York hospital from Turkey to train as a urologist. By arrangement, he had spent his first year in pathology to improve his English, to familiarize himself with the way an American hospital was run, and to grasp the rudiments of a residency training program. I had worked with him closely and rather liked him. To be sure, his fund of medical knowledge was meager, but his attitude was good. He was willing and worked hard, but in no sense did he have a grasp of scientific method. He could never become a pathologist. But he had good hands and a kind heart. During the 15 years I had been a hospital pathologist in New York, I had taken on a fair number of such young doctors for a first-year appointment before they were sure enough of themselves to proceed in their clinical specialty training, and most of them had turned out to be competent physicians, most of them passing their specialty boards without difficulty.

I looked at Dr. T., now a first-year resident in urology, as a long-lost friend. If anyone was going to catheterize me, I'd rather it were he.

"Yusuf, I had a hemorrhoidectomy this morning, and now I can't pee."

He approached my bed, placed his hand on my lower abdomen, and said, "You're distended. Your bladder is up to your belly button. How much IV did they give you?" I replied, "I don't know. I was out in the recovery room until about 1:30 p.m. Then they brought me back here."

Long pause. "Did they give you urocholine?"

"No. What's urocholine?"

"It's a drug. It makes you pee."

The name suggested to me that it acted on the autonomic nervous system, so I asked, "Does it act on the sympathetic or the parasympathetic nervous system?" Dr. T. replied, "I don't know how it acts. It makes you pee. Here, I go get some and give it to you." He went out. I reflected, yes, he doesn't know how it works, only that it works, and maybe that is all one needs to know—and it probably will work.

Dr. T. returned in a minute with a small bottle, a syringe, and an alcohol swab. I rolled over, and he injected it. "Here," he said, "I go see some patients. Back in twenty minutes. Then you pee." He was as good as his word. He came back in 20 minutes with a broad smile on his face and a 1000-cc urine flask in his hand. "They give you 2000 cc almost in the OR and recovery room. Too much." He got me off the bed and took me by the arm to the toilet. I lifted my johnny and braced myself against the wall behind the toilet, while he held the graduate. I strained for a minute, and then slowly a thin stream of clear urine began to pass. It was not like normal urination in which one can feel that one is actively voiding; it was like a passive flow through an inert, insensate urethra. At the end of five minutes by Dr. T.'s watch, I had passed a liter of clear fluid. He emptied it into the toilet. At the end of another four minutes I had passed another 800 cc (1800 cc in nine minutes, 200 cc a minute). Its specific gravity was 1.002. My bladder was empty and my discomfort was gone. I was exhausted. I thanked Dr. T., who took his departure, saying, "You have more trouble, you call me. I come." It had been a ridiculous, even a comical interlude, but I had escaped the catheter, and Dr. T.'s good hands and kind heart had been a blessing. In the years that have passed, I have often wished I had a photograph to commemorate the scene. I managed to eat a light, tasteless dinner and gradually became aware of a throbbing pain at the operative site. I accepted half a grain of codeine with pleasure, and later on some Seconal gave me a good night's sleep.

When I awakened on the morning of the first postoperative day, I was delighted to be able to void spontaneously, but the throbbing pain was there, and it soon became intense. My surgeon came by, and I described the urinary debacle of the previous evening. He was amused but not amused. He agreed they had given me more fluid than they should. I asked him about the anesthesia.

"Oh, they induced you with Pentothal, you remember. Then they gave you a muscle relaxant and intubated you, then an inhalation anesthetic." I asked him, "Which ones? Which agents?" He replied that he didn't know; he always left that to the anesthesia service. Then I told him that I had been unconscious in the recovery room for five hours after he had finished operating. He knitted his eyebrows and said, "That's too long. I'll have a chat with Dr. P. about that." He left orders for me to have half a grain of codeine on request. The morning passed in a haze of codeine and tolerable discomfort. About noon I put in a call to Dr. P., the chief of our anesthesia service, an old friend and a highly competent man. Later in the afternoon he came by, and I recounted the events of the previous day. "Don't make a federal case out of it," I told him, "but I think I was overanesthetized and overhydrated. When I was a resident, we did hemorrhoidectomies under spinal. The patients were conscious and back in their rooms half an hour after the surgeon finished. And I can't recall setting up an IV on a posthemorrhoidectomy patient." He agreed, "Yes, it was simpler then, but we've gotten very scientific, maybe too scientific. . . . But we did have problems with headaches after spinals. I guess I'll have to speak to my staff at our next meeting, and there has to be some way of controlling the nurses in recovery."

The next two days passed quietly with enough codeine to cover most of my pain. But the fourth postoperative day was the day of reckoning. I could sense that the crisis of my first postoperative bowel movement was at hand, and I steeled myself for the ordeal. I summoned a nurse and asked her to stand outside the toilet door. "If you hear a dull thud, come in, because I will have passed out." The ordeal was as painful as I had anticipated. I thought of Edward II and the red-hot poker, but with much bearing down and a silent scream, I succeeded in passing a small stool. I looked at it in the bowl; it was partly covered with some greenish material and some blood. I returned to my bed, and the nurse very gently cleaned my anus, something I hadn't required since I was 2 years old.

I spent the remainder of my hospital stay in the undignified fashion of having to relearn a skill I thought I had mastered 50 years before. I also recognized that for the time being I had lost the ability to distinguish among the presence of solid, liquid, or gaseous material at my anal sphincter, and I meditated upon how easy it would be to become the victim of a misplaced confidence. At no time was I free of discomfort, but codeine prevented excruciating pain, and Seconal enabled me to sleep reasonably well.

I was discharged after a week in hospital. My surgeon thoughtfully prescribed Seconal, and I was given a vial of 20 capsules of 1½ gr each. We never keep sleeping pills in the house because I've seen too many overdoses. He knew that I had plenty of codeine at home—good Lord, I had lived on it for months before the operation. It was good to get home and lie in my own bed. I felt well enough to cope with accumulated mail. But bowel movements were still quite painful, and my anus was still too tender for me to clean it in the customary way. I developed a system: First, I would draw a tub of hot water, adding some Vita-Bath. Then I would evacuate—slowly, carefully, and painfully. When my rectal ampulla seemed empty, I would lie down in the tub and gently cleanse the area of my affliction with a soft flannel cloth. As I prepared for bed on my first night home, I debated taking a capsule of Seconal and decided against it. I poured myself a healthy shot of brandy and slept like a baby. It is now 13 years later, and we still have most of the Seconal capsules left. I stayed at home for a week before I felt confident enough of my bowel movements to return to my hospital duties. I suppose the end point was when there was no more blood on the flannel cloth and I could use toilet paper in the ordinary way without discomfort. I had expected that the operation would keep me from work for a week, maybe 10 days, but recovery took 15 days, and a very unpleasant fortnight it was.

When I returned to duty, my colleagues thoughtfully showed me the slides they had prepared of my hemorrhoids, superb examples of venous thromboses in various stages of organization. I took photomicrographs of them and have used them in teaching conferences ever since. After all, one teaches from what one has learned, and my hemorrhoidectomy was, to use the cliché, "a learning experience."

One product of the experience was a couplet that modifies an all-too-familiar advertisement:

> Use Preparation Y,
> And kiss your hemorrhoids goodbye.

I wish one could.

CHAPTER 48

PHLEBITIS

ROBERT SCHEIG

Summer 1964 was excellent. I had just completed my first year as instructor in medicine at my alma mater, and my laboratory was going well. My boss was to be on sabbatical leave this year, so I was to be in charge of the clinical operation, the training of fellows, and the teaching program in my specialty of liver disease. I needed a vacation to recharge the batteries and to get rested before the advent of what should prove to be the busiest year of my life thus far.

We had a summer home on the ocean at Little Neck in Ipswich, Massachusetts. I had purchased a secondhand boat with a 65-horsepower motor and intended to learn about the ocean with my 9-year-old son. There was much to learn—boat handling, the tides, predicting the onset of bad weather, where and how to sink the mushroom to moor the boat, how to row a leaky dinghy. It was all glorious.

Now it was Labor Day and time to pull the boat and its mooring and trail the boat back to Connecticut. Being inexperienced, I volunteered to help others pull their moorings if they would help me pull mine, and so most of the day, I was in and out of the cold north shore waters, pulling moorings and putting boats on trailers. Finally everything was loaded and we began the four-hour drive home. The highways were packed with thousands of others returning from the holiday weekend while still others, like me, were hauling campers and boats to their winter's rest. It was stop and go most of the way. Halfway home I realized that I must have a charley horse, either from all the work in the cold ocean pulling boats and moorings or from the fancy footwork between brake and accelerator of my underpowered car. This diagnosis was reinforced when I finally reached home and almost fell while putting weight on my right leg when I stepped out of the car.

DR. ROBERT SCHEIG is a 55-year-old internist and gastroenterologist who currently is professor of medicine at the State University of New York at Buffalo and head of the Department of Medicine at the Buffalo General Hospital. He has a special interest in liver disease, ethanol, and fat metabolism.

When I awoke the next morning, the charley horse had not improved. Each step seemed to hurt the calf muscles as they were stretched. It was not until later in the day that I finally got around to feeling the leg and discovering that my superficial varicose veins were now extraordinarily tender and obviously thrombosed. I spent the next hour trying to figure out how I could treat myself as an outpatient before I realized that probably the quickest way of returning to work full speed would be to consult somebody with more experience than I had in these matters. My former on-call roommate during my residency had an established practice, and I had always told him that if I ever needed a doctor I would call him, and so I did. He told me I had to be admitted for anticoagulation.

It seemed strange to me that the man in white who came in to take my history was unknown to me since I thought I knew all of the house officers. I subsequently learned that the two interns on the team were afraid to work up "the professor" and had delegated that responsibility to a third-year medical student who was functioning as a subintern. For him, it was a nerve-racking experience, especially when it came to doing a rectal examination and putting in a heparin lock. My physician arrived a couple of hours later and outlined to me what would happen over the next week. In those days, the treatment even of superficial thrombophlebitis was strict bed rest, including the use of bedpan, warm soaks for one hour four times daily, intravenous heparin every four hours, and Dicumarol.

Several aspects of that hospitalization stand out vividly in my memory. Upon departing from his initial visit, my physician said, "By the way, Bob, you don't have cancer of the pancreas." I think that's one of the wisest things that he could have said, since he had read the worry in my mind. I had such faith in him that I believed him even though, intellectually, I knew that he had done no studies on which to base his authoritative and dogmatic statement.

I learned that the greatest torture physicians ever invented for patients is the unnecessary use of bedpans. There was a john in the room and within a day, the hospital no longer recorded any bowel movements from this patient. Old-fashioned adhesive tape not only irritates the skin but it hurts terrifically when removed after being placed on hirsute areas. I vowed never again, except in an emergency, to put an IV in and tape it down without first shaving the area to which the tape was to be applied. Despite plastic wrapping on the outside, it is impossible, apparently, to deliver hot soaks to as big an area as the lower leg without drenching the bed. Thus, for the week I was in the hospital, I never slept in a dry bed. It is equally impossible to train nurses that even with a plastic wrap on the outside, warm towels become cold with time and most uncomfortable. They also markedly increase micturition.

My lifetime reluctance to visit professional acquaintances when they are hospitalized stems from this hospitalization. With the best of intentions, everyone had to stop in to say "hello." There was a constant stream of visitors from daybreak to well past midnight. My hopes to catch up on some reading were thereby dashed. I unfortunately had offered to discuss any patient problems with my fellows. It seemed that each of them visited me minimally six times daily with problems, and they brought every liver biopsy up for me to review so that after a day, I had the permanent addition of a microscope to my room to save them from carting it back and forth from the laboratory.

During the day before I was to be discharged, I discovered that the phlebitis had now extended to a new area above the knee. I was so tired of being hospitalized that I prayed that none of my physicians would examine me before discharge and discover what would undoubtedly prolong my confinement. My prayers were answered. After the first day, no one had bothered to examine my leg, assuming that I—a physician—would accurately report the physical examination. It was time to go home. Except for going to the john, it was my first time out of bed in a week. Walking from the car to my house made me feel that I had just finished a 10-second hundred-yard dash. It took three days before the least effort did not cause me to break out in a profuse sweat and to feel exhausted.

There were several outcomes to this hospitalization. The difference between superficial and deep thrombophlebitis was less clear then than now, and so, believing that the risk of a pulmonary embolus in the future was a real one, I made out a will. During the hospitalization, a surgical consultation was obtained and the surgeon advised me to have my veins stripped if the varicosities recannulized and reappeared in the future. I had been a scrub nurse for two summers during my medical school days and the thought of this barbaric operation made my blood grow cold. Nevertheless, if necessary, I was willing to have it. However, my reluctance prompted me to go to the literature and ask the following questions: How often do varicose veins recur after stripping? Does the surgery decrease the risk of thrombophlebitis in the future? The answers to these two questions were not available in the medical literature then and are not available in the medical literature now. It continues to amaze me how uncritically surgical procedures are accepted by the medical community when the introduction of a new drug requires thousands upon thousands of trials before FDA approval is achieved.

I was told to go to a surgical supply store and get fitted for elastic stockings. No specific brand was recommended. My first stocking *seemed a half inch thick*, required a larger shoe size, and was hot and most uncomfortable to wear. It took three months before I discovered the Jobst stocking which I have worn ever since.

I have had about six bouts of superficial phlebitis since then. For the second, I again was hospitalized but, thereafter, I have learned that two aspirin every four hours for about three days is just as effective as the bed rest, the heparin, and the Dicumarol. So, apparently, has the medical community, since just today I was asked to see my secretary's father, who turned out to have superficial phlebitis. After appropriate consultations, we prescribed a nonsteroidal antiinflammatory drug and told the patient to stay off his feet. Of course, there is no prospective controlled study to support this form of therapy either.

I do believe that my own hospitalization has done two major things in regard to my own practice of medicine. It made me much more conscious of the little things, such as clean, rapid venipunctures, dry beds, early ambulation, and learning about or predicting the secret, scary concerns of the patient. It made me much more highly critical of the medical literature regarding therapy. Also, I don't make too many social visits to the sick unless they are relatives or very close personal friends, or unless I am invited.

CHAPTER 49

BLEEDING ULCER

ROBERT E. KRAVETZ

Even now, I am amazed at how tenaciously I clung to my role of physician when I had, in fact, become a patient, both acutely and critically ill. I never really relinquished control of the situation except during my stay in the intensive care unit.

It began as quite an ordinary day. I had been feeling stressed and pressured, but no more so than usual. I had seen my last patient just before five o'clock. Customarily, on the days when I was in my satellite office in Sun City, I would drive to my Phoenix office 30 minutes away, sort through my mail and messages, and then go home—I never arrived home that night.

Being a gastroenterologist, I thought it ironic that I should suffer from an irritable bowel syndrome. As I sat on the toilet, nothing seemed unusual until I noticed the unmistakable odor of bloody stools. Looking into the bowl, I saw them, loose and maroon-colored. My first thought was "Why me?" Life was going along fairly well and now this had to happen. We all use denial to avoid situations we would rather not face, and I was no different. I flushed the toilet and things looked normal again, but that illusion was transient.

I told myself that "Doctor Bob would take control of the situation and things would be just fine." "A maroon-colored movement," you say; "well, that means the bleeding is moderately brisk." The best approach to a rapid diagnosis would be a gastroscopy since I suspected that I was probably bleeding from an ulcer. It was now 5:30 p.m., and I had eaten lunch at noon, so I made myself NPO (nothing by mouth) and took a Reglan tablet to ensure gastric emptying prior to gastroscopy.

DR. ROBERT KRAVETZ, a 52-year-old practicing gastroenterologist in Phoenix, Arizona, is a governor of the American College of Gastroenterology and is also active in the affairs of the American College of Physicians. He has a special interest in improving physician-patient communication and has lectured extensively in the area of humanism to both medical and lay groups. Dr. Kravetz is involved in research in the area of the history of medical artifacts and is curator of a medical museum in Phoenix.

As I locked my office door, it never really occurred to me to drive to the Boswell Hospital located only five minutes away or to Thunderbird Hospital, which I passed on my way to Phoenix. I was quite intent upon preserving my normal routine and would drive the 30 minutes to Phoenix, stopping by my office to drop off my charts, take care of the messages, and then go to Baptist Hospital near my office to have blood drawn for a hematocrit. Then I would call one of my associates from the hospital and make arrangements for him to come and gastroscope me later that evening. It all seemed so simple and straightforward, and everything was completely under control.

As I drove along the freeway feeling rather calm, I really didn't give the bleeding much more thought. Then it occurred to me that perhaps I should stop by Baptist Hospital first to make the arrangements for the gastroscopy. After all, that would be so much more efficient and my associates could make their plans for the evening. On the other hand, my office was on the way to the hospital; maybe I should stop there first instead of backtracking. The decision I made may be the reason I am writing this story today, since I do believe that the other choice might have proved catastrophic in view of what followed.

When I arrived at the hospital, for I had decided to go there first, I parked directly in front of the emergency room as I had done so many times before. As I walked by the nurses' station in the emergency room on my way to the laboratory for my blood work, I glanced through the window and smiled. About 20 feet further a sudden wave of dizziness came over me, and I knew I would make it no further.

At this point, I gathered all my strength in an attempt to get back to the people sitting inside the nurses' station. The next thing I recalled was looking up at the ceiling and seeing the large overhead lights in the trauma room. I felt a bit giddy, but there was the very pleasant sensation of breathing fresh air, which actually was the oxygen I was receiving by nasal prongs. People were standing over me asking, "How do you feel? Are you all right?"

After my discharge from the hospital, I interviewed the emergency room nursing supervisor, into whose arms I had collapsed. To this day, I am grateful to her for her calm, quick thinking and action in mobilizing the help, since everyone was so shocked and taken by surprise by the acute events that unfolded. The following is her verbatim account of what took place:

> I saw you walking down the hall, and I remember saying to myself just briefly, "Gee, Dr. Kravetz looks pale," but you know you just have those transient thoughts and they pass. You walked right into the center of the nurses' station over to where the doctors were sitting. Doctor S. was there and I was next to him beside the chart rack. You put your hand on his shoulder and said, "Alan, I'm going to faint," and just fell

into Doctor S., who was sitting down. We all just looked at you as if you were kidding, then we realized that you were out. Alan was so startled; in fact, he really thought that you were kidding, but you were limp and he was just holding you. I grabbed you under the shoulders and rested your head in my arms. Then I looked at your face and immediately said, "Let's lay him down." You were still breathing, but your pupils were really dilated; you were damp with beads of sweat on your forehead, and your color was ghastly.

Doctors O. and D. were standing there also, and there was nobody else in the nurses' station. I told them to get a cart because I told them, "You can't treat him on the floor." I figured that once we laid you down you would wake up, but you didn't. That's when Alan grabbed your wrist and said, "Well, at least he has a pulse." They were trying to scramble to find a cart, and you were lying there on the floor.

Was I awake?

No, you were out completely, just breathing, with your tongue a little bit between your lips.

How did I look?

You looked like shit; your color was green; you were really more green and wet than anything else, just like a wet blanket. They had trouble getting the cart through the door.

I guess that's because people don't usually faint in that room.

That's right, they don't faint in our nurses' station. They may faint in the lobby or in our treatment rooms, but they don't faint in the nurses' station. As the doctors were trying to steer the cart through the doorway, I said to them, "Never mind, we're going to treat him here on the floor." I said, "Please get me the lifepack because that's the one that has the portable monitor."

The question was: What were you out from? You were diaphorectic and pale, but was it your heart, were you bleeding, or just what was happening? They managed to get the cart partly into the nurses' station and then the three doctors lifted you up onto the cart and we then moved you immediately into our Trauma II room. At the same time I started your IV.

I don't remember your starting the IV at all, Susan.

It's a good thing you don't remember because I started it with a number 16 gauge needle.

At this time you were still out and we had not obtained a blood pressure, but at least you were breathing. You were just ringing wet; you were glistening all over. I couldn't manage to get your IV taped down because the tape kept slipping off because you were so wet. Someone else put on the oxygen and Cindy was trying to draw blood from you real quickly. In a few moments, we had the monitor on you and we were starting to get your clothes off.

At about that time 500 cc of fluid was in you and you woke up. The first thing that you said as you turned to the side was "Make sure you fold my pants." The next thing you said was "My keys are in my pocket; would someone go out and please lock my Audi." I looked at Doctor S., who was standing there not believing what he was hearing. Then you said, "Alan, let me tell you what is wrong with me; I have been bleeding and I thought that I might be able to make it through until tomorrow, but I just could not." You then told him, "It is not necessary to insert a nasogastric tube as I am sure of the diagnosis." From then on, you were fully awake and with it, and you seemed to be doing better. Just before you woke up, your pressure was still only 84 systolic.

Susan, how long do you estimate that I was out?

It's hard to estimate, but I would say a good seven or eight minutes. It seemed like you were on the floor for an eternity because we couldn't seem to manage to get the cart into the nurses' station.

What did you all think?

I said to you, "You better not die in the nurses' station," but once Alan said, "He has a pulse, not much of anything else," then we figured you had to be bleeding. You were so singsong even when you did wake up; your voice seemed so tired and you seemed so fatigued, but you were still trying to talk and tell us what to do. You went from one octave right up to another and we could still see that you were deprived of oxygen, but you were at least better.

You gave us a real scare; it's different when it's a stranger. You do all the right things and everything else, but gosh, when it's someone you know, it's different. I said, "Don't you dare die on us, don't you dare." With people you don't know it's not that you care any less, but when it's someone you know, it brings it home that much closer. You looked so much better after you woke up. You really gave us a scare.

Arrangements had been made for my gastroscopy in the endoscopy room adjacent to the emergency room. Both of my associates had arrived and the endoscopy nurse told me that everything was ready. I really didn't want any sedation for, after all, hadn't I been colonoscoped without any medication? I wanted to know just what was going on and be aware of what was happening since I was so used to being involved in decision making.

During the procedure I became uncomfortable and was given intravenous Demerol. Gastroscopy was not bad except for the unpleasant sensation in my throat and the nausea from air being insufflated into my stomach as the procedure progressed.

I tried to concentrate on being somewhere else and to think of something pleasant, which is what I had always told my patients to do when I was endoscoping on them. It did work to some degree to lessen the discomfort, but having Nancy, our endoscopy nurse, hold my hand and put her arm around my shoulder and comfort me had an even greater therapeutic benefit.

"It's just a very small deep ulcer in the duodenal bulb," one of my associates told me. I said to myself, "My luck, such a tiny ulcer, why did it have to be so strategically located and erode into a vessel?" Now the gastroscopy was concluded and the instrument had been removed. By this time I was diaphoretic again and my systolic blood pressure had gone down to 70, probably due to some vagal reaction.

I am not sure whether my two associates were more distressed about this episode than I was. After conferring, they told me that they had decided to transfuse me with two units of blood because I had had such a significant reaction to my blood loss and my hematocrit was low. I told them, "You are not going to give me any blood—forget it." They insisted, and I finally agreed after much discussion. Now for the first time I was starting to take on the role of "patient."

From the emergency room I was admitted to the intensive care unit for observation. Therapy consisted of intravenous Tagamet and frequent antacids; blood was being drawn every six hours, and my vital signs were being monitored continuously. I really thought that the Tagamet could have been given orally without the addition of the antacids and that I could have my blood drawn every 12 hours instead of every six hours, but I decided not to say anything, and I had settled into becoming the model patient. There were no special requests on my part, and I did exactly everything I was told to do. In fact, the nurses told me what an excellent patient I was. There was no question, in my mind, that I was receiving extra attention and that this certainly made my stay there that much easier to tolerate.

For one of the few times in my adult life, I felt that I was being taken care of completely. Everything was being provided for my care. I did not have to make any decisions or take any responsibility for my thoughts or actions. It was an especially good feeling to be cared for, and secretly I still cherish those days that I spent in the hospital although not the reason why I had to be there.

As a physician, it seemed that the decision making and responsibility never ended for me. Even when I was not on call, there was always the concern about whether a patient was doing well, if I had overlooked any specific diagnosis or therapy that was essential, and whether there had been any complications to the procedure that had been performed. When the end of the day would come and I would arrive home, I continued to feel like a caretaker and a problem solver and sometimes I would feel that this responsibility was overwhelming me.

The question has often been asked about how one physician chooses another one to be his doctor and take care of his medical needs. In the case of my acute bleed, the answer was quite simple since I knew that I would contact my associates. I had worked with them for years and knew how competent they were and that I would be in the best of hands with this specific problem.

A surgeon was brought in on consultation, which I readily agreed to because it was always my practice to have one available when the bleeding was of such an acute and severe nature. I was not really concerned that I would need surgery since this was my first bleeding episode and I felt quite comfortable having him see me. The surgeon was a long-time friend and colleague; I chose him because I had worked with him for almost 20 years and I was extraordinarily confident of his skills. I also knew that he was conservative and that he had good clinical judgment, which was rather comforting to me since I was now the patient.

During my brief hospitalization, a number of my fellow physicians came by to say hello or visit with me. As I looked back, it was interesting to reflect upon the behavior of my colleagues. I appreciated those who just stopped by the door to ask very briefly about my welfare. It is amazing how such a simple gesture can take on such significance when you are now the patient. Some of them would step inside the room and stand by the bedside to make their inquiries and then move on. For a long time I had been aware of a study that compared patients' perceptions of how long their doctor spent with them when they stood by the bedside. Although the time spent in the study was exactly the same, the patient always perceived that more time was spent when the physician sat. The significant conclusion drawn from that study was that because it was perceived that the physicians had spent more time when sitting, it was also perceived that they were more interested and concerned about the welfare of their patients.

Indeed, I noticed that those visitors who sat at my bedside and chatted with me seemed to be spending more time with me and I felt that they were more interested in my well-being. I had always made it a practice to sit with my patients at the bedside, and after being in this position myself, I heartily endorse this type of patient visit because it creates a much more intimate physician–patient relationship and one of caring concern.

After discharge I remained away from the office another ten days and was out a total of only two weeks. Since my illness was really uncomplicated and readily diagnosed and treated, my recovery proceeded without any problems. Treatment was quite straightforward since I was in no pain or discomfort, and generally I felt confident I would make a complete and uneventful recovery.

My thoughts and plans about the future started to take form during this time. The unexpected forced respite from my practice gave me time to review my life—past, present, and future. Although there is no concrete evidence that stress plays a role in the pathogenesis of ulcers, it was taking its toll upon me in other ways and I knew that stress had to be diminished.

My two associates had already told me they would take all my calls for another month after my return to the office to ensure my full recovery. During this time, I continued to see patients in the office but was relieved of the burden of night and weekend coverage. I appreciate to this day their thoughtfulness and concern about my welfare.

In some way that was acceptable to both of my associates, I wanted to reduce some of my work load. Not only was I seeing the same number of patients as the others, but our on-call schedule was also equally divided. However, I had, from the beginning, managed most of the financial and business aspects of our practice, which had grown significantly over the years. I always had to bring some paperwork and problems home to solve in spite of carrying the same patient load as the others.

My request for minor changes in the night call schedule was rejected, and I felt both angered and hurt by this. I could see it from their point of view, but I felt that I was being fair and that my request was not unreasonable or without good cause. They did not seem to realize, as I did, that they could be afflicted by some illness or involved in some accident even at their younger ages. The problem will eventually be resolved, and meanwhile my office load has been reduced to allow me to take care of the other practice responsibilities. One thing that I did gain from my illness was to become more mellow and understanding of the viewpoints of others, but I must admit it has not been an easy lesson to learn.

Aside from the dramatic and acute onset of my illness, it was certainly not as serious as many of the other episodes related in this book. There has been no long-term impairment or consequences, but now the crucial question arose of how this event has reshaped and affected my life, and most important, what have I learned from this experience.

I have been greatly affected by what happened to me, perhaps out of proportion to the illness itself. But then, all of us respond differently to events in our lives, and my reaction may be because of where I view myself in my medical career and my life cycle at this time. Even prior to the bleeding episode, I had been plotting new directions in my life and reorienting my goals.

When one has built a highly successful and respected practice, received accolades and honors, material things take on much less meaning and importance. But what is important to me now is the direction my life will take, having been influenced by this event. I have come to terms with death and have become even more aware of how fragile life is. We all live our lives as though they will continue forever and death will come to others but never to us. The fantasy no longer exists for me. This realization has had some positive aspects to it. Life now has taken on a new and richer meaning, and I have learned to live it more fully and in the present, not regretting and reliving the past and constantly planning for the tomorrow that I know is promised to no man. How meaningful today has now become. How much more I can savor the experiences of these days and put everything into a more proper perspective.

Life goes on without any of us, although there is no question that the immediate family feels the loss greatly when we are taken from them. Practices continue and patients are still cared for as our presence and need seem to slowly fade as time passes. Physicians deal with death on a daily basis, and even though we think we are aware of our mortality, we really are not until we have had our own encounter with death, no matter how briefly.

We all make resolutions about how we will change, and yet we still tend to drift back into our old ways and old habits of rushing about, getting caught up in material things, and being so concerned about trivia that will be meaningless in a few days. How does one continue to maintain a proper perspective of life when old ways die so hard? We are ever so slow to change, but by reflecting upon what has taken place, our new direction can be maintained and our new roads continue to be traveled.

A patient once said to me, "I wish every physician could experience an illness, not too serious, but serious enough to know what it is like to be a patient." That statement has taken on significant meaning and importance, for I now view the patient–doctor relationship quite differently.

I believe that I am now a more compassionate and understanding physician, better able to view my patients' illnesses with greater empathy. No longer am I treating diseases, but rather I am now treating people who are unique with specific needs and different responses to their illness. Practice has become more enjoyable and rewarding, not in material ways, but in a richer personal satisfaction in what I am doing. I don't have "burnout" and the feeling of disillusionment with medicine that I hear so many of my colleagues talk about in the doctors' lounges.

I am still excited about new technologic advances in medicine and enjoy mastering the new material and techniques, for this does bring with it not only personal satisfaction but the knowledge that I can treat my patients better. I am so much more aware, however, of the "art of medicine" and realize how the art has been almost lost to, and overshadowed by, the "science of medicine" these days. The new direction that I have chosen in medicine is to learn more about "becoming a better practitioner of, and teacher of humanism." The eloquently stated words of Francis W. Peabody,[1] "Nothing is more important in the care of the patient than caring for the patient," have taken on a very personal meaning for me.

One other area that requires some comment is the question of revealing to our colleagues, patients, and acquaintances the details about our illness or even the fact that we were ill at all. I have not been reluctant to share my experience with others; I went so far as to write an open letter to our hospital administrator that appeared in the weekly newsletter about what I experienced and my appreciation to those who had cared for me:

> Dear Jim:
>
> I want you to know how special I feel Phoenix Baptist Hospital is. When I saw it from the other side, as a patient, I got an entirely different perspective of things.
>
> Fortunately, I was in the right place at the right time when I collapsed in the Emergency Room. My resuscitation and treatment were handled with the utmost expertise by Dr. S and the ER people to whom I am very much indebted. As I was lying there, I thought that there was no place where I could feel as comfortable and confident that I was getting the best medical care as in our ER.
>
> I have to say the same thing for the time that I spent in the Intensive Care Unit where everyone treated me so well and again I had that feeling that I was in an environment where I could relax completely knowing that if I did get into trouble that things would be handled expeditiously and with expertise.
>
> My very warmest thanks to everyone at the hospital who was involved with my care.
>
> Sincerely,

Physicians, all too often, because they feel compelled to maintain an image of always being strong and stable, deny their own vulnerability and needs. It is no shame to say that we are also human and have our weaknesses and imperfections. Our humanness makes us better physicians, and I am pleased to share that newly discovered quality with my patients, colleagues, and friends. I know now that I will not pass this way again, that my journey will be what I make it, and it will be better because of what I have experienced.

REFERENCE

1. F.W. Peabody, "The Care of the Patient," *Journal of the American Medical Association* 88 (1927); pp. 877–882; 252 (1984); pp. 813–818.

PART VIII

AIDS

CHAPTER 50

AIDS

STEPHEN K. YARNELL

One last thing, my son, be warned that writing books involves endless hard work, and that much study wearies the body.

—Ecclesiastes

"The physician is concerned (unlike the naturalist)...with a single organism, the human subject, striving to preserve its identity in adverse circumstances."[1] How is it when you are both the subject and object of concern? When you experience firsthand the striving to preserve oneself and bear the burden of the injunction "Physician heal thyself"?

Writing about the experience is hard work, and, being ill, my body is easily wearied. I wrote this account over a period of weeks—10 to 15 minutes at a time. Be warned that during this process, I was aware of neurologic deterioration manifest as a mild nomic aphasia associated with abnormal swings of moods. My ability to attend to the task and report the events may well be mildly to moderately impaired. With these caveats in mind, let me start, for want of a better place, in the middle.

A psychiatrist with a busy, hospital-based practice (on call every other night, every other weekend) does not have many opportunities to get away. So when a good friend, a dermatologist, asked my lover, Tom, and me to come and spend the weekend at his Palm Springs home, we jumped at the opportunity. The Friday morning of our weekend, I had an appointment with Dr. V., chief of an AIDS Clinic in San Francisco, to review my concerns about AIDS. I had gone to see

DR. STEPHEN YARNELL is a 43-year-old physician disabled for the past year. His community-based private practice of psychiatry was well developed prior to his illness. He had a clinical appointment with the University of California and was elected chief of psychiatry in his community hospital; the year before becoming ill, he was selected medical director for a new 20-bed behavioral science unit of the hospital.

him because I was in a high-risk group and several months earlier, I had developed herpes zoster. I approached the hospital with a mixture of dread and nostalgia, dread that I might be ill and nostalgia because I had trained as a student in the very same building that now housed the AIDS Clinic. I was made even more anxious by the efforts of the staff to make the clinic resemble a gay bar. The clerical staff wore outrageous clothes and earrings. The walls were postered with comical pictures of drag queens. As the medical procedures of taking my temperature, blood pressure, height, and weight progressed, I calmed myself. These latter things were familiar and comforting to me.

The exam room was stark 1940s. Dr. V., reassuringly normal in appearance, gave me a clean bill of health—no sign of the changes that precede the development of AIDS, not even ARC, he said. He told me not to worry and not to return. My feet had wings as I left the clinic, an animal escaping the abattoir and the smell of death.

We flew to Palm Springs, had dinner, and went to bed early. I was tired. The next day, I felt lazy and it was hot—I felt hot. I rested! Soon I realized I was feverish. I said little to our hosts and even tried playing tennis. I thought I had "the flu."

Monday, I called and made an appointment with Dr. O., my internist. I saw him the next day and reported my fever and general fatigue. He, too, thought it might be a viral "flu" and recommended rest, fluids, and Tylenol. For the next ten days, I took Tylenol and aspirin every three hours around the clock. I lost weight. I was off work (for one of the longest periods I can remember). My fever continued at 102° to 104°. I was sweating, shaking with chills, weak, and sick. I saw Dr. O. again.

On the first day of the two-day work-up, he sent me for X-ray, blood work, and induced sputum. A bronchoscopy was scheduled for 10:00 the following morning. I carried a morning sputum sample with me to the hospital. My parents came with me since I was too weak to drive my car. I was admitted to the outpatient surgery suite, NPO since midnight.

At 10:00 a.m. I was told that the procedure was delayed. At 11:00 a.m. I heard the nurse talking on the phone with Dr. O., I understood he would be in to see me at 1:00 p.m. I inferred that the sputum was positive for *Pneumocystis carinii* pneumonia (PCP) and that the bronchoscopy was not needed. My temperature was up. I asked for a Tylenol suppository. I resented the delay so that he could tell me in person. Why did I have to wait two hours NPO if there was to be no test? I didn't mention it because I remembered that doctors are thought of as the most critical patients, and I was afraid of making the nurses angry. But now I think it is important to emphasize the physical comfort of the patient.

Dr. O. told me the diagnosis—AIDS. He outlined treatment options for PCP and I elected to be treated at home with a 21-day course of Trimethoprim and Dapsone. I live in a two-story house with the bedrooms on the second floor. Dr. O. recommended buying a refrigerator for the bedroom because he predicted that I would become too weak to climb the stairs. My companion, Tom, fed me morning, noon, and night. I continued to lose weight. Nauseated, vomiting, and burning with rash from the medications, I learned how good phenothiazines are firsthand as I took Compazine suppositories alternating with Tigan. I listened to KJAZ, slept, and waited to get better. A month passed.

A social worker came to the house and took the information for my Social Security application. My father, loving as always, helped me through the interview as I lay in bed. He helped me with other forms as well—insurance, disability, etc. I had done these same forms for patients a thousand times, but now I couldn't do them—I was too weak. I couldn't drive my car. I couldn't make my bed. My mother cooked and brought food for me to eat. "Eat, eat," she would say, "you have to gain weight."

My mother and father were both emotionally upset. They had not discussed my gay life-style with me. The illness proved the final key for me as a closeted gay man. I found I had to struggle to maintain my identity. My resistance to well-meaning suggestions that I move "home" with them for care caused them angry feelings. My mother was quick to blame Tom and was initially hostile toward him. My mother, my father, Tom, and I had to rework our relationships with one another in a crisis climate.

The crisis initially focused on physical recovery but soon changed to a focus on treatment. My physician friends all had recommendations and suggestions. Experimental medication trials were on the news and in the newspaper. Dr. V. was the key for the West Coast as director of research for San Francisco.

I returned to see Dr. V. with high hopes that I might participate in a research program. He was sorry I was ill, but the research subjects had already been selected and all the programs of experimental treatment were filled. He told me there was no treatment option and I should wait for the results of the research. I might be treated later.

I talked with Dr. O., who suggested I write to Dr. Y. at NIH and volunteer for toxicity trials of newer drugs. Dr. Y. wrote back saying that I should again contact Dr. V. for AZT trials ongoing and that he would file my letter. I talked with my colleagues, who suggested many alternatives, but each was a blind alley. There was no treatment. The use of ribavirin, illegal in the United States, was discouraged by both Drs. O. and V.

I had not worked for over a month. My associates at work covered my practice as best they could, but it was too much. I tried to get a locum tenens coverage through a major firm; I discovered that it would cost more than my practice generated just to pay the fees of the firm and then I was expected to provide transportation and housing to the locum. I couldn't afford it.

My professional associate, Dr. P., and I agreed to find a psychiatrist to buy my practice and/or cover the patients' needs. A variety of people were suggested, contacts made, and my practice sold with the proviso that I could return if my health improved. Every person I shared the problem with was supportive and helpful. My professional colleagues called and expressed concern, offering to do anything they could. I was in daily contact with my loving secretary, Alice, who was a trooper throughout. She helped patients to get the emergency treatment they needed while the new doctor came on board.

I was initially very depressed. I cried and felt sorry for myself. I went to see a psychiatrist, who told me that my reactions were normal and predicted that I would improve. I did. Denial took over, my depression diminished, and I began to read science fiction to escape.

Work expands to fill all the available time—files need organizing, mail needs to be sorted and answered. At first, 10 to 15 minutes was all that I could spend before pain and exhaustion stopped me. But I was driven by the fear that no one but me could possibly sort through all the papers from my personal and professional life. My office paperwork was dumped in my dining room—for months we have eaten in the kitchen.

Christian Science and salvationist nostrums suddenly appeared. Friends urged church attendance. The articles on alternative health care suggested "A Course in Miracles"—I bought it while on vacation in Sun Valley. I started a group with other AIDS patients, studying "the course" (Christian Science dressed up as divine revelation to a professor of psychology). My cousin Emily, a math teacher, went with me to spiritual churches. She even took me to see her acupuncturist. Although there was a genuine increased interest in spiritual matters, I couldn't abandon the rational belief system developed over years of time. I was shaken and I needed support to maintain a rational perspective. I began attending the First Unitarian Church.

The Unitarian Universalist's humanist faith is one I accepted in college, and this church is one that can accept me as I am. I had stopped going when I moved from Berkeley, but I found comfort in going again. In a small group of persons joining the church, I found that my story was much like theirs. They were joining because of a loss or a feeling of isolation and dissatisfaction with their previous churches.

I was pleased to discover that the first meeting for me of the Hemlock Society was scheduled in my church. Again, the Unitarians support the exploration of liberal ideas that many find abhorrent. For me, the discussion of legislation that would decriminalize assisting at ethical suicide was uplifting. I wanted that freedom for myself if the disease process became intolerably painful.

Politics in California are always bizarre—Proposition 64 (LaRouche) would provide for isolation and quarantine of HIV positive persons on the basis that the disease is easily transmitted by casual contact. This is not true according to accepted medical authority. My efforts were to raise money to defeat the initiative. Every day the paper carried articles about AIDS and my interest turned to the articles as well as the weekly publications, *The New England Journal of Medicine* and *Science*, where I looked for the announcement of "the cure."

Afraid of infection, I fear the birds (TB, cryptosporidia), the cats (toxoplasmosis), my dog, my horse (mycoplasma avium), and people. For weeks I was reluctant to leave the house. I didn't ride my horse for several months. Walking in the park or at the beach was unpleasant because of the birds. My doctors gave contradictory advice—Dr. O. said to get rid of all the animals. Dr. V. said it didn't matter and enjoy what life I had left. My cousin asked if I couldn't get a bubble like the bubble boy. I chose to insulate and add central heat to the house so that I might be more comfortable in the coming winter. Chairs and rugs were sent to be cleaned. New labels were put on the old files. New files, labeled funeral, disability insurance payments, AIDS research, personal health, etc., were made in attempt to maintain control and organization.

Dr. P. suggested an analogy: I was like a ship that had been torpedoed and was in the process of sinking. As captain of the crew, my efforts were to maintain order and control the process if I could. Stumbling blocks I found particularly hard: The drugs recommended by my treating physicians were illegal in the United States and either I or my friends had to become criminals to bring them across the Mexican border. Experimental drugs shown to be helpful in early studies were not available and the process of becoming available has a schedule that is agonizingly slow once your remaining life is measured in months. In discussing my thoughts regarding ethical suicide, my doctor was reluctant to support me and asked that I not discuss it further with him. Laboratory studies continued to document a slow but progressive decline in T cells and granulocytes (white blood cells). My skin refused to respond to antigenic compounds. Throughout I feared that I might be doing something I should not be doing or that I was neglecting to do something that might make me better. There was little in the medical literature that was encouraging. Most articles were directed at protecting others from infection and assumed the deaths of all diagnosed with AIDS. Issues that previously held little interest for me now loomed large. Should I be buried? Would cremation be better? If so, are ashes better scattered or stored where family and friends can visit. Since I was not raised with a rigid faith, these questions are difficult to answer. That it doesn't matter is not a sufficient answer in the face of the reality of one's own imminent death. Who should have what remains behind? Family, of course, but what about friends? What about a lover for the past seven years who has no legal standing? Writing a will is very important. My will was written for the first time. I know I should have done it earlier, but I never got around to it. Also, a living will for the physicians caring for me and a durable power of attorney for my lover are important aids in maintaining a sense of responsible control over the events leading up to death.

Death is not so fearsome. To die in pain with a loss of dignity is what I fear. To die with loose ends is a problem. How do you prepare your taxes in advance? Just as I tidy up the deck garden on those days I'm well enough, I want to die cleanly and in a tidy manner. Do people send funeral notices? Should I write my own obituary and file it so that it will be ready for the papers? Where and what ceremony is appropriate?

The key factor about AIDS is that it is relatively slow. Lewis Carroll said of Alice falling into the well, "Either the well was very deep, or she fell very slowly, for she had plenty of time as she went down to look about her, and to wonder what was going to happen next."[2] There is plenty of time to reflect and think about the process, the events, the feelings involved. I am told I am dying, but there is no hurry about it.

Let me digress and return to a point of departure nearer the beginning. Some biographical information might help to frame the experience. I am the oldest of three sons. My father is a retired accountant. My mother and father have been married for 44 years. One of my brothers is 4 years younger than I am. He and his wife are artists. Another brother, 5 years younger, is finishing a residency in radiology at Hershey Medical Center. After taking his Ph.D. in chemistry at Stanford and working in the chemical industry for several years, he decided to become a physician. My brothers and their wives have been encouraging and supportive. I am a native Californian, born in Sacramento. I completed undergraduate training at Berkeley with honors in 1965. Medical school at the University of California San Francisco campus led to graduation with honors in 1969. Residency training at the Langley Porter Institute in San Francisco followed a medical internship at UCLA. At every step in my education, I was honored and respected.

The early days of practice were equally rewarding and fulfilling. On the basis of advice from the AMA, I began working in a suburb about 30 minutes from the city of San Francisco. Over several years, I became integrated into the medical community where I practiced. The local hospital served as a focal point for my involvement. Most rewarding was participation on the long-range planning committee of the hospital. A small group of friendly physicians and I formed a partnership and built a modern office building on the campus of the hospital. The hospital was redesigned. A new wing in psychiatry was opened and I became a medical director. My career was successful and secure.

My companion, Tom, is a registered engineer. We have lived together for seven years. Our sexual activity has been confined to our relationship. He is antibody negative. How it turned out this way, we have no idea. One explanation is that I was exposed before we met, and I have been carrying the disease since that time.

Both of us were frightened when the magnitude of the disease was first recognized. As a physician, I had a clear picture of the risks and I conveyed them to Tom. Although AIDS is a rare disease in the general population, in the circle of gay friends it rapidly became the primary cause of death, with a frequency far exceeding anything previously known. Every week or two, another friend was taken ill or died. This cast a pall over the dinner and cocktail parties in our community.

At first we avoided contact with persons with AIDS; the cause was unknown. It was reasonable to think that it was a transmissible agent. We were frightened. Later, when it was clear that casual contact could not transmit the newly identified viral agent known to cause the disease, we were able to spend time with friends who were sick.

One of my clearest memories is of a psychiatric consultation. I was called to see a young woman at the hospital. The internist, a specialist in infectious disease, thought that she was psychiatrically disordered. Her voice was "too loud" and her complaints didn't make any sense. I consulted and concluded that there was no psychiatric illness. I urged the internist to expand the work-up and include AIDS as a result of transfusion as a possibility. The tests were positive.

There was little I could do to help this woman with her psychiatric pain. She was unable to identify with the openly gay support groups available and felt isolated and alone. Her husband and family were frightened of the disease. I was frightened as well. I observed firsthand her decline and subsequent death. Throughout, I felt that this could be me; a year later it was me.

Looking back, I was the first to recognize that I was ill. I reacted as a physician. I studied the disease. I consulted colleagues more expert than myself. I selected for my treatment the best physicians in the area. By these well-worn habits, I was protected from the feelings of helplessness and hopelessness that lay in wait for me in my darker hours.

The physician's enemy is disorder. Maintaining control of life is his objective and, if that becomes impossible, control of death holds out the promise of victory over the forces of disorder and decay. Spiritual, emotional, and practical support from a community of family, friends, and professionals is all that counts. At the end as at the beginning, I am a human being in need of help from other human beings. My greatest joy is the increasing recognition of what others do for me out of love and respect. If this is what it means to find God for the humanist, then it isn't too late for me.

REFERENCES

1. Ivy McKenzie, quoted in Oliver Sacks, *The Man Who Mistook His Wife for a Hat and Other Clinical Tales* (New York: Simon & Schuster, 1985).
2. Lewis Carroll, *Alice's Adventures in Wonderland* (New York: Bantam Books, 1865).

EPILOGUE

The stories you have read here were not easy to collect. We doctors write case histories every day, but we rarely write stories about our patients, and too few of us write about our own illnesses. There are a few exceptions: an occasional portrayal in the *British Medical Journal*, *Lancet*, or *New England Journal of Medicine*. The most notable predecessor to this volume is the Miller and Pinner book, which appeared in 1947.[1] That book deserves rereading, although some of it is curiously dated in the 1980s, as if the viewpoints of physicians have altered almost as dramatically as the technology that supports them. Many of the writers in Miller and Pinner were psychiatrists, and some of the richest accounts in this book were also written by psychiatrists or those who had found help from them during their illness.

What doctors learn when they are sick and what they have told us in this book may help to improve the care we give and how we live as doctors. What our writers have not said has made the editors wonder about how the medical schools train students and house officers to give clinical care.

We have looked in these stories also for clues to how we may, somehow, come to terms with illness and disability, retirement, and impending death. For we share the idea of psychiatrist and poet that in all of us the fear of death is suppressed so that we can take joy in our life. Doctors may have that fear more strongly than most and repress it the best, which may be why they went into medicine. But it is always there, and illness frees it faster for the doctor than for most. If you disagree with this notion, reread the paper by Fox.

For most physicians, illness and disease have become such everyday experiences that there seems no reason to write up anything but its science. The tradition that led our predecessors to shun public expression of personality or grievance has only recently been discarded, but anecdotes are meaningless, too many still feel, and the personal story in newspaper or magazine seems eccentric or self-seeking. From the patient we extract the case. The sonogram shows the flow of blood but not the real heart. Only recently has the old idea come to life again that every person is his own poem, every life has a story. The stories in this book, which we have used as takeoffs for discussions with medical students, offer a contribution to the idea that life is a narrative, that each of us has a story and lives it—even if we cannot always express it.

There is a more practical reason why physicians so rarely write about getting sick. Practicing physicians usually need to maintain an aura of perfection, for the doctor who talks about being sick may lose his practice. Reliability and availability are key. The powerful chairman of an academic internal medicine department knew that having a myeloma took away his future: He could not be counted on to be there.[2] "My previous inborn sense of immortality [was] totally destroyed...the school leaders...also discounted my future....I had no future, the present was in disarray, and even my professional past, which had been the background for the work I was doing and was about to do more of, was made to look wasted." To play the role of healer, the practicing physician must seem immune to disease, a healer who will always be there.

Most healthy physicians are unlikely writers. More often, it is the alienated or the few whose creative impulses have been awakened by illness who write. Most of the time doctors view themselves like cars to be repaired. Find the structural defect, get the best doctor there is to repair it, and you will go another hundred thousand miles. Many of our physician-patient writers show such firm reliance on technology. The relief that comes from knowing—seeing—comes out most strongly in radiologists whose professional lives revolve around the depiction of disease, but surgeons, too, share that frenzy for a specific organic depiction of their troubles so it can be cut out.

The idea of body as machine, that interest in science over humanities, which permeates many of these stories, comes from our training and from our selection for medical school. Our grades in science and our ambition got us into medical school; achievement and energy count for more in that process than any tendency to introspection. Once in medical school, even philosophers and artists learn to measure, not to conjecture, to act and not to reflect. The pace in medical school and in professional life seldom leaves time for contemplation. Even away from the sick, medical research is almost always benchwork, creating, working with the latest recombinant DNA techniques. Armchair reflection in medicine is usually preceded by apology and rarely supported by grants; the macho ethos of medicine calls for doing, not for thinking. We are too familiar with suffering and learn too much about our fellows to let our imagination run, for if we did, we might never return to hospital or office. Richard Selzer, the surgeon, can find the mystic and poetic, even the bizarre, in his everyday work, but surgery does not call for so much imagination and Richard has retired to write. There is little poetry in doctors' accounts of their own illnesses because most physicians find little poetry in medicine. In love with health, we find no good in our enemy, which is disease. We have only to conquer. Cellular biology tells us that we are twists and turns in our DNA and RNA, that diseases are only pyrimidine bases misplaced. Clinical emphasis on *seeing* disease on videotape or hard copy underlines the definition of health as the perfect functioning of organs, each properly contributing to the body in a kind of healthy fascism. But people suffer in their minds, not in their microsomes. Doctors first learn that lesson when they are sick, a lesson that medical school and postgraduate training so seldom teach.

Doctors are often difficult patients, as these stories so readily attest, and as anyone who has ever taken care of another doctor will agree. Although they turn hypochondriacal in medical school, most doctors later postpone as long as possible any idea that they are sick, for most physicians learn to believe themselves invulnerable. As medical students, fearing one illness after another, we learn that most of our fears will not be borne out, that what looks like a wart will not prove a melanoma. But what erects the defenses of the physician at 25 may no longer hold true at 50.

Denial is also fostered by the attitude of many physicians toward their impaired colleagues.[3] The isolation of the academic physician with amyotropic lateral sclerosis[4] might seem idiosyncratic were it not for parallels in so many other accounts. Physicians recovering from alcoholism or other illness comment that silence has been the most common reaction of colleagues: "I didn't tell and they didn't ask." As we have told some of these stories to audiences of physicians and medical students, we have been struck by how often a physician has come up to comment vigorously on the sick doctor. Who puts up those signs, "No Visitors"? Outside the doctor's room they are like the bell of the leper proclaiming isolation. Why we doctors keep silent when a colleague is sick or getting old needs more discussion. Is it only that they give us a glimpse of ourselves? Denial comes from the defenses of invulnerability, the trained responses of medical school, and the distance of our colleagues.

Donning the hospital gown turns doctors into patients. Just as putting on a white coat as a third-year medical student symbolized entry into our mysteries, so the hospital gown stands for exile. The white coat provides a symbol of power and the hospital gown open at the back teaches more humility than even being on the other end of a proctoscope. It is the final surrender to patienthood, the beginning of what Hahn has called the "rituals of depersonalization."[5]

The trained detachment of our profession has a part in the physician's reaction to his or her own illness. We cannot allow ourselves to get involved with our patients. A young woman about to undergo a bone marrow transplant for leukemia after treatment of Hodgkin's disease, a patient for seven years, asked her new university physician, a kind man, to "Call me Roberta." "No," he said, "you are Mrs. S. and I am Dr. R." As we leave one sickroom, we physicians enter another. If you get too close, a little bit of you dies with each patient. Yet too rehearsed and too repeated, that protecting distance can become our manner and that manner becomes ourselves.

Denial comes out as detachment and both may lead to isolation, as these stories often show. The endocrinologist with amyotropic lateral sclerosis who had decided on a strategy to avoid disclosure of his illness, fearing that its disclosure would destroy his professional life, later lamented the isolation that ensued.[4] "I have received relatively few telephone calls or letters from the scores of colleagues I have met in more than 20 years of academic life." A colleague who died in Connecticut not too long ago told only his barber how sad he was that his colleagues avoided him. But we never knew whether his isolation came from his denial or the sorrow we could not face because we could not talk to him.

That otherwise very sensitive physician with myeloma doubted that anyone can understand the patient.[2] "Physicians and nurses, however much they strive to understand the total patient, may only comprehend something of his brain. . . . It is more difficult to get into a patient's heart. . . . It is impossible for a physician to reach inside a patient's soul. . . . No one can fully understand how the patient feels about his predicament. . . ." After so many years of teaching others how to take care of patients, he had no confidence that anyone can know the heart and soul of another. Empathy for him was a metaphor, not a reality.

How doctors react to being sick depends upon many factors, whether they are young or old, family doctor or specialist, practitioner or academician, and whether the disease is chronic or acute, potentially fatal or just a chronic burden. Of importance is whether the disease occurred before or after medical school. The youngster who has been chronically ill brings different conceptions with him to medical school. Some of the patients with inflammatory bowel disease in this volume keep statistics, as if for them the good life was not baseball but enemas.

What did that routine do to their concept of medical practice? of themselves?

In this book you have seen how most sick doctors try hard to be "good" patients and not to complain. Many of us physicians no longer know how to deal with emotion in patients or in ourselves. The good patient is docile, he may suffer, but he does not complain. The impersonal nature of our hospitals and offices reaffirms that message. It is so much easier to examine the X-ray or scan than to listen to the patient or to tell him that he may suffer. Controlled trials reinforce the foolish idea that all doctors are equivalent, that only the procedure or drug changes, an individual is only one of a series, Auden reminds us. A person is unique.

The equanimity that doctor-patients try to portray sometimes seems a pose. Physicians know the complications; we are aware of the disasters. Occasionally we doctor-patients rebel, cry out, leave the hospital early, or ask for second or third opinions. That special sense of fear remains and summons denial. But most doctors who are sick try to suffer in silence even if our knowledge makes us worry more than others. Try as we may to be "good," doctors are sometimes "bad" patients because we know the worst. The general surgeon with regional enteritis is more depressed than most because he has seen only the extremes of perforation, obstruction, and abscess.

Many modern physicians ignore symptoms for more objective evidence of disease. They have little patience for minor complaints that provide information less reliable than the hard copy of image or laboratory number. But when they fall sick, from the new perspective of patient, most doctors are delighted to discover new diagnostic clues in their own symptoms. They learn how a patient feels and a doctor reacts.

Yet sick doctors are lonely behind those No Visitors signs. They are always on watch, vigilant for what they know can, and does, go wrong. On guard to protect themselves, still they try hard to pretend to be the good patients that doctors want. For they know that just as they are watching, their colleagues are watching them. It is not easy to be a doctor and a patient all at once, as so many of these stories show.

When the sick doctor finally looks for help, the doctor taking care of him or her finds no easy task. The doctor-patient usually thinks he knows the diagnosis, even if it is the wrong one. Ordinary patients have confidence in their physician's skill, but the medical training of physician-patients gets in their way. They never really accept, never really are given, the chance to be just a patient. Moreover, for the doctor's doctor there is always a sense of fraternity, an immediate merger of identities with physicians. We know him or her. We know what he or she wants and knows. They know what we know and what we may hide from other patients. To talk of cancer chemotherapy with the physician who has studied, and even understood, the literature is to find that the net of hope we spread under other patients has holes we cannot patch.

That is a problem. Immediately the sick physician becomes us. We view his illness as our illness, we merge—as the psychoanalyst might put it—in a final confrontation with our own illness. Our past, our present, and our future confront us in the body of the sick physician. It is such a reversal of the natural order of things. Even reading about a doctor's travails with disease is different for a doctor from reading about what another patient might have to say, for we know the doctor understands what is going on better than the layman. He sees the present and the future all together. The physician-patient gives and takes the history, observer and observed, the quintessential whole person. Yet a kind of "doubling" takes place: He is a physician looking at himself as he might a patient, but he is the patient changing and stressing and modifying his sensations and reporting symptoms to portray what he thinks is going on. Whether the treating physician is honored at being consulted or threatened by someone who knows so much varies. How he responds to his feelings may influence whether he helps the physician-patient postpone diagnostic studies, to deny what is going on, or mobilizes too many studies in an effort to reassure him or her. Does the doctor-patient receive better or worse care for that? It is hard to be sure, but taking care of sick colleagues raises questions about whether doctors and patients can, or should, be friends, whether doctors should take gifts from patients, or whether bills should be sent, just as to any other patient.

For other people, getting sick is a mysterious amalgam of anxiety, fear, discomfort, and hope. When doctors get sick, the setting does not change, but they are suddenly on the other side of the doctor's desk. In the hospital the doctor lies on the bed, no longer standing beside it. The view has changed—and he is no longer in control. Yet the physician-patient wants to remain in control and the doctor's doctor knows it. The radiologist reads his own films, the gastroenterologist scrutinizes his cecum, with a little help. The physician trying to remain in control of his own care forgets the clouded judgment of the sick and how wrong their choices may be. That may be one reason why physicians travel so far to get "the best," so that they can finally give up control when they have made a choice. Yet that reliance on authority, on the "very best," lends itself to the overrating of the chosen doctor even as it absolves the doctor-patient of responsibility of getting better. The doctor who tries to control his own care and fails can then blame his physicians for the failings of his body—or of his spirit. "I put them in charge and they made mistakes."

Most doctor-patients stress the alienation of being a patient. Sacks remembered his months as a patient.[6] "But if I rejoiced in the blessing of the sun, I found I was avoided by the non-patients in the gardens—the students, nurses, visitors who came there. I was set apart, we were set apart, we patients in white nightgowns and avoided clearly, though unconsciously, like lepers. . . . I realized how I myself, in health, in the past, had shuddered away from patients quite unconsciously, never realizing it for a moment." Isolation grows even stronger when the patient has cancer. Sanes[7] found that "the patient with . . . cancer . . . faces social death, death as an active, contributing, accepted member of society...[a cancer patient] is already as good as dead." Others have the feeling that their colleagues continue to regard them as different even after they have recovered, for they had been tainted with the scent of death, the smell of weakness.

Guilt keeps the doctor-patient from rest far longer than it should. For work has been his life. We doctors define ourselves by our work and when things are not going right, we usually try to work harder than ever. Listen to a retired doctor answer the phone as "Dr. ______" and you will realize how vital to most of us is the identity of doctor. Is that more than habit? Over and over again in this volume sick doctors boast, "I was able to work," and recall how much pleasure they took in fulfilling their function. Yet to read how a physician barely able to get around continues his daily tasks is to wonder what all of us, his colleagues, were thinking. Some of the stories we have read, however inspiring to us as physicians, make us want to know that physically impaired physicians practice under some scrutiny.

Why don't sick doctors just stop working? It is more than expenses and income. Doctors are compulsive, with an exaggerated sense of responsibility; our helpfulness erects defenses against aggressiveness and feelings of worthlessness. Illness becomes something that has to be fought, particularly if our self-esteem grows only from being loved and needed. We need to keep working to be ourselves.

AUTONOMY, PATERNALISM, AND TRUTH TELLING

Autonomy may be lauded for modern patients, but it is not something sick physicians usually choose for themselves once they have found a doctor. Sick doctors want to be taken care of, even if they try to remain in control; we find the most relief when someone else takes over. Here we are, a group with special knowledge, and often trying to exert control beyond the bounds of reason, and yet almost to a man or woman sick doctors who express an opinion suggest that they want to be taken care of so that they can give up their lonely vigil. Most of them want to be cared for, have decisions made for them.

In the end, sick doctors must trust their doctors to make decisions for them, to be loyal to them. In that we may represent a special case, for it is so easy for doctors to identify with sick doctors that we are special patients, surer than most that our interests will be served. But that should surely be the goal of medical practice for all: to be so loyal to our patient's interests that we can make those right decisions.

Franz Ingelfinger's story is well known.[8] "I received from physician friends from throughout the country a barrage of well intentioned but contradictory advice....As a result not only I, my wife, my son and daughter-in-law (both doctors) and other family members became increasingly confused and emotionally distraught. Finally, when the pangs of indecision had become nearly intolerable, one wise physician friend said, 'What you need is a doctor.'...When that excellent advice was followed, my family and I sensed immediate and immense relief."

Paternalism is much demeaned these days, but we come away from the reading of these doctors' stories with a stronger conviction than ever[9] that the doctor who is loyal to the patient's cause, loyal to the patient's wishes, even if it must sometimes be as he imagines them to be, can bring more help, peace of mind, even, than the doctor who spreads his wares to let the patient choose, even than the doctor who holds the sick patient up as an equal partner. These stories often show that sick people have bad judgment.

The past decade has seen "telling the truth" sometimes seem more important for doctors than taking care of patients. But unvarnished truth is not always welcome to sick doctors, who prefer it covered by an ineluctable compassion. We want faith, hope, and kindness. We want to be taken care of. All sick doctors come down on the side of hope and optimism, consolation that recognizes how hard it is to know the truth. No one suggests that doctors should lie to their patients, but most of them seem to agree that hope, consolation, and an optimistic outlook can do no harm.

ADJUSTMENT TO ILLNESS

Does a physician become a "better person" after an illness? Getting sick gives doctors a taste of retirement, makes them face the empty time when, no longer active physicians, they will no longer be needed. Physicians do not seem to adjust to disease and disability more easily than others because of their special knowledge. Doctors are, after all, just like everyone else when we are sick. Maybe psychiatrists fare better; they are the only medical writers for whom the psyche is so explicit. Those physicians who have been to psychiatrists seem to derive a deeper and richer experience from having been sick. Yet when doctors get sick, they are as sorry for themselves as other patients, it appears. With so much professional experience in the blindness of fortune, doctors might be philosophical about the arrows of misfortune, but that only rarely proves true. Burdened with spiritual arrogance, we doctors spend our days working for others, receiving gratitude, money, and prestige. It is difficult to return home at night without feeling that we have served the Lord all day, and sometimes all night. Even if modern doctors regard themselves more as conduits of power than sources of healing, we react to the loss of authority.

Sometimes doctors reassess their goals and careers, their relationships to family and friends after illness, but that is not always true. Indeed, one of the problems with medical practice in the 1980s may be the strong hold that the medicomaterialist, engineer-scientist view has on us physicians. Many accounts of personal changes seem perfunctory. Many doctors recover and seem to return to their activities without any obvious self-assessment.

Do doctors become more compassionate after they have been sick? You can find almost any answer in this book. Doctors want compassion from their physicians even when they may not have shown it to their own patients. One recurrent theme is that "I was kind, with time to be compassionate to my own patients, explained and was helpful, but why is my physician not doing the same for me?" Although Nietzsche suggests that pity is not the emotion that most people want from their friends, our doctors crave compassion.

As few of our writers mentioned anything about doctor bills, they were unique among patients since they give, expect, and usually get professional courtesy. Rarely did they share the experience of other patients arriving home after hospitalization, tired but glad to be alive, only to start receiving bills from the internist, the cardiologist, the infectious disease consultant, the neurologist they didn't remember seeing, and then the surgeon, the first assistant, the anesthesiologist, and more. Payment to doctors for their services beyond insurance payments apparently never troubled any of our contributors.

SUMMING UP

In the end, the doctors' accounts of their own illnesses are just the beginning of our conversation. We have to bring our own interpretation, for while suffering may give strength to the philosophical, and illness creativity to the poet, sickness so threatens the physician's identity that we have to ponder how we can make the transition from doctor to patient, from doctor to person, even.

The experience of the modern physician is so much in the physical world and so little in the mind that talking about physician-patients may help to free us physicians from our own anxieties and fears, to give us a wider glimpse of ourselves. These stories provide texts for discussion not only of how to be a patient but of how to be a doctor.

The vigilance of the sick doctor in the hospital against what may go wrong suggests that we should examine hospital and office routines and that we should tell our own patients to be on their guard, to complain and question, even to call us on the phone from their beds if something does not seem right. In the era of DRGs, we doctors may even need to be patient-advocates against the medical economic system.

These stories show how isolated a sick doctor can be. Society gives us a high place, for we have special powers and can know the secrets of the heart. But the price may be loneliness, isolation by affluence and by self-importance. We need to find ways to make medical education more humanistic, to train physicians to become practitioners of an art as much as mechanics repairing machines. We doctors are only what our training has made us. Talking about the humanities, philosophy, and literature might remind us of how much beyond cellular mechanics our students need to learn. The humanities will not improve the technical care of our patients, but they may help to civilize that care. We must look for no final answers, but simply for conversations so that all of us who can take care of the sick can reflect instead of run.

We have not learned what makes the difference in how a doctor reacts to illness. Religion does not seem to help most physicians very much, but we may be a select group in that. Inborn nature, character, the premorbid personality may bring acceptance. Specific factors such as the age at getting sick or the age of one's children, all the accomplishments of ambition, are important. But to come to terms with illness, for doctors at least, seems to require letting go of the past and getting on with the future, regardless of regret for what might have been and how short that future may seem. For the young doctor, a chronic illness like ulcerative colitis can be grist for the mill, to use in the future. You can be more than just a patient. You may long for what you cannot have, you may rage against the doctor's pills, but you must go on. For the old with fatal disease, regrets for youth and health must not take the central place. "How do I want to spend the rest of my time?" is a more important question than, "Why did this happen to me?"

The surgeon Mack gives us clues.[10] Fifty years old, he had just been divorced when a small cancer was discovered in his right lung.

He paid no attention to the dismal prospect but thought a great deal and read Simonton. "I no longer saw myself as a person with cancer who had to struggle to survive day by day. I was well. I had lived through cancer and been cured. I had beaten it, and I no longer had to deal with the problem. Although I regretted the changes in my life that were necessitated by my limited postoperative lung function, I felt very fortunate." Denial perhaps, but his denial helped him to function, which is what we doctors want.

Even two years later when metastases in his bones required chemotherapy and more radiation, Mack would persist. "For the past three years I have taken a constant oral dose of methotrexate—25 mg every five days....I had become a patient with Stage III disease, with a very small chance of two years' survival...and virtually no chance of living for five years." But he was determined to live. "I could sit back and let my disease and my treatment take their course, or I could pause and look at my life and ask, What are my priorities? How do I want to spend the time that is left?...I became convinced that adding hope, love, and positive expectations and trying to shape a slower more gentle life could do no harm and might be beneficial." Mack does not deny his very real problems. "I get tired of taking pills, of bloody noses, mouth ulcers, and lack of energy. There are many days when I yearn to be out jogging, hiking the hills, or playing squash....I get tired of being frightened by each new symptom, feeling sorry for myself...[but] mostly I am grateful for all the choices I have made that allow me to rejoice in being alive."

The physicians who are sustained by an optimism that may seem illusory leave messages for those of us who remain for a while. Any physician, young or old, who can escape the self-concern of the sick, the ready solipsism that turns to selfishness, offers the best model.

You will have your own thoughts about these stories. The answers are not as important as the reflections and conversations about our patients and ourselves. One message from the sick doctors tells us that hope helps as much as truth, and that imagination, drama, passion, and even poetry are as important in medical practice as they are in the rest of life. The tales of sick doctors can temper our mechanical, knife-sharp abilities and certainties with more uncertainty and with civility. The sick doctors remind us that we are all links in a chain and that just as we are fathers and sons, mothers and daughters, we are doctors and will someday be patients, and that our lives run along a precipice that separates life from death.

REFERENCES

1. M. Pinner, and B. F. Miller, eds., *When Doctors Are Patients* (New York: W. W. Norton, 1952), p. 231.

2. S. Papper, "Care of Patients with Incurable, Chronic Neoplasm—One Patient's Perspective," *American Journal of Medicine* 78(1985), pp. 271–276.
3. J. N. Chappel, "Physician Attitudes toward Distressed Colleagues," *Western Journal of Medicine* 134(1981), pp. 175–180.
4. D. Rabin, P. L. Rabin, and R. Rabin, "Compounding the Ordeal of ALS—Isolation from My Fellow Physicians," *New England Journal of Medicine* 307(1982), pp. 506–509.
5. R. A. Hahn, "Between two worlds: Physicians as patients," *Medical Anthropology Quarterly* 16(1985), pp. 87–98.
6. O. Sacks, *A Leg to Stand On* (New York: Summit Books, 1984), p. 163.
7. S. Sanes, *A Physician Faces Cancer in Himself* (Albany: State University of New York Press, 1979).
8. F. I. Ingelfinger, "Arrogance," *New England Journal of Medicine* 303 (1980), pp. 1507–1511.
9. H. M. Spiro, "Loyalty as Guide," in *Doctors, Patients and Placebos* (New Haven: Yale University Press, 1986), p. 227.
10. R. M. Mack, "Lessons from Living with Cancer," *New England Journal of Medicine* 311(1984), pp. 1640–1644.

GLOSSARY

These are not dictionary definitions. They are explanations of medical terms and doctors' jargon.

ANAPHYLAXIS A sudden, dangerous collapse of the patient caused by sensitivity to a substance to which the patient has been exposed.

ANGINA PECTORIS Chest pain caused by diminished flow of blood to the heart muscle. It is usually brought about by exertion and relieved by rest.

ANGIOGRAPHY Injection of a radioopaque material into an artery for purposes of imaging. Helpful in determining location of obstructions of arteries.

ARRHYTHMIA Abnormal heart rhythm.

AVASCULAR NECROSIS OF THE HIP Sometimes seen as a complication of prednisone (steroid) therapy. It may require total hip replacement.

BETA BLOCKER A type of medication used in coronary artery disease, hypertension, and other disorders.

CALCIUM ANTAGONIST A type of medication used primarily in coronary artery disease and hypertension.

CEREBRAL CONCUSSION Loss of consciousness from a blow to the head.

CHEMONUCLEOLYSIS A new procedure in which a disc-dissolving substance is injected into a disc in an attempt to avoid surgery.

CLOMIPHENE A medication used to induce ovulation in women having difficulty becoming pregnant.

COLECTOMY Surgical removal of the large bowel.

COLONOSCOPY Direct vision of the large bowel by a long, flexible tube that has a light on one end and viewpiece on the other.

CPR Cardiopulmonary resuscitation.

CROHN'S DISEASE A chronic inflammatory disease of the small and large bowel. Its main symptoms may be diarrhea and pain. Its cause is unknown. Complications may lead to fistulas and intestinal obstruction.

D&C DILATATION AND CURETTAGE Removal of a part of the lining of the uterus for microscopic examination or to complete an incomplete miscarriage.

DIAZEPAM Generic name of Valium.

DIC-(DISSEMINATED INTRAVASCULAR COAGULATION) A dreaded disorder of the blood-clotting mechanism that can occur in several clinical settings.

DUCK A hand-held container for men to use when urinating in bed. It is impossible to use without spilling urine on the bedclothes.

DYSPHAGIA Difficulty in swallowing.

ESR Erythrocyte sedimentation rate. A nonspecific blood test that may help to detect disease.

ECT (ELECTROCONVULSIVE THERAPY) Procedure that sends a carefully monitored pulse of electricity through the brain for treatment of severe depression. How it works is not known, but it may be life saving in ending depression before suicide occurs.

ECTOPIC PREGNANCY Pregnancy in which the fetus grows outside of the uterus, usually in the fallopian tube. Surgery is usually required.

EKG Electrocardiogram.

EPIGASTRIUM The area of the abdomen just below the lower rib cage and the lower end of the breast bone.

EXTRASYSTOLES Extra heartbeats that may not be important, although a run of them may be significant.

FASCINOMA Interns' jargon for a fascinating case.

GASTROSCOPY A procedure in which a long, flexible tube that has a light on the end is introduced into the stomach, and sometimes the duodenum, for direct vision.

GULLAIN-BARRÉ SYNDROME An acute inflammation of one or more groups of nerve cells in which patients may rapidly become paralyzed.

HEMODIALYSIS Running the blood of a patient, most often one with kidney failure, through an "artificial kidney" that separates certain toxic substances from the blood.

HYPO Patient jargon for a hypoglycemic reaction, which is a symptom of lowered blood sugar caused by too much insulin.

IM Intramuscular.

LUMBAR PUNCTURE Placement of a needle in the lower back for withdrawal of cerebral spinal fluid for examination. The needle must be skillfully inserted to be useful.

LYME DISEASE An inflammatory disorder caused by a tick bite, typically occurring in the summer. Named after Lyme, Connecticut.

LYMPHANGIOGRAM Injection of material into the lymph vessels of the feet so that lymph nodes higher up in the body can be imaged to determine malignant involvement.

MALIGNANT FIBROUS HISTIOCYTOMA A malignancy of the soft tissues, so rare that most physicians will not have encountered a case during their careers.

MALIGNANT MELANOMA A type of cancer that is curable but, when surgical treatment fails, is a particularly virulent disease.

MENIERE'S DISEASE A disorder of the inner ear, characterized by recurrent attacks of dizziness, tinnitus, and deafness.

METS Medical jargon for metastases.

MITRAL COMMISSUROTOMY A repair of the mitral valve of the heart.

MULTIPLE SCLEROSIS A disease of the nervous system, the cause of which is unknown. Its symptoms vary greatly but may include weakness, visual loss, and incoordination. Its course involves periods of improvement and worsening.

MYCOSIS FUNGOIDES A chronic malignant disease, related to lymphoma, that primarily involves the skin. Therapy is not always successful.

MYOCARDIAL INFARCTION Medical term for heart attack.

NONSTEROIDALS Pain relievers for a variety of inflammatory discomforts. Considered to have fewer potential side effects than steroids.

ORCHIECTOMY Removal of a testis.

PHANTOM PAIN Pain "felt" in an amputated limb.

PLATELETPHORESIS Separation of blood into its component parts so that the platelets can be harvested and used when specifically needed.

PNEUMOHEMOTHORAX A collection of air and blood between the lungs and rib cage. Usually indicates a serious accident.

PNEUMOTHORAX A collection of air between the lungs and the rib cage that can vary from minor and undetected to severe respiratory distress.

PULMONARY EDEMA Excess fluid in the lungs. Associated with a number of disorders but primarily with heart failure.

PULMONARY EMBOLUS A clot that travels an artery of the lung. It may cause sudden death if it is extremely large.

PYLOROPLASTY A revision of the pylorus that is sometimes done for ulcer treatment.

PYLORUS The far end of the stomach, occurring just before the duodenum.

RETROSTERNAL Behind the breast bone.

SCOTOMA A blind spot in the visual field.

SPLENECTOMY Removal of spleen.

STERNUM Breastbone.

STICKS Briticism for canes.

TLC Tender loving care. Required by physician-patients no less than by "normal" patients.

TALWIN A narcotic used for pain relief. It may have peculiar side effects.

THROMBOPHLEBITIS A clot in a vein that occurs most frequently in the leg. It is dangerous when a piece of the clot breaks off and is carried to the lung. See also pulmonary embolus.

TRICYCLICS A type of medication used for depression.

ULCERATIVE COLITIS An inflammatory disease of the large bowel, which causes bloody diarrhea. It is usually chronic and requires a great deal of medical attention. Its cause is unknown. Ulcerative colitis is one of the diseases that transforms a person into a patient.

VENTRICULAR TACHYCARDIA An abnormal heart rhythm of rapidly recurring extra beats. It is dangerous when sustained.

VIRAL MYOCARDITIS An infection of the heart muscle caused by a virus that can significantly weaken the heart.

MIX
Papier aus verantwortungsvollen Quellen
Paper from responsible sources
FSC® C105338

If you have any concerns about our products,
you can contact us on
ProductSafety@springernature.com

In case Publisher is established outside the EU,
the EU authorized representative is:
Springer Nature Customer Service Center GmbH
Europaplatz 3, 69115 Heidelberg, Germany

Printed by Libri Plureos GmbH
in Hamburg, Germany